Allergy and Asthma: Practical Diagnosis and Management

Allergy and Asthma: Practical Diagnosis and Management

Editor: Jake Bennett

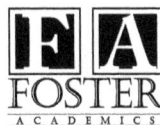

FA FOSTER
A C A D E M I C S

www.fosteracademics.com

www.fosteracademics.com

FA
FOSTER
ACADEMICS

Cataloging-in-Publication Data

Allergy and asthma : practical diagnosis and management / edited by Jake Bennett.
    p. cm.
Includes bibliographical references and index.
ISBN 978-1-63242-691-8
1. Allergy. 2. Asthma. 3. Allergy--Diagnosis. 4. Asthma--Diagnosis. 5. Allergy--Treatment.
6. Asthma--Treatment. 7. Immunology. I. Bennett, Jake.
QR188 .A46 2019
616.97--dc23

Foster Academics,
118-35 Queens Blvd., Suite 400,
Forest Hills, NY 11375, USA

ISBN 978-1-63242-691-8 (Hardback)

Contents

Preface

This book has been a concerted effort by a group of academicians, researchers and scientists, who have contributed their research works for the realization of the book. This book has materialized in the wake of emerging advancements and innovations in this field. Therefore, the need of the hour was to compile all the required researches and disseminate the knowledge to a broad spectrum of people comprising of students, researchers and specialists of the field.

The hypersensitivity of the immune system causes allergies. Asthma is one such example. It is a long-term inflammatory disease of the airways of the lungs, which is characterized by bronchospasm and reversible airflow obstruction. Some of the signs and symptoms of asthma are coughing, shortness of breath, wheezing and chest tightness. It is believed to be caused by a combination of environmental and genetic conditions. Environmental factors such as exposure to allergens and air pollution can trigger asthma. The diagnosis of asthma is based on an examination of symptoms and response to therapy and spirometry. There is no known cure for asthma. Triggers such as irritants and allergens can be avoided and managed by inhaling corticosteroids. For uncontrolled symptoms, antileukotriene agents and long-acting beta agonists may also be used. This book is a compilation of chapters that discuss the most vital concepts and emerging trends in the diagnosis and treatment of asthma. The various studies that are constantly contributing towards advancing the understanding of this disease are examined in detail. This book, with its detailed analyses and data, will prove immensely beneficial to professionals and students involved in this area at various levels.

At the end of the preface, I would like to thank the authors for their brilliant chapters and the publisher for guiding us all-through the making of the book till its final stage. Also, I would like to thank my family for providing the support and encouragement throughout my academic career and research projects.

Editor

Antigen-induced airway hyperresponsiveness and obstruction is related to caveolin-1 expression in airway smooth muscle in a guinea pig asthma model

Mayra Álvarez-Santos[1], Patricia Ramos-Ramírez[1], Fernando Gutiérrez-Aguilar[1], Sandra Sánchez-Hernández[1], Ricardo Lascurain[2], Raúl Olmos-Zuñiga[3], Rogelio Jasso-Victoria[3], Norma A Bobadilla[4,5] and Blanca Bazan-Perkins[1*]

Abstract

Background: Caveolin-1 is a fundamental signalling scaffold protein involved in contraction; however, the role of caveolin-1 in airway responsiveness remains unclear. We evaluated the relationship between caveolin-1 expression in airway smooth muscle (ASM) and antigen-induced airway responsiveness and obstruction in a guinea pig asthma model.

Methods: Airway obstruction in sensitised guinea pigs, induced by antigenic (ovalbumin) challenges administered every 10 days, was measured. Antigen-induced responsiveness to histamine and the expression of caveolin-1 and cavin 1, 2 and 3 were evaluated at the third ovalbumin challenge. The control group received saline solution instead of ovalbumin.

Results: After the first challenge, antigen exposure induced a transient airway obstruction and airway hyperresponsiveness, high levels of IL-4 and IL-5 in lung and airway globet cells proliferation at the third antigenic challenge. Caveolin-1 mRNA levels in total lung decreased in the experimental group compared with controls. Flow cytometric analysis of ASM from the experimental group showed a high number of cells expressing caveolin-1 compared with controls. This increase was confirmed by western blot. Airway obstruction and hyperresponsiveness correlated with the degree of increased caveolin-1 expression in ASM cells ($P < 0.05$; r = 0.69 and −0.52, respectively). The expression of cavins 1, 2 and 3 in ASM also increased in the experimental group compared to controls. Immunohistochemical findings reveal that differences in ASM caveolin-1 were not evident between groups. Nevertheless, a marked decrease in caveolin-1 and caspase 3 was observed in the pulmonary vascular smooth muscle of asthma model compared with controls. Histological analysis did not reveal differences in smooth muscles mass or subepithelial fibrosis levels in airways between groups. However, an enlargement of smooth muscle mass was observed in the pulmonary microvessels of experimental animals. This enlargement did not induce changes in pulmonary or systemic arterial pressures.

Conclusions: Our data suggest that caveolin-1 expression in ASM has a crucial role in the development of antigen-induced airway obstruction and hyperresponsiveness in a guinea pig asthma model. In addition, the asthma model in guinea pigs appears to induce a contractile smooth muscle phenotype in the airways and a proliferative smooth muscle phenotype in pulmonary vessels.

Keywords: Airway hyperresponsiveness, Airway obstruction, Airway smooth muscle, Asthma, caspase 3, Caveolin-1, Cavin, Pulmonary arterial smooth muscle

* Correspondence: perkins@iner.gob.mx
[1]Instituto Nacional de Enfermedades Respiratorias Ismael Cosío Villegas, Departamento de Hiperreactividad Bronquial, Calzada de Tlalpan 4502, Mexico
Full list of author information is available at the end of the article

Background

Airway smooth muscle is a central structure in asthma pathogenesis. An important characteristic of asthma is that numerous stimuli can trigger intense and rapid bronchospasm in a phenomenon called airway hyperresponsiveness [1,2]. Currently, the precise mechanism by which the development of hyperresponsiveness is induced remains unknown. Nevertheless, airway remodelling features such as fibrosis and smooth muscle hypertrophy/ hyperplasia have been recognised as playing a part [2].

Caveolin-1 is a hairpin-loop protein that forms omega-shape invaginations in the plasma membrane, which are known as caveola [3]. In asthma, a shortage of caveolin-1 has been observed in the airways of asthmatic patients [4]. Similar results have been noted in the lungs of ovalbumin-challenged mice, where a reduction of caveolin-1 mRNA expression has been observed [5,6]. In contrast, increased levels of caveolin-1 are found in the airway smooth muscle of antigen-challenged in mice [7] and the lungs of guinea pigs subjected to an asthma model [8].

In airways, caveolin-1 is involved in the downregulation of fibrosis and smooth muscle proliferation [9,10]. However, the role of caveolin-1 in airway hyperresponsiveness is unclear. The development of airway hyperresponsiveness in allergen (ovalbumin)-challenged mice without caveolin-1 has been observed [7,11], and Hsia and colleagues [12] have found the absence of caveolin-1 induced airway hyperresponsiveness in endotoxin (lipopolysaccharide)-challenged mice. Moreover, the role of caveolin-1 in airway hyperresponsiveness has become highly controversial due to the view that caveolin-1 is related to the regulation of contractile mechanisms [9,13,14], including, proteins that participate in intracellular Ca^{2+} mobilisation [15,16]. For example, M3 muscarinic, bradykinin, and H1 histamine receptors and store-operated Ca^{2+} entry-regulatory mechanisms colocalise with caveolin-1 [17]. Additionally, the recruitment of Ca^{2+} sensitisation components such as RhoA and PKCα is caveolin-1-dependent [18,19]. Furthermore, caveolin-1 is a key regulator of store-operated Ca^{2+} entry by increasing Orai1 expression in airway smooth muscle [20].

Since 2005 some proteins named cavins has been associated with caveola biogenesis and organization [21]. In particular, cavin 1 (RNA pol I transcription factor), cavin 2 (serum deprivation protein response) and cavin 3 (SDR- related gene product that binds to C kinase) are widely expressed in tissues, included smooth muscles [22]. Recently, it has been observed a decrease in expression of cavins in airways of caveolin-1 knock-out mice, although its role in airway contraction its unknown [7].

Experimental asthma models are fundamental in asthma research. Particularly, guinea pigs asthma model are susceptible to develop early and late allergic responses after allergen challenge and also can be used as a model for chronic allergic asthma [23,24]. Asthma model in guinea pig is useful since the lung pharmacology and the response to inflammatory mediators is similar to humans in comparison to rats and mouse [25,26].

In the current study, we determined the relationship between caveolin-1 expression and the pathophysiological characteristics of asthma and found that caveolin-1 expression increases in airway smooth muscle and that this increase is related to antigen-induced obstruction and hyperresponsiveness. In contrast, pulmonary vascular smooth muscle showed low expression of caveolin-1, which was accompanied by smooth muscle cell proliferation.

Methods

We used outbred male guinea pigs weighing 0.35-0.4 kg from Harlan Mexico (strain HsdPoc:DH). The animals were maintained in our institutional laboratory animal facilities with filtered air conditioned at $21 \pm 1°C$ and 50-70% humidity, 12/12-h light/dark cycles, sterilised pellets (2040 Harlan Teklad Guinea Pig Diet) and water available *ad libitum*. All animals were handled according to protocols approved by the Scientific and Bioethics Committee of the Instituto Nacional de Enfermedades Respiratorias.

Study design

To determinate the role of caveolin-1 in airway smooth muscle pathophysiology during asthma, ovalbumin sensitised guinea pigs were exposed to three antigenic challenges, each administrated every 10 days (Figure 1). During each challenge, the broncho-obstructive index was measured. At the third antigenic challenge, the development of antigen-induced airway hyperresponsiveness was evaluated by performing dose–response curves to histamine before and after an antigenic challenge. Animals were then sacrificed to obtain lung and tracheal samples. In lung samples, caveolin-1 mRNA was measured by RT-PCR. Additionally, changes in the amount of collagen in the airway lamina propria and the extent of airway and pulmonary microvessel smooth muscle layers were analysed via light microscopy. Caveolin-1 expression was examined using immunohistochemistry. Caveolin-1 expression in smooth muscle cells from tracheae was measured by flow cytometry. Tracheal smooth muscle strips were used to evaluate the expression of caveolin-1 and cavins 1, 2 and 3 by western blot. Systemic and pulmonary arterial pressures were measured at the third challenge. Control animals received sham manoeuvres performed with saline solution.

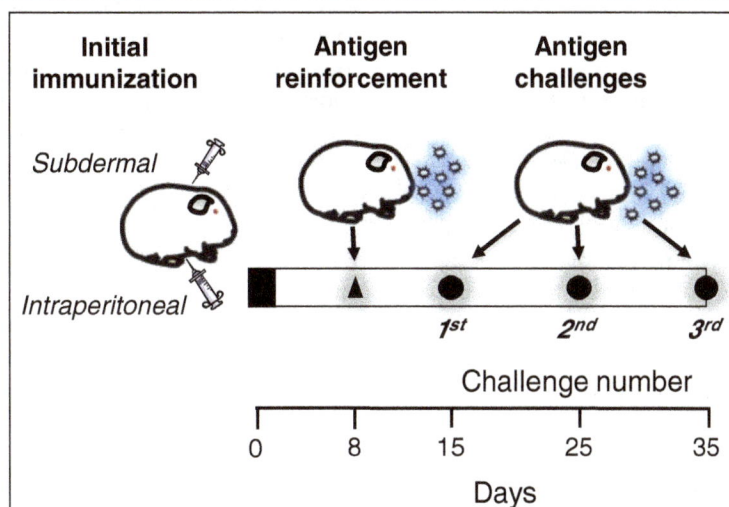

Figure 1 Experimental design. After initial immunisation and reinforcement with antigen (ovalbumin), guinea pigs received three antigen challenges. At third challenge the evaluation of broncho-obstructive index, dose–response curves to histamine as well as immunological, histopathological and vascular function analysis were performed.

Asthma model

Guinea pigs were sensitised and challenges were performed according to previously described methods [23,27]. The antigen sensitisation of guinea pigs was performed by intraperitoneal (0.5 mg/ml) and subdermal (0.5 mg/ml) injections with a combination of 60 μg/ml ovalbumin plus 1 mg/ml aluminium hydroxide dispersed in saline solution (Figure 1). The doses used in sensitisation and challenges in this asthma model were adjusted to reduce anaphylactic shock during challenges. Antigen sensitisation was reinforced eight days later with ovalbumin aerosol (3 mg/ml saline) delivered over five minutes. Aerosols were produced by a US-1 Bennett nebuliser (flow, 2 ml/min; Multistage liquid impinger, Burkard Manufacturing Co., Rickmansworth, Hertfordshire, UK) releasing mixed particles with sizes of <4 μm (44%), 4–10 μm (38%), and >10 μm (18%). From day 15 onward, guinea pigs were challenged over one minute with an ovalbumin aerosol every 10 days (1 mg/ml during the first challenge and 0.5 mg/ml in subsequent challenges) (Figure 1).

Acute airway obstructive responses after ovalbumin inhalation challenges were recorder using a barometric plethysmograph. A whole-body single-chamber plethysmograph for freely moving animals was used (Buxco Electronics Inc., Troy, NY, USA) to evaluate pulmonary function. The signal from the chamber was processed with computer-installed software (Buxco Bio System XA v1.1) to calculate several respiratory parameters, including the broncho-obstructive index, Penh. We calculated this index using the following equation [28]:

$$Penh = ((Te\text{-}Rt)/Rt)\ (PEP/PIP)$$

where Te = expiratory time (s), Rt = relaxation time (s), PEP = peak expiratory pressure (cmH_2O), and PIP = peak inspiratory pressure (cmH_2O). The software was adjusted to include only breaths with a tidal volume of 1 millilitre or more, with minimal inspiratory time of 0.15 seconds, maximal inspiratory time of 3 seconds, and maximal difference between inspiratory and expiratory volumes of 10%. This guinea pig model of allergic asthma does not develop a noticeable late airway response. We corroborated that this sensitisation procedure induces the increment of Th2 (CD4 + IL13+) lymphocytes in bronchoalveolar lavage.

Antigen-induced airway responsiveness

In guinea pigs, airway hyperresponsiveness was measured after antigen challenge in sensitised (n = 18; asthma model) and non-sensitised (n = 13; control group) animals [27]. Airway responsiveness was evaluated on day 35 (third ovalbumin challenge) by exposing each animal to increasing non-cumulative doses of histamine aerosols (0.001 to 0.32 mg/ml; Sigma Chemical Co., St. Louis, MO, US) after an initial broncho-obstructive index acquisition before and after ovalbumin administration. Each histamine dose was delivered over 1 minute, and the average of the broncho-obstructive index over the following 10 min was obtained. The interval between doses was 10 min. The dose–response curve finished when the broncho-obstructive index reached three times its baseline level. Once the index returned to the initial baseline value (<50% increment), the ovalbumin challenge was administered. A second curve was measured three hours later. Control group received saline instead ovalbumin administration.

Dissection of airway smooth muscle strips for flow cytometry and Western blot studies

Twenty-four hours after concluding histamine curves, some sensitised ($n = 10$) and non-sensitised ($n = 9$) guinea pigs were overdosed with an intraperitoneal injection of pentobarbital sodium (65 mg/kg), and their tracheae were dissected to obtain airway smooth muscle strips.

Isolation of airway smooth muscle cells

The strips of 7 sensitised and 6 non-sensitised guinea pigs were incubated at 37°C for 10 min in 5 ml of Hanks' solution (Gibco, Gaithersburg, MD, US) with 2 mg cysteine and 0.05 U/ml papain (Sigma Chemical Co., St. Louis, MO, US). The strips were then washed in Leibovitz's solution (Gibco, Gaithersburg, MD, US) and placed in a physiological saline solution (PSS, mM) containing 118 NaCl, 25 NaHCO$_3$, 4.6 KCl, 1.2 MgSO$_4$, 1.2 KH$_2$PO$_4$ and 11 glucose (Sigma Chemical Co., St. Louis, MO, US). Smooth muscle strips were cut (0.5 x 5 mm), and fragments weighing 200 mg total were placed in 2.5 ml PSS with collagenase type I (1 mg/ml; Sigma Chemical Co., US) and dispase II (4 mg/ml; Sigma Chemical Co., St. Louis, MO, US) at 37°C. Ten minutes later, the fragments were transferred to similar PSS containing fresh enzymes. Tissue was dispersed mechanically until isolated cells were observed. Leibovitz's solution was added to stop the enzymatic activity.

Flow cytometry

For the detection of caveolin-1 production in the isolated airway smooth muscle cells, a three-color immunofluorescence approach was used following a previously described method [29]. Isolated myocytes were incubated with 10 μg/ml brefeldin-A (Sigma Chemical Co.; St. Louis, MO, US) for four hours to inhibit new cytokine release. After staining, cells were washed, fixed with 4% p-formaldehyde for 10 min at 4°C, washed, and permeabilised with 0.1% saponin in PBS with 10% BSA and 1% NaN$_3$. Afterwards, cells were gently shaken in the dark for 15 min at room temperature and 1 μl/1x10^6 cells were labelled with caveolin-1 antibody (BD Biosciences Pharmingen, San Diego, CA, US). Then, cells were incubated during 30 min with secondary antibody FITC mouse (BD Biosciences Pharmingen, San Diego, CA, US). Finally, cells were analysed for the expression of markers, on a FACScan flow cytometer (Becton Dickinson, San Diego, CA, US) using software, and 10,000 events were counted. To analyse the staining of intracellular caveolin-1, the blasts were initially gated by their physical properties (forward and side scatter). A second gate was then drawn based on the fluorescence characteristics of the gated cells, assessing fluorescence intensity by histograms. Intensity of fluorescence staining is expressed as the mean fluorescence intensity. Control stains were performed using fluorochrome-conjugated isotype-matched antibodies. Background staining was <1% and subtracted from experimental values.

Western blot analysis

Smooth muscle strips from guinea pig tracheae ($n = 3$, each group) were placed in lysis buffer (1% Triton X-100, 50 mM Tris, pH 7.4, 150 mM NaCl, 0.1 mM EDTA and EGTA, 1.0 mM phenylmethylsulfonyl fluoride, 10 μg/ml aprotinin and leupeptin, 1.0 mM Na$_3$VO$_4$, and 50 mM NaF; Sigma Chemical Co.; St. Louis, MO, US) and homogenised (Polytron PT3100, Kinematica, Switzerland). Tissue protein (40 μg) from each sample was loaded in different lanes of a 12% SDS-polyacrylamide gel. In an additional lane, a control protein (GAPDH; Sigma Chemical Co.; US) was also added. After electrophoretic separation under reducing conditions, proteins were transferred to a nitrocellulose membrane and quenched with Tris-buffered saline (TBS) containing 5% non-fat milk and 0.1% Tween-20. Membranes were subjected to overnight incubation (12 h, 4°C) with rabbit polyclonal antibodies raised against caveolin-1 (BD Biosciences Pharmingen, San Diego CA, US), cavin-1 (Anti/PTRF/Cavin-1, Millipore, Billerica MA, USA), cavin-2 (SDR, Thermo Scientific, Rockford IL, USA) and cavin-3 (PRKCDBP, Thermo Scientific, Rockford IL, USA), and then washed three times with TBS-Tween-20 (0.1%). Caveolin and cavins were detected by adding horseradish peroxidase-labelled anti-mouse antibodies. Immunoblots were developed using an enhanced chemiluminescent reactant (LumiGLO, Cell Signalling; US) and an optimal exposition of the nitrocellulose sheets to X-ray films (Biomax ML Film, Kodak, Rochester, NY US). Caveolin-1 and cavin immunoblots were analysed by densitometry using Kodak digital science ID software version 2.03 (Eastman Kodak, Rochester, NY, US).

RNA isolation

Total RNA from the right lung of some sensitised and non-sensitised ($n = 3$, each group) guinea pigs was isolated following the guanidine isothiocyanate-caesium chloride method [30]. Total RNA was examined by 1% agarose gel electrophoresis, and the RNA concentration was determined by UV light absorbance at 260 nm to evaluate the integrity of RNA (Beckman DU640, Fullerton, CA, US).

RT-PCR

The relative level of caveolin-1 mRNA expression was assessed in left lung homogenates by semiquantitative

RT-PCR, as previously described [31]. Briefly, all primer sequences were custom ordered from GIBCO BRL (Gaithersburg, MD, US). Sense caveolin-1 primers were amplified to obtain a fragment of 230 bp, bases 1 to 230 (sense 5'-ATG TCT GGG GGT AAA TAC GT-3' and antisense: 5'-CCT TCT GGT TCC GCA ATC AC-3). A fragment of GAPDH was also amplified to evaluate or reduce nonspecific effects of experimental treatment and to semi-quantify caveolin-1 expression. RNA samples were treated with DNAse to evaluate genomic DNA contamination relative to samples passed through a PCR procedure without adding reverse transcriptase. RT-PCR was carried out using 2.5 µg of total RNA from lung homogenate. Before the RT-PCR reaction, total RNA was heated at 65° C for 10 min. RT-PCR was performed at 37°C for 60 min in a total volume of 20 µl using 200 U of the Moloney murine leukaemia virus reverse transcriptase (GIBCO BRL, Gaithersburg, MD, US), 100 pM of random hexamers (GIBCO, BRL Gaithersburg, MD, US), 0.5 mM of each dNTP (Sigma, St. Louis, MO, US), and 1× RT buffer (75 mM KCl, 50 mM Tris · HCl, 3 mM $MgCl_2$, 10 mM DTT, pH 8.3). Samples were heated at 95°C for 5 min to inactivate the reverse transcriptase and diluted to 40 µl with PCR-grade water. One-tenth of RT-PCR individual samples from each group was used for caveolin-1 or GAPDH amplification in 20-µl final volume reactions containing 1× PCR buffer (10 mM Tris · HCl, 1.5 mM $MgCl_2$, 50 mM KCl, pH 8.3), 0.1 mM of each dNTP, 0.2 µCi of [α32P]-dCTP (3,000 Ci/mmol, 9.25 MBq, 250 µCi), 10 µM of each primer, and one unit of Taq DNA polymerase (GIBCO, BRL Gaithersburg, MD, US). Samples were overlaid with 30 µl of mineral oil and PCR cycles were performed in a DNA thermal cycler (M.J. Research, Watertown, MA, US), with the following profile: denaturation for 1 min at 94°C; annealing for 1 min at 55°C and a 1-min extension step at 72°C. The last cycle was followed by a final extension step of 5 min at 72°C. Control gene was co-amplified simultaneously in each reaction. Amplification kinetics were performed following our standard procedure [31]. To analyse PCR products, one-half of each reaction was electrophoresed in a 5% acrylamide gel. Bands were stained with ethidium bromide, visualised under UV light, cut out, suspended in 1 ml of scintillation cocktail (Ecolume, ICN, Aurora, OH, US), and counted by liquid scintillation (Beckman LS6500, Fullerton, CA, US). The amount of radioactivity recovered from the excised bands was plotted in a log scale against the number of cycles. To semi-quantify caveolin-1 and the control gene, all reactions were performed at least in quadruplicate.

Conventional histology and automated morphometry analysis

Left caudal lung lobes of some guinea pigs ($n = 6$, each group) were dissected and fixed by manual perfusion of 10% neutral buffered formaldehyde solution via intra-arterial route until the lung lobe was exsanguinated. Lung fragments obtained by sagittal cutting were embedded in paraffin, and 4 µm-thick lung sections were stained with Masson trichrome stain. The surface areas ($µm^2$) of airway smooth muscle and lamina propria, as well as the vascular smooth muscle of adjacent vessels, were determined through the use of automated morphometry (Qwin, Leica Microsystems Imaging Solutions, Cambridge, UK). Data were adjusted by length of the corresponding basement membrane, and their average was considered the final result. All measurements were conducted in six bronchi, six bronchioles and six arterioles (~100 µm diameter) chosen randomly from each animal. Total epithelial cells in six bronchi of each guinea pig were counted and the percentage of globet cell was obtained. The bronchus and bronchiole were identified by the presence or absence of cartilage in the airway wall, respectively.

ELISA

Anti-human interferon-γ (IFN-γ; R&D System, Minneapolis, USA), interleukin-4 (IL-4; R&D System, Minneapolis, USA) and IL-5 (clone TRFK5; BD Pharmingen, USA), antibodies were used in lung homogenates of sensitized and non sensitised guinea pigs ($n = 6$, each group) to measure cytokines by ELISA as previously described [27].

Immunohistochemistry and immunofluorescence

The same paraffin-embedded lung tissue blocks used for the morphometric study were used for immunohistochemistry ($n = 6$, each group) and immunofluorescence ($n = 2$, each group). Sections (3 µm) were deparaffinised (55°C, 30 min) and rehydrated through submersion in graded alcohols (xylene, 1:1 xylene-alcohol, alcohol, and 70% alcohol for 10 min each, followed by rinsing in distilled water). Antigen retrieval was performed with 10 mM citrate buffer, pH 6, for 5 min in a microwave oven. Samples were treated with hydrogen peroxide (3%) to quench endogenous peroxidase, and nonspecific sites were blocked later with horse serum (2%). Sections were incubated at 4°C overnight with an antibody to caveolin-1 (BD Biosciences Pharmingen, San Diego CA, US). To detect the specific binding of this primary antibody, an R.T.U. Vectastain Universal Quick Kit was used (Vector Laboratories, Inc., Burlingame, CA, USA) in which tissues were incubated sequentially with blocking serum, a pan-specific secondary antibody, and streptavidin/peroxidase complex. Finally, 3-amino-9-ethyl-carbazole (BioGenex,

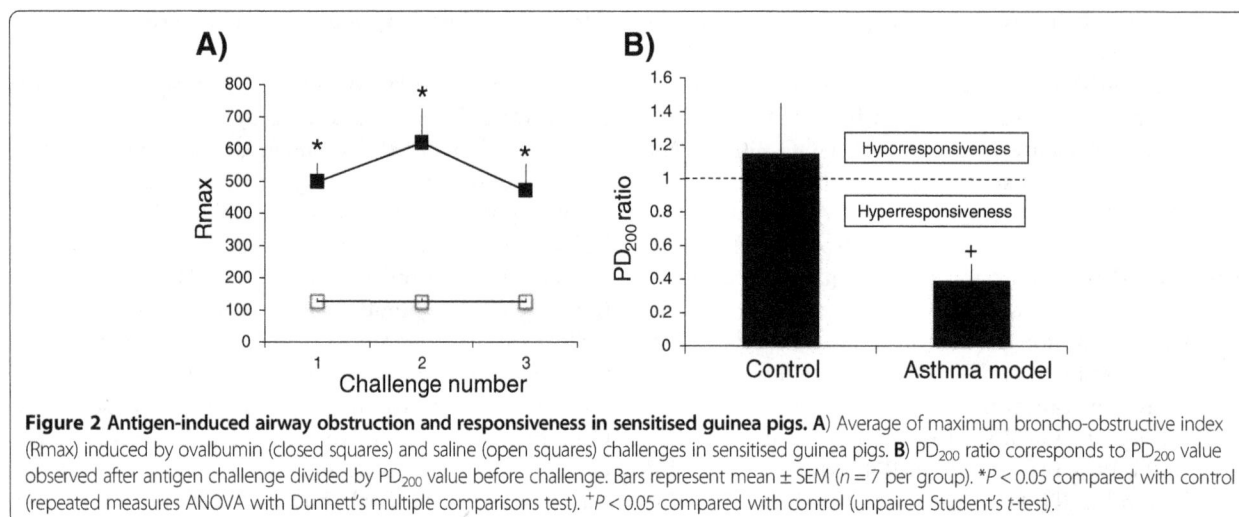

Figure 2 Antigen-induced airway obstruction and responsiveness in sensitised guinea pigs. A) Average of maximum broncho-obstructive index (Rmax) induced by ovalbumin (closed squares) and saline (open squares) challenges in sensitised guinea pigs. **B)** PD_{200} ratio corresponds to PD_{200} value observed after antigen challenge divided by PD_{200} value before challenge. Bars represent mean ± SEM ($n = 7$ per group). *$P < 0.05$ compared with control (repeated measures ANOVA with Dunnett's multiple comparisons test). +$P < 0.05$ compared with control (unpaired Student's t-test).

San Ramon, CA, USA) was used as a chromogen. Sections were counterstained with Mayer's haematoxylin. Slides were rinsed twice with 0.1% Tween-20 phosphate-buffered saline during the whole process. To control for the non-specific binding of the secondary antibody, sections from the same lung were processed without the primary antibody. No positive staining was observed in non-specific binding controls. The rabbit IgG (Southern Biotech, Birmingham, AL, USA) isotype control was negative.

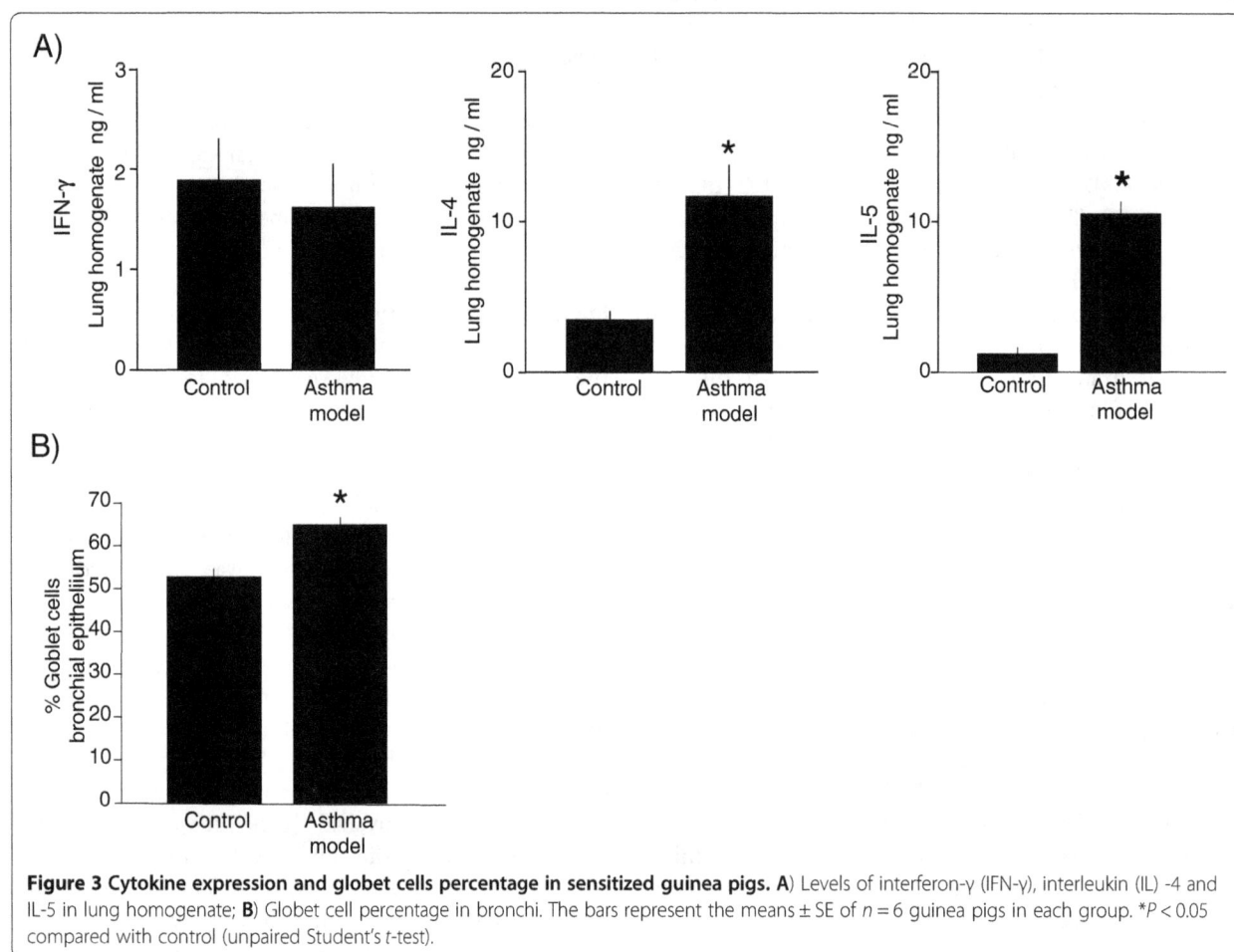

Figure 3 Cytokine expression and globet cells percentage in sensitized guinea pigs. A) Levels of interferon-γ (IFN-γ), interleukin (IL) -4 and IL-5 in lung homogenate; **B)** Globet cell percentage in bronchi. The bars represent the means ± SE of $n = 6$ guinea pigs in each group. *$P < 0.05$ compared with control (unpaired Student's t-test).

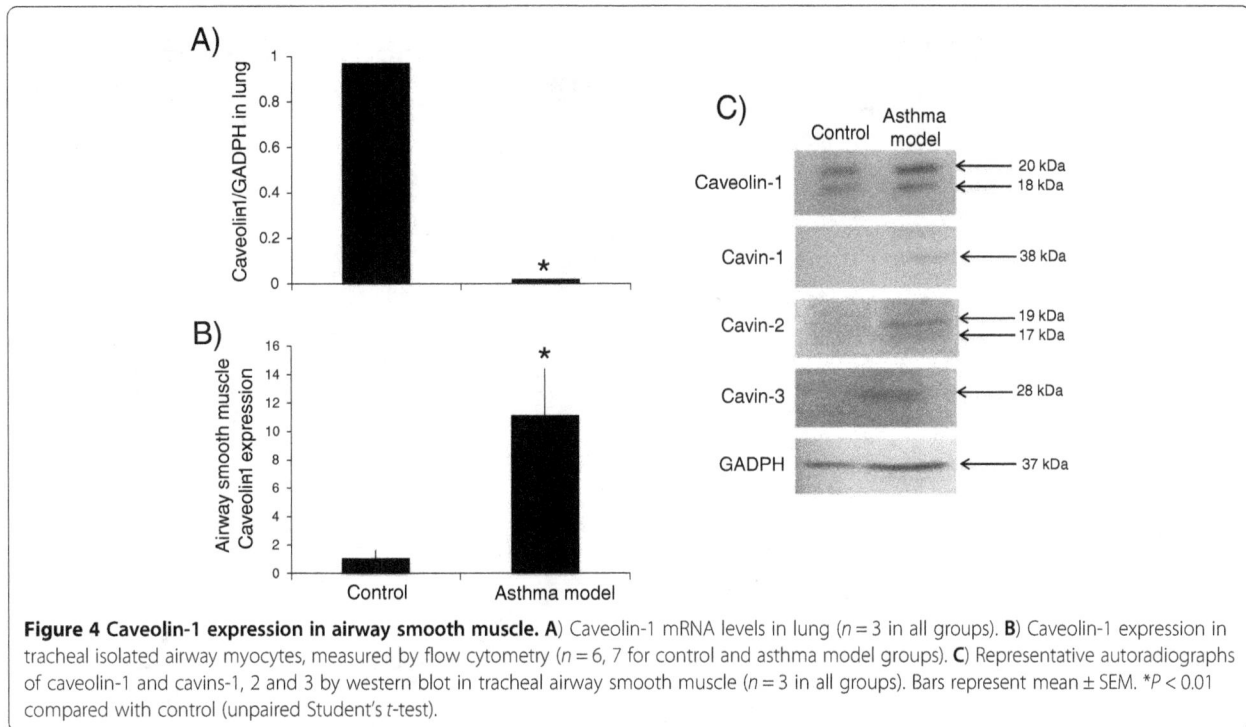

Figure 4 Caveolin-1 expression in airway smooth muscle. A) Caveolin-1 mRNA levels in lung ($n = 3$ in all groups). **B)** Caveolin-1 expression in tracheal isolated airway myocytes, measured by flow cytometry ($n = 6, 7$ for control and asthma model groups). **C)** Representative autoradiographs of caveolin-1 and cavins-1, 2 and 3 by western blot in tracheal airway smooth muscle ($n = 3$ in all groups). Bars represent mean ± SEM. *$P < 0.01$ compared with control (unpaired Student's t-test).

For the detection of caspase 3 by immunofluorescence, paraffin-embedded tissue was cut 4–6 m thick and tissue sections were placed in slides and incubated for 30 min at 55°C. Tissue slides were deparaffinized in xylenes twice for 10 min each. Hydrate sections gradually through graded alcohols using 2 changes for 10 min each of the following solutions: 100% ethanol, 95% ethanol, and deionized water. For antigen unmasking, slides were covered with 10 mM sodium citrate buffer, pH 6.0, and heat at 95°C for 5 min. Slides were then cooled in TBS-T buffer for 20 min at room temperature. To suppress non-specific binding of antibodies, tissue slides were incubated with 0.2% BSA in PBS for 20 min at 4°C. After that, immunofluorescence staining was carried out by overlaying each slide with 20 μl of rabbit polyclonal anti-caspase 3 antibody (Abcam, San Francisco, CA, USA) for 2 h at 4°C. After washing in TBS-T buffer for 5 min, a secondary incubation was performed with fluorescein isothiocyanate (FITC)-labeled goat anti-rabbit IgG (Jackson ImmunoResearch Laboratories Inc. Amish Country, PA, USA) for 30 min at 4°C. After twice washing, slides were counterstained with fluoroshield mounting medium with DAPI (Sigma-Aldrich Co, St. Louis, MO, USA) for nuclei staining (blue channel). All incubations were carried out in a humidified dark chamber. In other experiments, tissue slides were incubated only with FITC-labeled secondary antibody, which was used as background staining control. Finally, tissue slides were examined by fluorescence microscope with

appropriate filters (Leica DM-LS 2000, Mannheim, Germany), and analyzed by ImageJ64 software (http://rsb.info.nih.gov/ij/).

Hemodynamic

After 12 h of fasting, some guinea pigs ($n = 8$ for sensitised, and $n = 4$ for non-sensitised) were anaesthetised with isofluorane (1.5%, Sofloran, México, DF) delivered by a precision vaporiser (Isotec 3, Ohmeda, Steeton, West Yorkshire, UK) carried in oxygen. Their heart rates were monitored with an automatic non-invasive device Datascope Passport Model EL (Datascope Corp, Mahwah, NJ, USA), and after deep anaesthesia, animals were ventilated through a trachea cannula that was connected to both, a ventilator (Harvard, Rodent Model Ventilator 683) and the vaporiser. Then, the right carotid artery was dissected, and a catheter was introduced to measure the systemic arterial pressure and diastolic arterial pressure. A similar procedure was performed to introduce a catheter into the pulmonary artery through the right ventricle to determine the pulmonary arterial pressure. Datascope Passport monitored all pressures.

Materials

Ovalbumin (chicken egg albumin) grade II and all stains for microscopy were purchased from Sigma Chemical Co. (US). Aluminium hydroxide was purchased from J.T. Baker, USA. Pentobarbital sodium was acquired from Pfizer, Mexico.

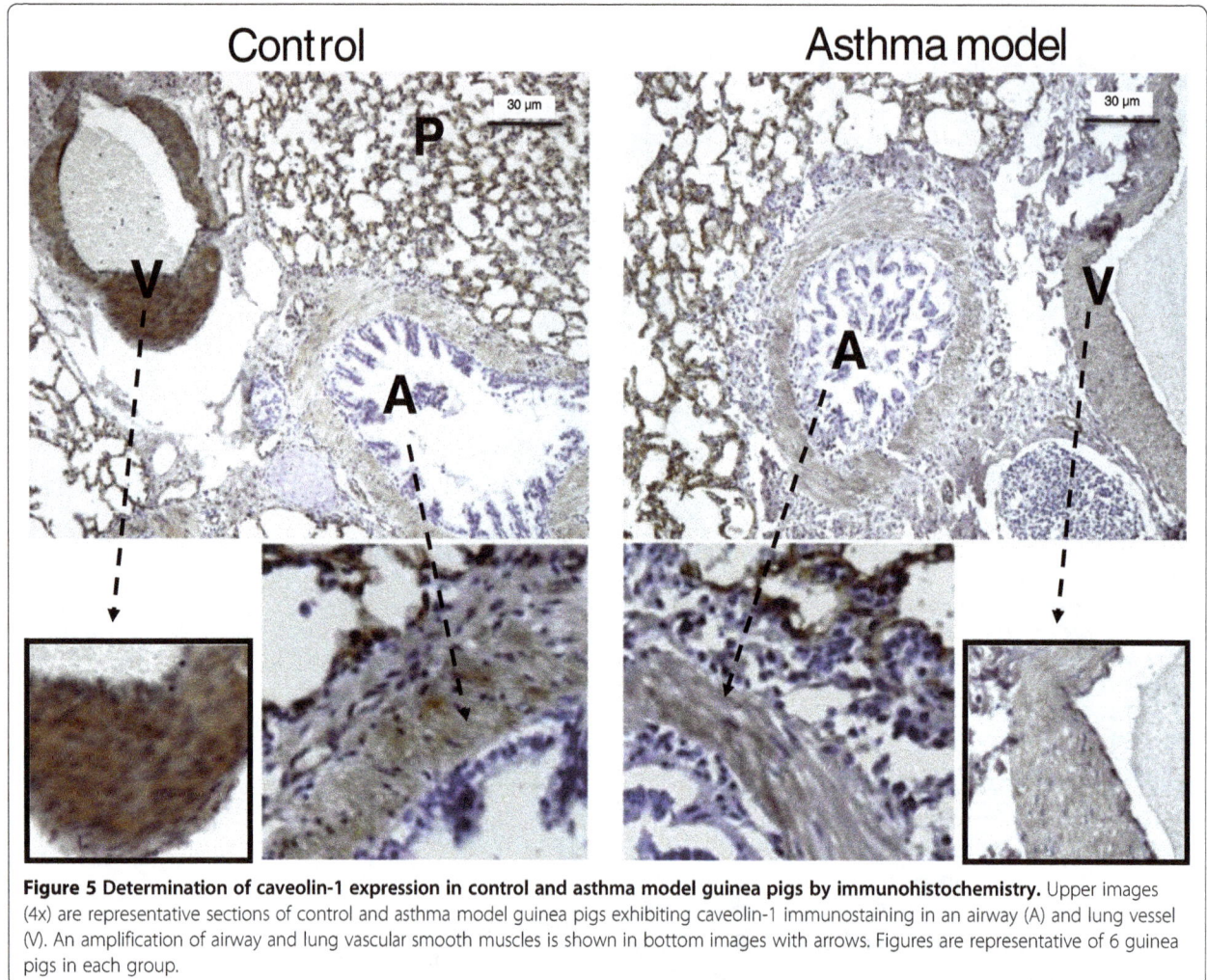

Figure 5 Determination of caveolin-1 expression in control and asthma model guinea pigs by immunohistochemistry. Upper images (4x) are representative sections of control and asthma model guinea pigs exhibiting caveolin-1 immunostaining in an airway (A) and lung vessel (V). An amplification of airway and lung vascular smooth muscles is shown in bottom images with arrows. Figures are representative of 6 guinea pigs in each group.

Statistical analysis

Airway responsiveness to histamine was evaluated by means of the provocative dose 200% (PD_{200}), i.e., the interpolated histamine dose that caused a three-fold increase of basal broncho-obstructive index. Change in histamine responsiveness induced by antigen challenge was evaluated by the PD_{200} ratio, i.e., PD_{200} value observed after OVA challenge divided by PD_{200} value before challenge. In multiple comparisons, one-way or repeated-measure ANOVA followed by Dunnett's tests was used. Comparison between control and asthma model groups was evaluated by means of Student's unpaired t-test. Associations between caveolin-1 and airway responsiveness and obstruction were assessed through Spearman's correlation coefficient. Statistical significance was set at two-tailed $P < 0.05$. Data in the text and figures are expressed as the mean ± SEM.

Results and discussion
Antigen-induced airway obstruction and responsiveness

The guinea pig has served as a helpful model in the study of asthma, with some advantages over other models such as the rat and mouse, because it shares various pharmacological characteristics of human asthma, besides the strong airway obstructive response that guinea pigs exhibit after agonist stimulation [32]. Responses to antigen challenge in guinea pig asthma models are characterised by a rapid and transient airway obstruction in sensitised animals [23,27]. In the current study, the values of basal airway obstruction index were similar between control and experimental groups (data not shown). Saline challenge did not modify the basal obstruction index in the control group, but ovalbumin challenge induced a transient increase in the index that reached statistical significance in comparison with the control group ($P < 0.05$; $n = 18$ asthma model, and $n = 13$ control group; Figure 2A).

An important pathophysiological feature of asthma is the development of airway hyperresponsiveness. In this study, the basal histamine PD_{200} value was similar between the control and experimental groups (data not shown). In the control group, the histamine PD_{200} value after saline challenge was similar to the basal PD_{200}

value. In the experimental group, the PD_{200} value after ovalbumin challenge was lower than the basal PD_{200} value. In the control group, the PD_{200} ratio was significantly lower than that obtained in the control group ($P < 0.05$; $n = 18$ asthma model, and $n = 13$ control group; Figure 2B), implying that all guinea pigs sensitised with the antigen showed hyperresponsiveness to histamine.

Inflammatory markers in asthma as the Th2 cytokines IL-4 and IL-5 [33] significantly increases in lung homogenates of asthma model guinea pigs in comparison with controls ($P < 0.05$; $n = 6$ each group; Figure 3A). In contrast IFN-γ, a Th1 cytokine, has similar levels in both groups (Figure 3A). In addition, a significantly increment of globet cells was observed in bronchi epithelium of asthma model group (P < 0.05; $n = 6$ each group; Figure 3B) suggesting that this model of acute asthma induces structural changes in airway epithelium.

Caveolin-1 expression in asthma model

In comparison with other cells, smooth muscle expresses high levels of caveolin-1 in the plasma membrane [34]. In airway smooth muscle, the signalling platform associated with caveolin- 1 takes important roles in the recruitment of various signalling proteins involved in contraction. For example, caveolin-1 is involved in Ca^{2+} homeostasis via the presence of voltage gated L-type Ca^{2+} channels, the plasma membrane Ca^{2+} ATPase, calsequestrin and calreticulin in caveolin-enriched membranes [15]. Other components that

play a role in airway smooth muscle contraction, such as M3 muscarinic, bradykinin, H1 histamine, phospholipase Cβ1, Gαq and store-operated Ca^{2+} entry-regulatory mechanisms, co-localise with caveolin-1 [17,35]. Moreover, TNF-α, a fundamental cytokine in asthma pathogenesis [36], induces RhoA activation, enhances force responses to acetylcholine, and increases Ca^{2+} responses to acetylcholine, histamine and bradykinin through caveolin-1 upregulation [18,37,38]. Certainly, caveolin-1 is associated with key molecules that participate in airway smooth muscle contraction.

In agreement with other studies [4-6], we found that caveolin-1 is downregulated in the lung homogenates of experimental animals, as shown in Figure 4A. The level of caveolin-1 mRNA in the lung homogenate of controls was significantly higher in comparison to the experimental group ($P < 0.01$; $n = 3$ in all groups); nevertheless, flow cytometric studies in isolated myocytes demonstrated that the number of cells that express caveolin-1 increased significantly in the experimental group compared to controls ($P < 0.01$; $n = 6$ and 7 for control and asthma model groups, respectively; Figure 4B). Similar results in the airway smooth muscle bundles of experimental group animals obtained by immunohistochemistry analysis have been described previously [8]. In our study, we observed that functional changes in the asthma model correlated with the number of smooth muscle cells that expressed caveolin-1. The PD_{200} ratio

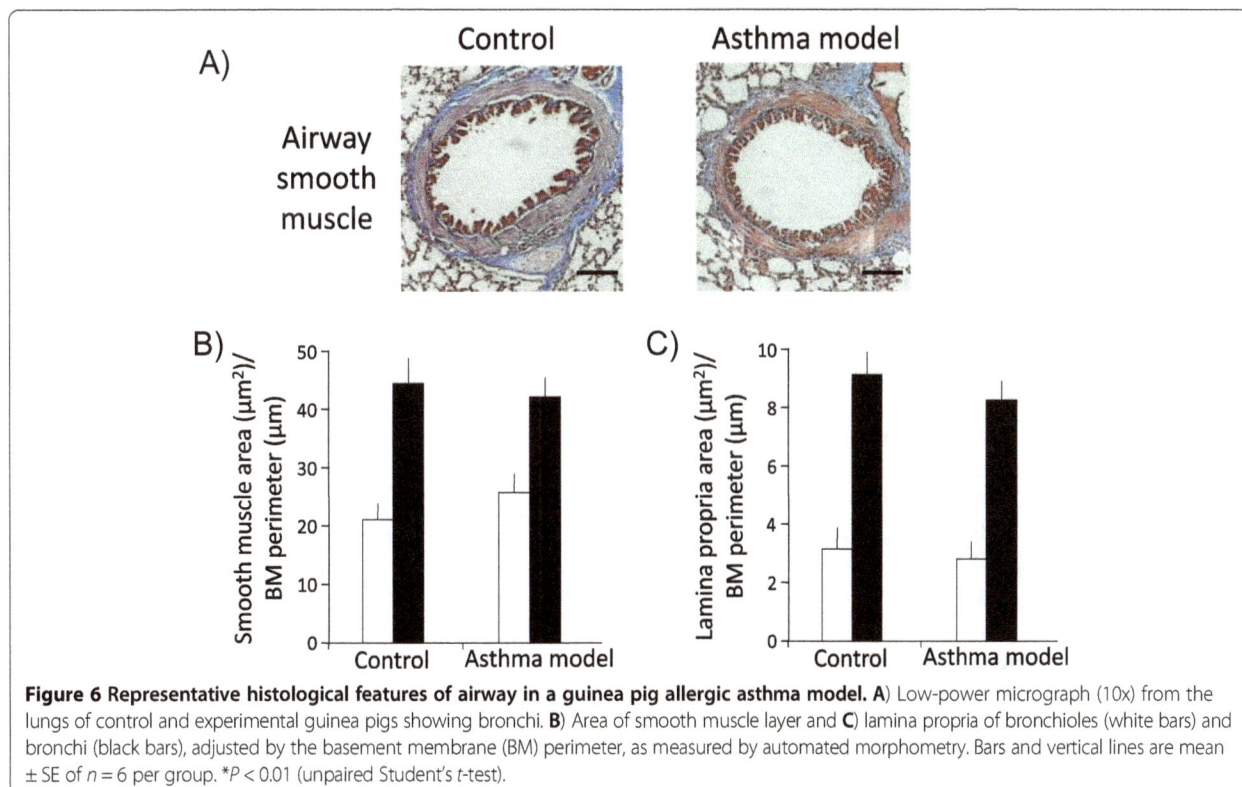

Figure 6 Representative histological features of airway in a guinea pig allergic asthma model. A) Low-power micrograph (10x) from the lungs of control and experimental guinea pigs showing bronchi. **B**) Area of smooth muscle layer and **C**) lamina propria of bronchioles (white bars) and bronchi (black bars), adjusted by the basement membrane (BM) perimeter, as measured by automated morphometry. Bars and vertical lines are mean ± SE of $n = 6$ per group. *$P < 0.01$ (unpaired Student's t-test).

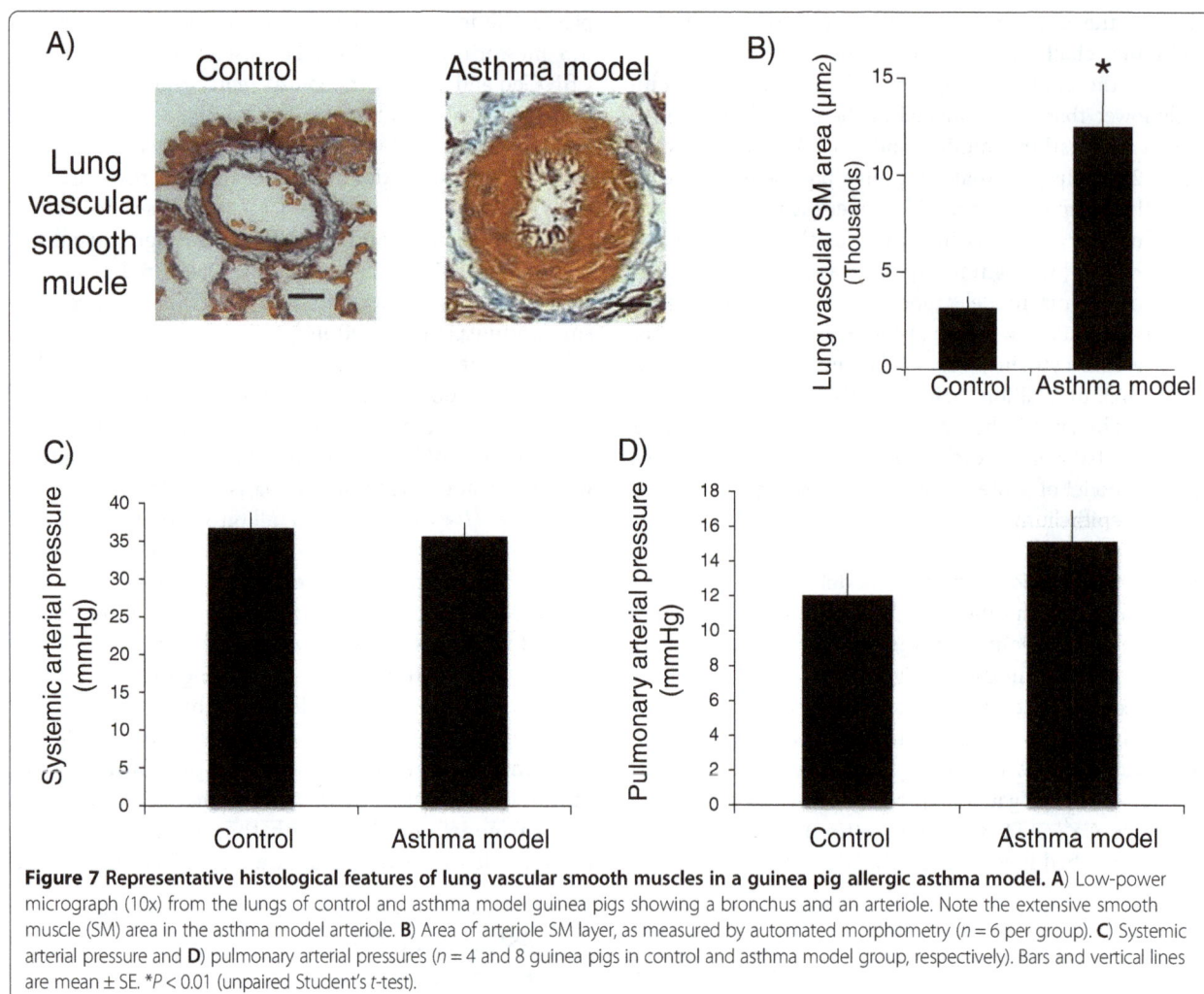

Figure 7 Representative histological features of lung vascular smooth muscles in a guinea pig allergic asthma model. A) Low-power micrograph (10x) from the lungs of control and asthma model guinea pigs showing a bronchus and an arteriole. Note the extensive smooth muscle (SM) area in the asthma model arteriole. **B)** Area of arteriole SM layer, as measured by automated morphometry ($n = 6$ per group). **C)** Systemic arterial pressure and **D)** pulmonary arterial pressures ($n = 4$ and 8 guinea pigs in control and asthma model group, respectively). Bars and vertical lines are mean ± SE. *$P < 0.01$ (unpaired Student's t-test).

was inversely correlated with airway smooth muscle caveolin-1 (r = –0.517, $P < 0.05$; $n = 13$), implying that a greater number of cells positive for caveolin-1 corresponded to greater antigen-induced airway responsiveness. In addition, the Rmax correlated with the number of cells positive for caveolin-1 (r = 0.691, $P < 0.01$; $n = 13$), indicating that antigen-induced airway obstruction is directly associated with caveolin-1 in airway smooth muscle cells.

Western blot analysis detected two specific bands for caveolin-1 at approximately 18 to 20 kDa, and the expression of both bands increased in the experimental group (Figure 4C; $n = 3$ all groups). In addition, cavins 1, 2 and 3, a group of proteins that, along with caveolin-1, regulates caveolae organisation and function [3], were found in controls but were more highly expressed in the experimental group (Figure 4C; $n = 3$ in all groups). Previously, cavins 1, 2 and 3 have been found to increase in the airway smooth muscle of ovalbumin-sensitised mice [7]. Although the role of cavins in asthma is unknown, TNF-α induced the upregulation of cavins in airway

smooth muscle, suggesting that inflammation may regulate cavin expression [39].

Immunohistochemical images did not reveal noticeable changes in caveolin-1 staining between controls and asthma model groups in airway smooth muscle or parenchyma (Figure 5; $n = 6$ all groups); nevertheless a strong reduction of caveolin-1 expression in vascular smooth muscle of the experimental group was observed in comparison with controls (Figure 5). In view that only pulmonary vascular smooth muscle showed a strong reduction in caveolin-1 expression in asthma model, and the other structures did not exhibit changes, it is possible that the intense decrease in caveolin-1 mRNA levels in total lung homogenates (Figure 4A) of the asthma model was likely produced by the downregulation of caveolin-1 in this smooth muscle.

Airway and lung vascular smooth muscle structure

Airway remodelling has been proposed as an important factor associated with caveolin in the development of airway hyperresponsiveness. For example, in a previous study [23] of a model of chronic asthma in guinea pigs (nine antigen challenges), we found an association between subepithelial fibrosis and airway hyperresponsiveness. Caveolin-1 contributes to remodelling by producing suppressive effects in airway smooth muscle proliferation [9], likely through the inhibition of constitutive p42/p44 MAPK activity [40] and by inducing type I collagen in lung tissue [5]. Airway hyperresponsiveness is a consequence of airway remodelling induced by the lack of caveolin-1 in knock-out mice [7,11].

To evaluate airway remodelling in guinea pigs, Masson trichrome staining was used to distinguish airway and lung vascular smooth muscle layers based on their strong red cytoplasmic staining (Figures 6A and 7A). Automated morphometric analysis of smooth muscle mass and subepithelial fibrosis of bronchioles and bronchi did not show significant differences between control and asthma models (Figure 6B and C; $n = 6$ in control and $n = 7$ in asthma model groups). In addition, we did not observe an association between the degree of hyperresponsiveness and the level of subepithelial fibrosis ($r = 0.25$; $n = 13$) or airway smooth muscle mass ($r = 0.18$; $n = 13$). Nevertheless, widening of the airway adjacent vessels was observed ($P < 0.05$; $n = 6$ per group; Figure 7A and B). The total numbers of smooth muscle nuclei in bronchioles in the experimental and control groups were similar (29 ± 2.3 and 28 ± 2.5 nuclei, respectively; $n = 6$ per group, data

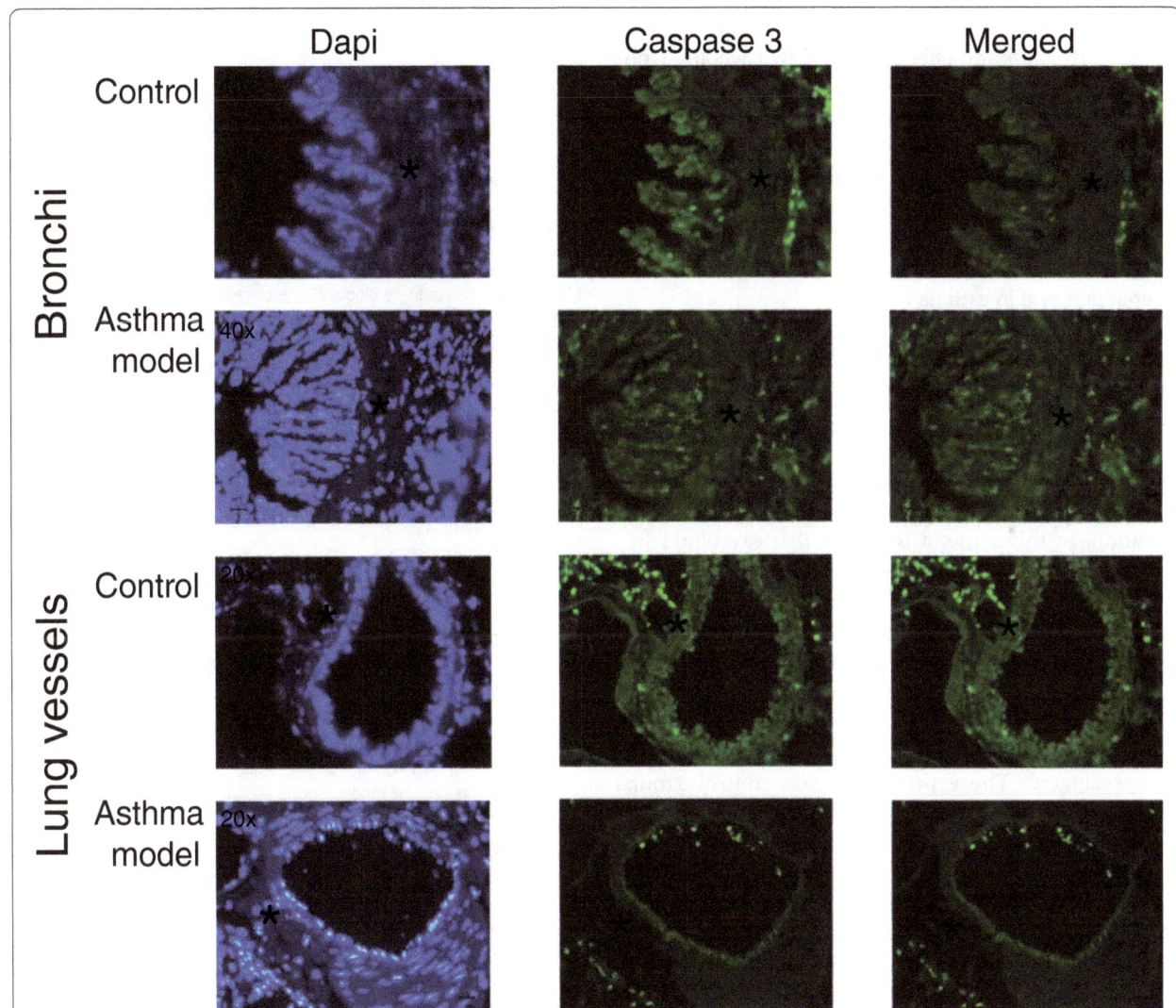

Figure 8 Immunofluorescence microscopy showed a significant reduced fluorescent staining for caspase 3 in smooth muscle from blood vessels. Lung tissue sections from guinea pig were incubated with rabbit polyclonal anti-caspase 3 antibody, followed by FITC-labeled goat anti-rabbit IgG. Nuclei were counterstained with DAPI and they are shown in blue. Caspase 3 positive (apoptotic) cells are uniformly distributed in bronchi either in samples from model asthma or control (upper panels observed by 40x magnification) as well as in blood vessel from control (medium panel, 20x magnification). In contrast, a significant decrease of apoptotic cells in blood vessel smooth muscle cells is observed in asthma model. Representative images of at least two independent experiments. * corresponds to smooth muscle bands in bronchi and lung vessels.

not illustrated); however, an increase in the number of total smooth muscle cell nuclei from airway adjacent vessels was observed in experimental guinea pigs compared with controls (51 ± 10.4 and 12 ± 1.2 nuclei, respectively; $P < 0.01$; $n = 6$ per group, data not shown). In addition, caspase 3 expression determinate by immuno-fluorescence in bronchi smooth muscle did not show noticeable change in asthma model and control groups; nevertheless, an evident diminution of caspase 3 expression was observed in lung smooth muscle from vessels in asthma model group ($n = 2$; Figure 8). It suggests that apoptosis is inhibited in vascular smooth muscle in asthma model, a tissue that also shows a decrement of caveolin-1 expression (Figure 5) and an enlargement of tissue area (Figure 7B). According to the above, these findings are in agreement with the antiproliferative and proapoptotic effects induced by caveolin-1 observed in almost cell types [41]. Then, in conclusion these results suggest that pulmonary vascular smooth muscle, but not airway smooth muscle, is capable to show remodelling changes in acute asthma model in guinea pigs and that caveolin-1 is associated with this phenomenom.

Arterial pressure in asthma model

A feature of the contractile, but not proliferative, airway smooth muscle phenotype is the abundance of caveolae, suggesting that caveolin-1 may have an inhibitory role in airway smooth muscle proliferation [9]. In contrast, the intense diminution of caveolin-1 observed in smooth muscle from airway adjacent vessels in experimental guinea pigs appears to be related to the increase in proliferation. In this sense, it is known that caveolin-1 has a fundamental role in regulating the proliferation of vascular smooth muscle [42]. In mice, the absence of caveolin-1 has been shown to modify arterial filling and increase pulmonary vascular resistance [43]. To determinate the putative physiopathological effect of vascular smooth muscle hyperplasia on our experimental guinea pigs, systemic and pulmonary arterial pressures were evaluated. The experimental and control groups did not show differences in systemic or pulmonary arterial pressures ($n = 4$ in control, and $n = 8$ in asthma group; Figure 7C and D). Vascular smooth muscle hyperplasia is observed in asthma patients [44], but this hyperplasia is unrelated to pulmonary hypertension because it includes not only hyperplasia of the smooth muscle but also enhanced vascular contractility and impaired vasodilation [45].

Conclusions

Our results suggest that the development of antigen-induced airway obstruction and hyperresponsiveness is associated with caveolin-1 expression in airway smooth muscle in a guinea pig model of asthma. It appears that the model induces the development of two different phenotypes, one contractile in airway smooth muscle and the other proliferative in pulmonary vessels. In addition, although the asthma model induced a strong caveolin-1 downregulation in vascular smooth muscle accompanied by myocyte proliferation, this phenomenon did not induce pathophysiological consequences such as changes in arterial pressure.

Competing interests

The authors declare that they have no competing interests.

Authors' contributions

MAS, PRR, SSH, RL, FGA, ROZ, RJV performed the experiments and acquired data. BBP and NAB analysed the data. BBP conceived of and designed the experiments and wrote the paper. All authors read and approved the final manuscript.

Acknowledgements

Mayra Alvarez-Santos was supported for his graduate studies by the Posgrado en Ciencias Biológicas, Universidad Nacional Autónoma de México (UNAM) and CONACyT for providing a scholarship number 294207. We thank Instituto Nacional de Enfermedades Respiratorias for the economic support given to this project.

Author details

[1]Instituto Nacional de Enfermedades Respiratorias Ismael Cosío Villegas, Departamento de Hiperreactividad Bronquial, Calzada de Tlalpan 4502, Mexico. [2]Departamento de Bioquímica, Facultad de Medicina, Universidad Nacional Autónoma de México, México, DF, Mexico. [3]Departamento de Cirugía Experimental, Instituto Nacional de Enfermedades,Respiratorias Ismael Cosío Villegas, Calzada de Tlalpan 4502, Mexico. [4]Molecular Physiology Unit, Instituto de Investigaciones Biomédicas, Universidad Nacional Autónoma de México, México, Mexico. [5]Instituto Nacional de Ciencias Médicas y Nutrición Salvador Zubirán, Department of Nephrology, México, Mexico.

References

1. Buc M, Dzurilla M, Vrlik M, Bucova M. Immunopathogenesis of bronchial asthma. Arch Immunol Ther Exp (Warsz). 2009;57:331–44.
2. Cockcroft DW, Davis BE. Mechanisms of airway hyperresponsiveness. J Allergy Clin Immunol. 2006;118:551–9. quiz 560–551.
3. Fridolfsson HN, Roth DM, Insel PA, Patel HH: Regulation of intracellular signaling and function by caveolin. FASEB J 2014.
4. Bains SN, Tourkina E, Atkinson C, Joseph K, Tholanikunnel B, Chu HW, et al. Loss of caveolin-1 from bronchial epithelial cells and monocytes in human subjects with asthma. Allergy. 2012;67:1601–4.
5. Chen CM, Wu MY, Chou HC, Lang YD, Wang LF. Downregulation of caveolin-1 in a murine model of acute allergic airway disease. Pediatr Neonatol. 2011;52:5–10.
6. Le Saux CJ, Teeters K, Miyasato SK, Hoffmann PR, Bollt O, Douet V, et al. Down-regulation of caveolin-1, an inhibitor of transforming growth factor-beta signaling, in acute allergen-induced airway remodeling. J Biol Chem. 2008;283:5760–8.
7. Aravamudan B, Vanoosten SK, Meuchel LW, Vohra P, Thompson M, Sieck GC, et al. Caveolin-1 knockout mice exhibit airway hyperreactivity. Am J Physiol Lung Cell Mol Physiol. 2012;303:L669–681.
8. Gosens R, Stelmack GL, Bos ST, Dueck G, Mutawe MM, Schaafsma D, et al. Caveolin-1 is required for contractile phenotype expression by airway smooth muscle cells. J Cell Mol Med. 2011;15:2430–42.
9. Halayko AJ, Tran T, Gosens R. Phenotype and functional plasticity of airway smooth muscle: role of caveolae and caveolins. Proc Am Thorac Soc. 2008;5:80–8.
10. Le Saux O, Teeters K, Miyasato S, Choi J, Nakamatsu G, Richardson JA, et al. The role of caveolin-1 in pulmonary matrix remodeling and mechanical properties. Am J Physiol Lung Cell Mol Physiol. 2008;295:L1007–1017.

11. Gabehart KE, Royce SG, Maselli DJ, Miyasato SK, Davis EC, Tang ML, et al. Airway hyperresponsiveness is associated with airway remodeling but not inflammation in aging Cav1−/− mice. Respir Res. 2013;14:110.

12. Hsia BJ, Pastva AM, Giamberardino CD, Potts-Kant EN, Foster WM, Que LG, Abraham SN, Wright JR, Zaas DW: Increased Nitric Oxide Production Prevents Airway Hyperresponsiveness in Caveolin-1 Deficient Mice Following Endotoxin Exposure. *J Allergy Ther* 2012, Suppl 1.

13. Bergdahl A, Sward K. Caveolae-associated signalling in smooth muscle. Can J Physiol Pharmacol. 2004;82:289–99.

14. Gosens R, Mutawe M, Martin S, Basu S, Bos ST, Tran T, et al. Caveolae and caveolins in the respiratory system. Curr Mol Med. 2008;8:741–53.

15. Darby PJ, Kwan CY, Daniel EE. Caveolae from canine airway smooth muscle contain the necessary components for a role in Ca(2+) handling. Am J Physiol Lung Cell Mol Physiol. 2000;279:L1226–1235.

16. Gosens R, Stelmack GL, Dueck G, Mutawe MM, Hinton M, McNeill KD, et al. Caveolae facilitate muscarinic receptor-mediated intracellular Ca2+ mobilization and contraction in airway smooth muscle. Am J Physiol Lung Cell Mol Physiol. 2007;293:L1406–1418.

17. Prakash YS, Thompson MA, Vaa B, Matabdin I, Peterson TE, He T, et al. Caveolins and intracellular calcium regulation in human airway smooth muscle. Am J Physiol Lung Cell Mol Physiol. 2007;293:L1118–1126.

18. Hunter I, Nixon GF. Spatial compartmentalization of tumor necrosis factor (TNF) receptor 1-dependent signaling pathways in human airway smooth muscle cells. Lipid rafts are essential for TNF-alpha-mediated activation of RhoA but dispensable for the activation of the NF-kappaB and MAPK pathways. J Biol Chem. 2006;281:34705–15.

19. Taggart MJ, Leavis P, Feron O, Morgan KG. Inhibition of PKCalpha and rhoA translocation in differentiated smooth muscle by a caveolin scaffolding domain peptide. Exp Cell Res. 2000;258:72–81.

20. Sathish V, Abcejo AJ, Thompson MA, Sieck GC, Prakash YS, Pabelick CM: Caveolin-1 regulation of store-operated Ca2+ influx in human airway smooth muscle. *Eur Respir J* 2012.

21. Vinten J, Johnsen AH, Roepstorff P, Harpoth J, Tranum-Jensen J. Identification of a major protein on the cytosolic face of caveolae. Biochim Biophys Acta. 2005;1717:34–40.

22. Hansen CG, Nichols BJ. Exploring the caves: cavins, caveolins and caveolae. Trends Cell Biol. 2010;20:177–86.

23. Bazan-Perkins B, Sanchez-Guerrero E, Vargas MH, Martinez-Cordero E, Ramos-Ramirez P, Alvarez-Santos M, et al. Beta1-integrins shedding in a guinea-pig model of chronic asthma with remodelled airways. Clin Exp Allergy. 2009;39:740–51.

24. Smith N, Broadley KJ. Optimisation of the sensitisation conditions for an ovalbumin challenge model of asthma. Int Immunopharmacol. 2007;7:183–90.

25. Ricciardolo FL, Nijkamp F, De Rose V, Folkerts G. The guinea pig as an animal model for asthma. Curr Drug Targets. 2008;9:452–65.

26. Ressmeyer AR, Larsson AK, Vollmer E, Dahlen SE, Uhlig S, Martin C. Characterisation of guinea pig precision-cut lung slices: comparison with human tissues. Eur Respir J. 2006;28:603–11.

27. Ramos-Ramirez P, Campos MG, Martinez-Cordero E, Bazan-Perkins B, Garcia-Zepeda E. Antigen-induced airway hyperresponsiveness in absence of broncho-obstruction in sensitized guinea pigs. Exp Lung Res. 2013;39:136–45.

28. Hamelmann E, Schwarze J, Takeda K, Oshiba A, Larsen GL, Irvin CG, et al. Noninvasive measurement of airway responsiveness in allergic mice using barometric plethysmography. Am J Respir Crit Care Med. 1997;156:766–75.

29. Lecoeur H, Ledru E, Gougeon ML. A cytofluorometric method for the simultaneous detection of both intracellular and surface antigens of apoptotic peripheral lymphocytes. J Immunol Methods. 1998;217:11–26.

30. Sambrook J, Russell DW, Sambrook J. The condensed protocols from Molecular cloning : a laboratory manual. Cold Spring Harbor, N.Y.: Cold Spring Harbor Laboratory Press; 2006.

31. Bobadilla NA, Herrera JP, Merino A, Gamba G. Semi-quantitative PCR: a tool to study low abundance messages in the kidney. Arch Med Res. 1997;28:55–60.

32. Canning BJ, Chou Y. Using guinea pigs in studies relevant to asthma and COPD. Pulm Pharmacol Ther. 2008;21:702–20.

33. Woodruff PG, Modrek B, Choy DF, Jia G, Abbas AR, Ellwanger A, et al. T-helper type 2-driven inflammation defines major subphenotypes of asthma. Am J Respir Crit Care Med. 2009;180:388–95.

34. Gabella G. Quantitative morphological study of smooth muscle cells of the guinea-pig taenia coli. Cell Tissue Res. 1976;170:161–86.

35. Sharma P, Ghavami S, Stelmack GL, McNeill KD, Mutawe MM, Klonisch T, et al. beta-Dystroglycan binds caveolin-1 in smooth muscle: a functional role in caveolae distribution and Ca2+ release. J Cell Sci. 2010;123:3061–70.

36. Brightling C, Berry M, Amrani Y. Targeting TNF-alpha: a novel therapeutic approach for asthma. J Allergy Clin Immunol. 2008;121:5–10. quiz 11–12.

37. Sathish V, Abcejo AJ, VanOosten SK, Thompson MA, Prakash YS, Pabelick CM. Caveolin-1 in cytokine-induced enhancement of intracellular Ca(2+) in human airway smooth muscle. Am J Physiol Lung Cell Mol Physiol. 2011;301:L607–614.

38. Sathish V, Yang B, Meuchel LW, VanOosten SK, Ryu AJ, Thompson MA, et al. Caveolin-1 and force regulation in porcine airway smooth muscle. Am J Physiol Lung Cell Mol Physiol. 2011;300:L920–929.

39. Sathish V, Thompson MA, Sinha S, Sieck GC, Prakash YS, Pabelick CM. Inflammation, caveolae and CD38-mediated calcium regulation in human airway smooth muscle. Biochim Biophys Acta. 1843;2014:346–51.

40. Gosens R, Dueck G, Gerthoffer WT, Unruh H, Zaagsma J, Meurs H, et al. p42/p44 MAP kinase activation is localized to caveolae-free membrane domains in airway smooth muscle. Am J Physiol Lung Cell Mol Physiol. 2007;292:L1163–1172.

41. Jin Y, Lee SJ, Minshall RD, Choi AM. Caveolin-1: a critical regulator of lung injury. Am J Physiol Lung Cell Mol Physiol. 2011;300:L151–160.

42. Sedding DG, Braun-Dullaeus RC. Caveolin-1: dual role for proliferation of vascular smooth muscle cells. Trends Cardiovasc Med. 2006;16:50–5.

43. Maniatis NA, Shinin V, Schraufnagel DE, Okada S, Vogel SM, Malik AB, et al. Increased pulmonary vascular resistance and defective pulmonary artery filling in caveolin-1−/− mice. Am J Physiol Lung Cell Mol Physiol. 2008;294:L865–873.

44. Harkness LM, Kanabar V, Sharma HS, Westergren-Thorsson G, Larsson-Callerfelt AK: Pulmonary vascular changes in asthma and COPD. *Pulm Pharmacol Ther* 2014.

45. Yildiz P. Molecular mechanisms of pulmonary hypertension. Clin Chim Acta. 2009;403:9–16.

2

Interleukin-25 and eosinophils progenitor cell mobilization in allergic asthma

Wei Tang[1,2], Steven G. Smith[1], Wei Du[2], Akash Gugilla[1], Juan Du[2], John Paul Oliveria[1], Karen Howie[1], Brittany M. Salter[1], Gail M. Gauvreau[1], Paul M. O'Byrne[1] and Roma Sehmi[1*]

Abstract

Background: Eosinophil-lineage committed progenitor cells (EoP) migrate from the bone marrow and differentiate locally to provide an ongoing source of mature eosinophils in asthmatic inflammatory responses in the airways. Sputum levels of EoP are increased in asthmatics compared to normal controls suggesting an exaggerated eosinophilopoietic environment in the airways. Understanding what factors promote EoP traffic to the airways is important to understand the diathesis of asthma pathology. Interleukin (IL)-25, is an epithelial-derived cytokine that promotes type 2 inflammatory responses. We have previously shown that levels of IL-25 and expression of the IL-25 receptor (IL-17RA and IL-17RB) on mature eosinophils are greater in allergic asthmatics compared to atopic non-asthmatics and non-atopic normal controls. In addition, these levels were increased significantly increased following allergen inhalation challenge and physiologically relevant levels of IL-25 stimulated eosinophil degranulation, intracellular IL-5 and IL-13 expression and primed migration to eotaxin. The current study, examined the role of IL-25 on allergen-induced trafficking of EoP in atopic asthmatics.

Methods: Asthmatics (n = 14) who developed allergen-induced early and late responses were enrolled in the study. Blood was collected at pre- and 24 h post-challenge. At each time point, surface expression of IL-17RA and IL-17RB on EoP was evaluated by flow cytometry. Migration assays examined the effect of IL-25 on EoP chemotactic responses, in vitro. In addition, IL-25 knockout ovalbumin (OVA) sensitized and challenged mice were studied to evaluate in vivo mobilization effects of IL-25 on newly formed EoP and mature eosinophils.

Results: There was a significant increase in numbers of blood EoP expressing IL-17RB, 24 h post-allergen inhalation challenge in allergic asthmatics. Pre-exposure to IL-25 primed the migrational responsiveness of EoP to stromal cell-derived factor 1α. In OVA-sensitized mice, knocking out IL-25 significantly alleviated OVA-induced eosinophil infiltration in the airway and newly formed eosinophils were reduced in the lung.

Conclusions: The findings of this study indicate a potential role for IL-25 in allergen-induced trafficking of EoP to the airways and local differentiation promoting tissue eosiniophilia in asthmatic responses.

Keywords: Asthma, Allergen challenge, Eosinophils progenitor, IL-25, IL-25 receptors, BrdU, CD34

Background

Asthma is a chronic disease of the airways characterized by reversible airflow obstruction, airway inflammation and airway hypperesponsiveness. Tissue eosinophilia and type 2 cytokine producing cells including T-helper (Th) 2 cells and group 2 innate lymphoid cells, are the predominant components of the airway inflammatory cell infiltrate in subjects with allergic asthma [1].

Interleukin-25 (IL-25; IL-17E) is a pro-inflammatory cytokine that belongs to the IL-17 cytokine family and, unlike other members of the IL-17 family, plays a pivotal role in the maintenance of type 2 immune responses [2]. IL-25 has been shown to directly activate eosinophils, by up-regulation of the adhesion molecule ICAM-1, stimulate the release of pro-inflammatory chemokines such as monocyte chemoattractant protein-1, IL-8, macrophage

---

*Correspondence: sehmir@mcmaster.ca

[1] Division of Respirology, Department of Medicine, McMaster University, Hamilton, ON L6M 1A6, Canada

Full list of author information is available at the end of the article

inflammatory protein-1 and IL-6, as well as delay apoptosis [3, 4]. The IL-25 receptor consists of two subunits, IL-17RA (the signaling sub-unit) and IL-17RB (the specific cytokine binding subunit) that form the functional heterodimeric receptor, IL-17RA/RB [5]. In a previous baseline cross-sectional study, we have shown significantly increased expression of IL-17RA and IL-17RB on mature eosinophils and plasma levels of IL-25 in asymptomatic mild allergic asthmatics compared with atopic non-asthmatics and non-atopic normal subjects [6]. In addition, we reported significant increases in plasma levels of IL-25 and intracellular IL-25 eosinophil levels, as well as IL-17RA/RB and IL-17RB receptor expression on mature eosinophils, 24 h following allergen-inhalation challenge in allergic asthmatics [7]. Furthermore in vitro experiments showed that at physiologically relevant concentrations, IL-25 stimulated eosinophil degranulation and primed the migrational responses of mature eosinophils.

A considerable body of evidence supports the view that in allergic asthma, eosinophil-lineage committed progenitor cells (EoP) traffic from the bone marrow to the lungs via the peripheral circulation and that the local tissue-driven differentiation of these cells may contribute to the development and maintenance of tissue eosinophilia [8]. The effect of IL-25 on the traffic of bone marrow-derived hemopoietic progenitor cells (HPC) and more specifically eosinophil-lineage commmited progenitor cells (EoP) to the lungs in allergic asthmatic responses has not been reported to date.

In this study, we examined IL-25 and IL-25R expression on EoP in asthmatic subjects following allergen-inhalation challenge. In addition, we employed an OVA-sensitized mouse model to investigate whether traffic of mature eosinophils and newly formed eosinophils to the site of inflammation was influenced by IL-25.

Methods
Study design
Fourteen subjects with mild allergic asthma, aged between 19 and 52 years, were enrolled in the study. All volunteers were atopic with one or more positive skin prick tests; a forced expired volume in 1 s (FEV_1) greater or equal to 70% of predicted; and dual airway responses to inhaled allergen as determined by a fall in $FEV_1 \geq 15\%$ within the first 2 h, followed by second fall in FEV_1 between 3 and 7 h after allergen inhalation challenge (Table 1). All subjects were steroid naïve and only intermittently used β_2-agonists. Subjects attended the laboratory for three consecutive visits. On visit 1 (day 1), a medical history and physical examination were performed and subjects underwent a skin prick test, spirometry, methacholine inhalation challenge. On visit 2 (day

Table 1 Baseline subject characteristics

Sex	Age	Ag inhaled	%FEV1 (%predicted)	PBaseline PC_{20} (mg/ml)
M	19	Cat	81	0.31
M	25	HDM	114	10.31
F	19	Cat	117	20.80
F	49	HDM	97	1.07
M	44	Grass	73	16.00
F	41	Ragweed	94	0.83
F	47	Cat	90	0.60
F	20	Tree	92	3.19
M	52	HDM	100	6.99
M	27	Ragweed	97	2.71
F	21	Horse	98	16.00
F	19	Ragweed	80	5.82
M	49	HDM	90	16.00
F	24	HDM	116	0.38
F	25	HDM	108	15.48

Subject characteristics: all subjects were skin prick test positive; had a forced expired volume in 1 s ($FEV1$) $\geq$ 70% predicted; FEV_1—forced expiratory volume in 1 s; all patients PC_{20}—provocative concentration of methacholine causing a 20% drop in FEV_1; *HDM* house dust mite; *Ag* allergen

2), subjects underwent allergen inhalation challenge and spirometry was measured hourly up to 7 h post-challenge. At Visit 3 (day 3), spirometry and methacholine challenge was performed 24 h after inhalation challenge. Flow cytometric assessments were performed on blood samples collected before and 24 h post-allergen challenge. All subjects gave written informed consent, and the study was approved by the Hamilton Health Science Research Ethics Board (HIREB # 12-583).

Allergen inhalation challenge
Allergen inhalation was performed as previously described [9]. The allergen producing the largest diameter skin wheel was diluted in saline for inhalation. The concentration of allergen required to achieve a 20% decrease in FEV_1 (the allergen PC_{20}) was predicted using the methacholine PC_{20} and the titration of allergen determined from the skin prick test. The early asthmatic response (EAR) was recorded as the greatest fall in FEV_1 between 0 and 2 h after allergen inhalation, whereas the greatest drop in FEV_1 between 3 and 7 h was recorded as the late asthmatic response (LAR) as previously described [9].

Cell preparation and Immunofluorescence staining
For identifying $CD34^+$ hemopoietic progenitor cells, 20 mL heparinized venous blood was diluted with McCoys 5A (Invitrogen, USA), then layered on Lymphoprep (Axis-Shield, USA) and centrifuged (2200 rpm,

20 min). Mononuclear cells were removed and washed with McCoy's 5A (centrifugation at 1500 rpm for 10 min at 4 °C) and re-suspended in FACS buffer, then immunostained with CD34-Alexa Fluor 700, CD45-Pacific Blue, CD125-APC, IL17RA-FITC and IL17RB-PE or corresponding isotype controls (BD Bioscience and R&D systems). Cells were incubated for 30 min at 4 °C then washed with FACS buffer and fixed in 1% PFA prior to flow cytometric acquisition.

Flow cytometry acquisition

Data were acquired using a 15-color LSR II flow cytometer equipped with 3 lasers (Becton–Dickinson Instrument Systems) with FACSDiva software program (Becton–Dickinson Biosciences). Following acquisition of 300,000 events, data analyses were performed using FlowJo software version 9.3.2. (Tree Star Inc.) to enumerate IL-25 receptor components expression; for gating strategy details see Additional file 1: Fig. S1 for hemopoietic progenitor cells (HPC; CD34^{high}CD45^{dull}) and eosinophil-lineage committed progenitor cells (EoP; CD34^{high}CD45^{dull}CD125^{high}) as previously described in detail [10].

Progenitor cell migration—trans well migration assay

The migrational response of progenitors was assessed in transwell chambers (24-well cell clusters, 6.5 mm Transwell® with 5 μm pore polycarbonate membrane insert filters; Corning Costar, NY, USA) as previously described [10]. Briefly, peripheral blood mononuclear cells isolated, as described above, were depleted by adherence to plastic (2 h, 5% CO2 and 37 °C) and CD34$^+$ cells enriched by positive selection using MACS immunomagnetic beads (Miltenyi Biotec, CA, USA). Cell purity of CD34$^+$ cells was > 95%, viability > 90%. The chemoattractant, SDF-1 (CXCL12; 10 ng/mL; R&D Systems) or diluent (IMDM plus 10% FBS) was loaded into the lower well and CD34$^+$ cells (5 × 10^4) were added to the upper transwell inserts. Cells in the lower well (representing migrated responding cells) were immunostained as HPC (CD34$^+$CD45$^+$) or EoP (CD45$^+$CD34$^+$CD125$^+$) and enumerated by flow cytometry, as described above. Migrated cells were expressed as a percentage of the total cells added to the top transwell. Cells were pre-incubated with IL-25 (R&D Systems) for 18 h (37 °C, 5% CO$_2$) prior to the migration assay.

OVA sensitized mice

Wild type C57BL/6 mice were purchased from Shanghai SLAC laboratory Co., Ltd. (Shanghai, China). IL-25 knockout mice on the same background were purchased from Qinghua University animal center (Beijin, China). Mice were aged between 6 and 8 weeks-old, weighing

between 20 and 22 g, and were housed at 18–25 °C, humidity 50–60%, 0.03% CO$_2$, 12/12 h light/dark cycle and food/water were available ad libitum and refreshed every 3 days. For both wild type and IL-25KO mice, the sensitized animals (OVA sensitized and OVA challenged; n = 6) received an intraperitoneal injection of 100 μg ovalbumin (OVA; Sigma Aldrich; Merck KGaA) and 2 mg alum (Sigma Aldrich; Merck KGaA) in PBS on days 0, 7 and 14. On days 25, 26 and 27, the mice were challenge with aerosolized 1% OVA in PBS for 30 min. For both wild type and IL-25KO mice, Sham control mice (Sham sensitized and Sham challenged, n = 6) received PBS intraperitoneally with alum on days 0, 7 and 14, and were challenged with aerosolized PBS on days 25, 26 and 27. BrdU (1 mg) was given by intraperitoneal injection twice per day, on days 25 and 27, 30 min prior to challenge with OVA as previously described [11, 12].

Bronchoalveolar lavage fluid (BALF), blood and bone marrow sampling

BALF collection was performed 24 h after the final OVA or PBS challenge. Lungs were lavaged with 1 mL PBS through the trachea and BALF was collected. Blood (0.5–0.8 mL) was drawn prior to BALF collection into heparin from each mouse. Bone marrow was harvested from the femur and tibia into heparin as previously described [12]. Smears of blood and bone marrow samples were made to perform eosinophil counts following standard staining with hematoxolin and eosin.

Measurement of eosinophil number in BALF

Cells were seeded in PBS medium (Beyotime Institute of Biotechnology, Haimen, China) at 1 × 10^5 cells/mL and stained with Fast Wright and Giemsa Stain kit (Nanjing Jiancheng Technology Co., Ltd., Nanjing, China), according to manufacturer's protocol. Eosinophils were counted with a light microscope and expressed as percent eosinophils.

Inflammatory index measurement

The lung inflammation index score after OVA or diluent challenge was measured as previously described [13]. The index is: 0 equals no inflammatory infiltration; 1 equals a minimal inflammatory cell infiltration; 2 equals a layer of inflammatory cells annular infiltration; 3 equals 2–4 layers of inflammatory cell ring infiltration; 4 equals more than 4 layers of inflammatory cells annular infiltration.

Immunohistochemistry (IHC) semi-quantitative analysis

The expression levels of BrdU in lung tissues were quantified by Image-Pro Plus 6.0, expressed as mean optical density (OD), which equals intensity of optical density divided by area of lung tissues observed under microscope ($400\times$). Newly produced eosinophils were identified as BrdU positive and eosin positive cells.

Statistical analysis

Statistical analysis was performed using GraphPad Prism5 software (GraphPad Software Inc.). This study is powered on sputum eosinophil progenitor cells in mild asthmatics, and changes 24 h post-allergen were the primary outcome. Assuming within subject variability from previously published data in mild asthmatics [9], the sample size required to detect the "minimal important differences" between baseline and 24 h post-allergen measurements was calculated. Based on repeated measures ANOVA analyses, using the sample size module of NCSS statistical package with $\beta = 0.20$ (power = 80%) and $\alpha = 0.05$ (likelihood of type 1 error = 5%) and a minimum important difference = 0.72, SD = 0.59, the sample size is calculated to be n = 14. Normally distributed data are expressed as mean $\pm$ SEM. The methacoline PC_{20} is expressed as geometric mean and geometric standard error of the mean (GSEM). For HPC and EoP IL-25 receptor expression and migration experiments, a repeated measures ANOVA was used. Post-hoc comparisons were performed using the Tukey's multiple comparison tests. $p < 0.05$ was considered significant for all analyses.

Results

Following allergen inhalation challenge, all asthmatic subjects developed an early and late bronchoconstrictor responses; the maximal early fall in FEV_1 (within 0–2 h post-allergen) was $33.67 + 8.22\%$ and the maximal late fall in FEV_1 (3–7 h post-allergen inhalation) was $22.47 + 8.43\%$ (Table 2). This was associated with a significant increase airway eosinophilia (Table 2) and total number of number of blood HPC and EoP (HPC: 1663 ± 657 vs. 723 ± 244 per 10^6 WBC, $p < 0.01$; EoP: 1188 ± 442 vs. 519 ± 140 per 10^6 WBC, $p < 0.01$) 24 h post-allergen compared to pre-allergen levels. Further phenotypic analyses of HPC and EoP demonstrated significant increases in expression of IL-25 specific binding sub-unit (IL-17RB), 24 h post-allergen compared to pre-allergen baseline levels (Fig. 1). In contrast, these changes were not observed for the signaling sub-unit IL-17RA or combined receptor complex IL-17RA/RB on either HPC or EoP (Fig. 1).

In pilot studies, we found that IL-25 over a wide concentration range (0.1 – 1000 pg/ml) has no effect on the migrational responses of EoP compared to diluent control, in vitro (data not shown). However, pre-incubation with IL-25 (optimal concentration 1 pg/ml), compared to diluent, significantly enhanced the subsequent migrational response of both HPC and EoP to a sub-optimal

Table 2 Subject lung function and sputum

	Allergen challenge
EAR (% change in FEV_1)	$- 33.67 \pm 2.12$[#]
LAR (% change in FEV_1)	$- 24.47 \pm 1.77$[#]
Methacoline PC_{20} (mg/mL)	
Pre-Ag	7.77 ± 1.88
24 h post-Ag	2.20 ± 0.51*
Total sputum cells ($\times 10^6$ cells/mL)	
Pre-Ag	3.62 ± 0.64
24 h Post-Ag	6.59 ± 1.27*
Sputum eosinophils (%)	
Pre-Ag	4.68 ± 1.63
24 h Post-Ag	12.26 ± 2.68*,#
Blood eosinophils (per 10^9 WBC)	
Pre-Ag	38 ± 6
24 h Post-Ag	64 ± 9*

Data are presented as geometric mean $\pm$ SEM. There was a significant difference the EAR and LAR % change in FEV_1, methacoline PC_{20}, total sputum cells, and sputum and blood eosinophils post-allergen

FEV_1 forced expiratory volume in 1 s; $PC20$ provocative concentration of methacoline causing a 20% drop in FEV_1, Ag allergen, EAR early asthmatic response, LAR late asthmatic response, WBC white blood cells, HPC hemopoietic progenitor cells, EoP eosinophil progenitors

*$p < 0.05$ comparison to baseline and #$p < 0.05$ comparison to diluent

concentration of SDF-1α (10 ng/ml) (HPC: 64 ± 13 vs. 35 ± 6 and EoP: 73 ± 8 vs. 39 ± 10 respectively, $p < 0.0001$) (Fig. 2). Pre-treatment with an IL-25 neutralizing antibody (previously optimized at 2.4 ng/ml) significantly inhibited the priming effect of IL-25 on SDF-1α stimulated migration of HPC and EoP (Fig. 2).

In IL-25 knock out (KO) mice that were OVA-sensitized, a partial but significant attenuation of airway inflammation following allergen -challenge was observed (Additional file 2: Fig. S2). The inflammatory index in the control mice compared to wild type OVA challenged and IL-25 KO OVA challenged mice were 0.50 ± 0.51 vs. 1.63 ± 0.77 vs 0.93 ± 0.54 respectively ($p < 0.001$ for all comparisons to control mice) (Fig. 3). Furthermore, OVA challenge significantly increased the percentages of eosinophils in wild type compared to control mice in BALF (7.83 ± 4.84 vs. $3.40 \pm 0.43\%$) and bone marrow samples (5.33 ± 0.85 vs. $2.7 \pm 0.25\%$) (Fig. 4). Compared to the wild type mice, eosinophils levels were significantly attenuated in the OVA challenged IL-25 KO mice in BALF (7.83 ± 4.84, vs. $3.06 \pm 1.78\%$, $p < 0.01$) (Fig. 4).

The proportion of BrdU + eosinophils expressed as a percentage of the total eosinophils in BAL and bone marrow was significantly reduced in OVA challenged IL-25 KO mice compared to wild type mice (BAL: 12.5 ± 6.51 vs. $51.7 \pm 7.56\%$, $p < 0.01$; bone marrow: 2.4 ± 1.28 vs. $69.1 \pm 6.11\%$, $p < 0.001$) (Fig. 5). In the lungs, BrdU expression after OVA challenge was

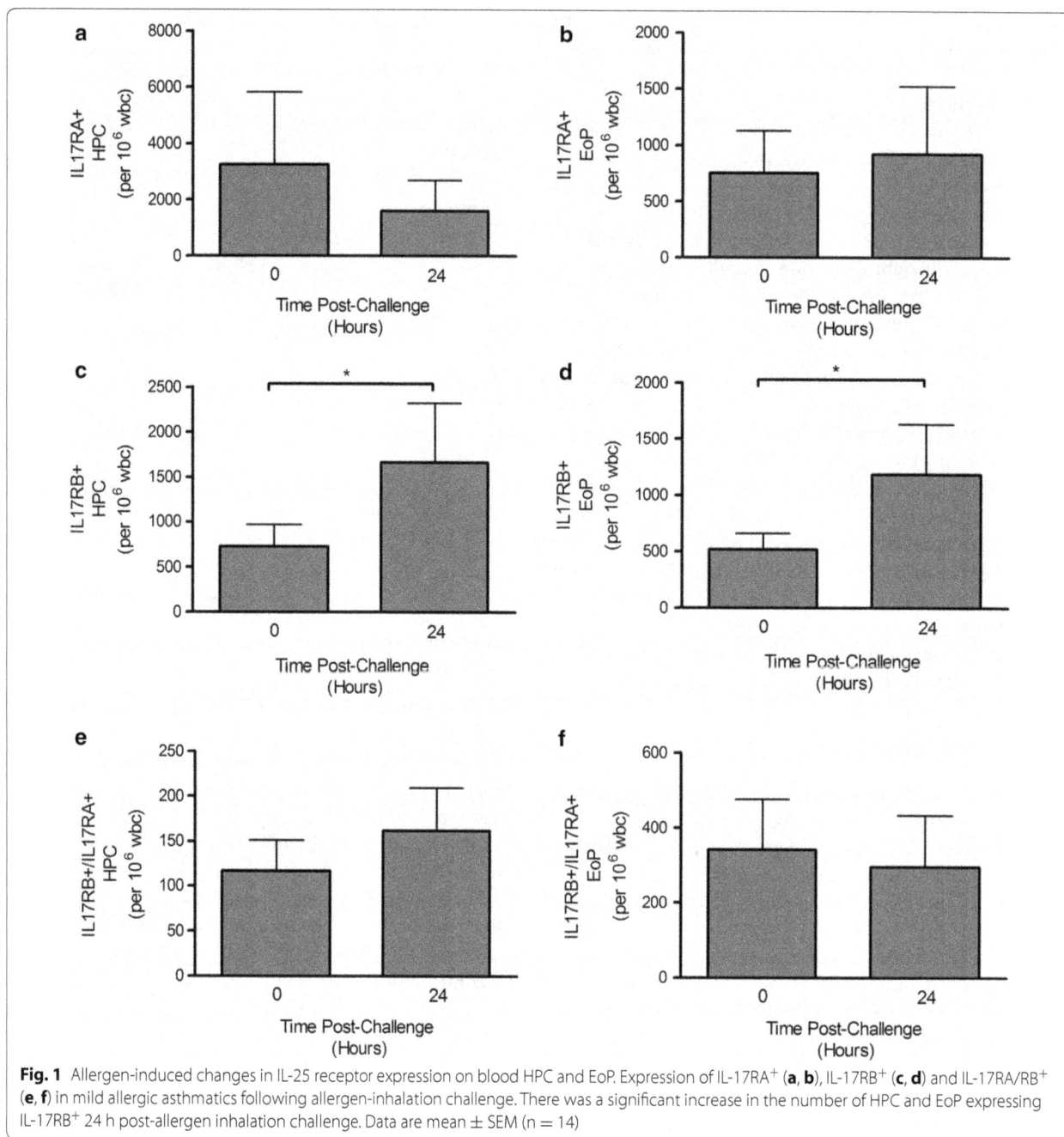

Fig. 1 Allergen-induced changes in IL-25 receptor expression on blood HPC and EoP. Expression of IL-17RA$^+$ (**a**, **b**), IL-17RB$^+$ (**c**, **d**) and IL-17RA/RB$^+$ (**e**, **f**) in mild allergic asthmatics following allergen-inhalation challenge. There was a significant increase in the number of HPC and EoP expressing IL-17RB$^+$ 24 h post-allergen inhalation challenge. Data are mean $\pm$ SEM (n = 14)

significantly decreased in IL-25 KO mice compared with wild type mice (mean density, 0.013 $\pm$ 0.010OD vs. 0.020 $\pm$ 0.013OD; p < 0.01), (Fig. 6).

Discussion

This study has demonstrated that following allergen-inhalation challenge in allergic asthmatic subjects, IL-17RB is up-regulated on the surface of HPC, as well as EoP in the blood. In addition, IL-25 primes migrational

responses of blood-derived HPC and EoP to the progenitor chemoattractant, SDF-1α. These findings suggest that in response to inhaled allergen, upregulation of IL-25 receptor binding sub-unit expression on EoP in peripheral blood may promote increased occupancy of IL-25 on its specific receptor and stimulate priming of migrational responsiveness, thereby facilitating the homing of eosinophil precursors to the airways. Furthermore, in OVA-sensitized mice, knocking out IL-25 significantly

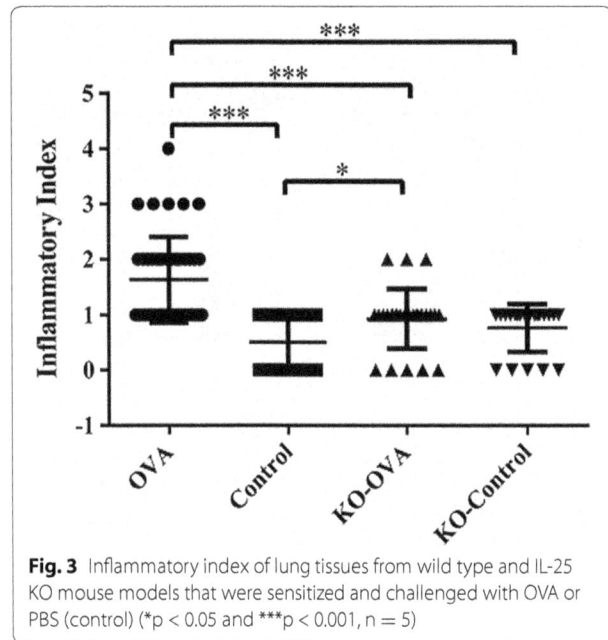

Fig. 2 IL-25 priming of (**a**) HPC and **b** EoP migration, in vitro. Pre-incubation overnight with IL-25 primed the migrational responsiveness of both HPC and EoP stimulated by SDF-1α. SDF-1α alone induced migration. Data are presented as mean ± SEM (n = 6) (*p < 0.05 comparison to diluent; #p < 0.05 comparison to SDF-1α alone)

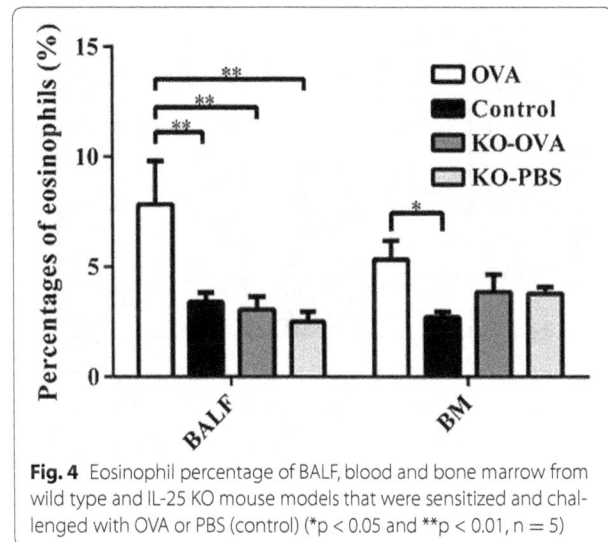

Fig. 3 Inflammatory index of lung tissues from wild type and IL-25 KO mouse models that were sensitized and challenged with OVA or PBS (control) (*p < 0.05 and ***p < 0.001, n = 5)

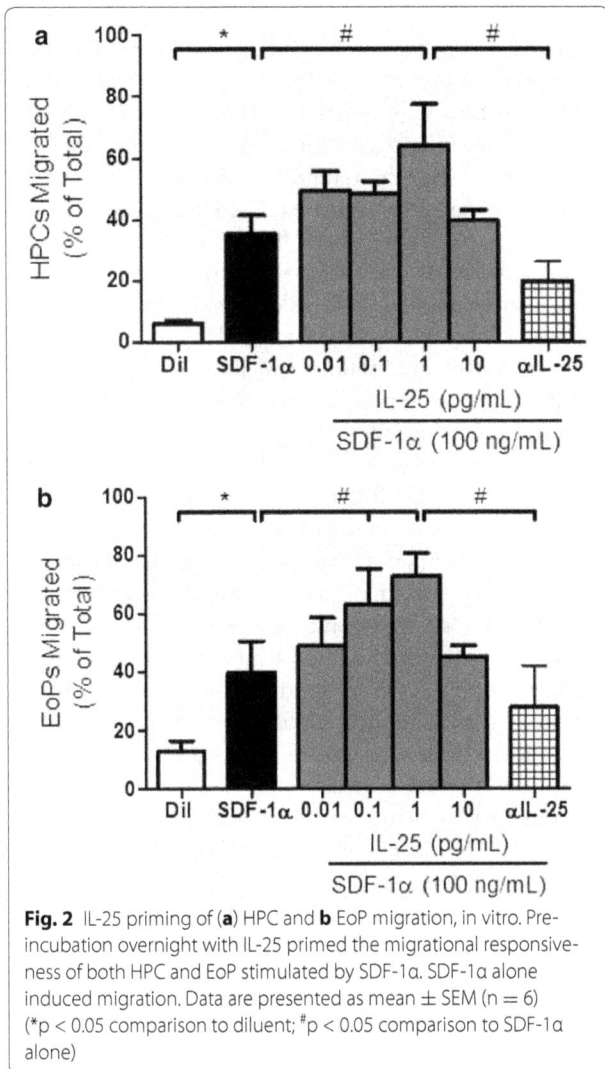

Fig. 4 Eosinophil percentage of BALF, blood and bone marrow from wild type and IL-25 KO mouse models that were sensitized and challenged with OVA or PBS (control) (*p < 0.05 and **p < 0.01, n = 5)

alleviated lung inflammation, airway eosinophil infiltration and lung homing of newly produced eosinophils.

The biological effects of IL-25 are mediated by IL-25 receptor, which is composed of sub-units IL-17RA and IL-17RB. IL-25 is the high affinity ligand for IL-17RB, while IL-17RA shares the common ligand for IL-17A [5, 14]. Polymorphisms in the IL-17RB gene in humans have been linked with asthma susceptibility [15]. In a previous study, we have shown that IL-25 receptor expression on eosinophils is markedly higher in allergic asthmatics compared with atopic non-asthmatic and normal subjects [6]. In addition, we showed that the level of plasma IL-25 significantly increases following allergen inhalation challenge in allergic asthmatics [7]. In humans, IL-25 is produced by structural cells, such as epithelial and endothelial cells, and inflammatory cells, such as eosinophils, basophils and mast cells. IL-25 has been shown to

link innate and adaptive immunity by enhancing type-2 cytokine production, including IL-5 and IL-13 [2].

The current study suggests that IL-25 plays a role in the recruitment of immature eosinophils to the airways in asthma. Our previous research has shown that EoP traffic from the systemic circulation into inflamed tissue sites, the migration orchestrated by locally produced chemokines, such as SDF-1α [16]. In line with these findings, our current data demonstrate that, although IL-25 did not directly stimulate migrational responses of EoP, pre-exposure to IL-25 enhanced the subsequent migrational response to SDF-1α. As such, it can be postulated that IL-25 may contribute to eosinophilic inflammation

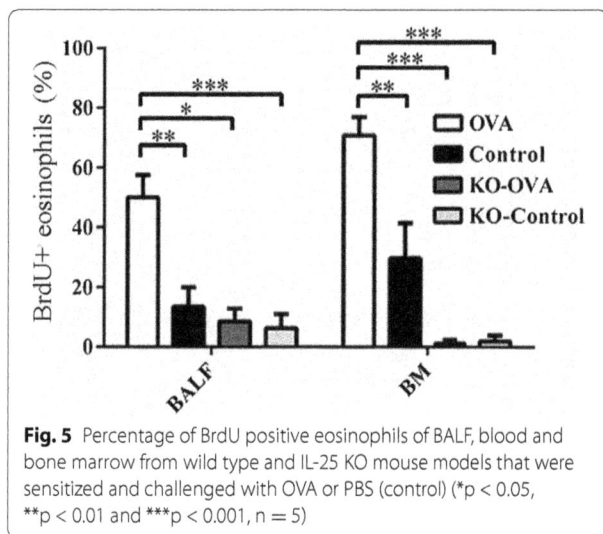

Fig. 5 Percentage of BrdU positive eosinophils of BALF, blood and bone marrow from wild type and IL-25 KO mouse models that were sensitized and challenged with OVA or PBS (control) (*p < 0.05, **p < 0.01 and ***p < 0.001, n = 5)

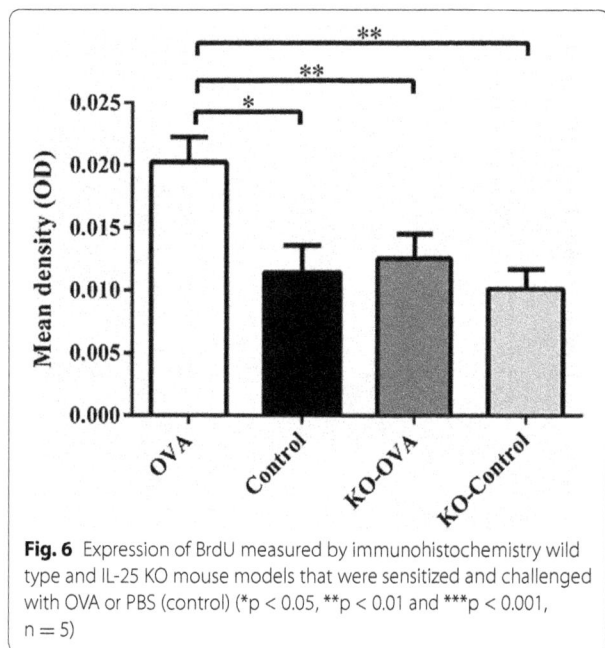

Fig. 6 Expression of BrdU measured by immunohistochemistry wild type and IL-25 KO mouse models that were sensitized and challenged with OVA or PBS (control) (*p < 0.05, **p < 0.01 and ***p < 0.001, n = 5)

observed in the lung following allergen exposure through the priming of migrational responses of immature and mature eosinophils.

We have previously shown a significant increase in HPC and EoP in the sputum 24 h post-allergen challenge, which was associated with a significant increase in the expression of receptors for epithelial derived cytokines including TSLP (TSLPR and CD127) and IL-33 (ST2) on HPC and EoP [10]. Furthermore, pre-exposure to TSLP and IL-33 primed the migration of progenitor HPC and this effect was inhibited by blocking antibodies to TSLPR and ST2, respectively, suggesting that lung-homing of

HPC maybe orchestrated by epithelial-derived cytokines, including TSLP and IL-33 [10]. Our current data support the view that the epithelial-derived cytokine IL-25 can prime the migrational response of these cells and promote lung-homing. In contrast to findings with TSLP and IL-33, we show here for the first time that IL-25 can prime the migrational responses of HPC *and* EoP while the latter cytokines only had effects on HPC [10]. A limitation of the study was that we performed these receptor up-regulation analyses in the blood as opposed to sputum samples as have been described in the above mentioned study. However, our findings in blood-derived eosinophil progenitor cell populations were similar to changes in sputum. Furthermore, the priming experiments with IL-25 were in agreement with the priming experiments performed with TSLP and IL-33 in blood derived cells suggesting similarity in the underlying mechanism.

The pro-inflammatory effects of IL-25 has been well demonstrated in animal models. Exogenous administration of IL-25, or transgenic expression induces type 2 asthma-like inflammation in the airways in mice [17, 18]. Conversely, anti-IL-25 antibody reduces airway inflammation in animal models of allergic asthma [19, 20]. In addition, IL-25-deficient mice have significant suppression of the number of eosinophils and the levels of pro-inflammatory mediators in bronchoalveolar lavage fluids (BALF) [21]. In this current study, OVA challenge of sensitized IL-25-deficient mice not only decreased mobilization of mature eosinophils, but also newly formed eosinophils. In IL-25 KO mice, the attenuation of newly produced eosinophils (BrdU + eosinophils) was observed the airways (BALF) and bone marrow samples suggesting that IL-25 may be involved in the formation of newly produced eosinophils in the bone marrow, as well as in the airways. We acknowledge that by labeling with BrdU, this study only enumerated newly formed eosinophils and not EoP per se. As such, it is unclear as to whether these newly formed eosinophils matured within the bone marrow and migrated to the airways, or if EoP migrated to the airways and differentiated locally within the tissue to mature eosinophils. However, we have previously shown that EoP traffic to the site of inflammation and have the potential of forming eosinophils in situ [22, 23] thus supporting the view that the BrDU + eosinophils arose as a result of local differentiative processes.

Conclusions

In summary, IL-25 high affinity receptor part (IL-17RB) expression on EoP is increased in the peripheral blood of subjects with asthma after allergen challenge. IL-25 also enhanced the migrational response of eosinophil progenitors. IL-25 knockout mice showed decreased eosinophilic inflammation in the bone marrow and airways.

Finally, in IL-25 KO mice there was decreased mobilization of newly produced eosinophils after OVA challenge. These results suggest that increases in IL-25 and expression of its receptor on EoP are important in the trafficking of these cells from the bone marrow to the airways during allergen-induced airway responses in asthma and that IL-25 may be a useful drug target to attenuate allergen-induced airway responses.

Abbreviations

Ag: allergen; PB: peripheral blood; FEV_1: forced expired volume in 1 s; PC_{20}: concentration required to achieve a 20% decrease in FEV_1; EAR: early asthmatic response; LAR: late asthmatic response; ELISA: enzyme-linked immunosorbent assay; HPC: hemopoietic progenitor cell; EoP: eosinophil-lineage committed progenitor cell; SDF-1α: stromal cell derived factor 1α; IL-25(IL-17E): interluekin-25; OVA: ovalbumin; BM: bone marrow; IHC: immunohistochemistry; BrdU: bromodeoxyuridine; KO: knock out; HE: hematoxylin–eosin.

Authors' contributions

WT participated in the design of the study. WT, SS and AG performed the progenitor cell migration assays as well as flow cytometric acquisition. WD and SG performed FACS analyses and the statistical analysis.WD, JD performed the animal experiment as well as IHC staining. KH coordinated the asthma patients study and performed inhalation challenges and lung function testing. GMG, PMO and RS conceived of the study, and participated in its design and coordination and drafted and edited the manuscript. All authors read and approved the final manuscript.

Author details

[1] Division of Respirology, Department of Medicine, McMaster University, Hamilton, ON L6M 1A6, Canada. [2] Department of Respirology and Critical Medicine, Ruijin Hospital, Shanghai Jiaotong University School of Medicine, Shanghai, China.

Acknowledgements

The authors would like to thank all the subjects who volunteered for this study. We thank Sue Beaudin, Tara Scime and Heather Campell for expert technical expertise. We thank for Prof. Xiaohu Wang from Qinhua University Beijin China for providing the IL-25 knockout mice.

Competing interests

The authors declare that they have no competing interests.

Funding

This study was partially supported by grants from the Chinese National Natural Science Foundation (No. 81400012); Interdisciplinary Program of Shanghai Jiao Tong University (Project Number: 2015164); Shanghai Key Discipline for Respiratory Disease (2017ZZ02014). Steven Smith was a recipient of Father Sean O'Sullivan postdoctoral research fellowship award.

References

1. Kubo M. Innate and adaptive type 2 immunity in lung allergic inflammation. Immunol Rev. 2017;278(1):162–72.
2. Saenz SA, Taylor BC, Artis D. Welcome to the neighborhood: epithelial cell-derived cytokines license innate and adaptive immune responses at mucosal sites. Immunol Rev. 2008;226:172–90.
3. Cheung PF, Wong CK, Ip WK, Lam CW. IL-25 regulates the expression of adhesion molecules on eosinophils: mechanism of eosinophilia in allergic inflammation. Allergy. 2006;61(7):878–85.
4. Wong CK, Cheung PF, Ip WK, Lam CW. Interleukin-25-induced chemokines and interleukin-6 release from eosinophils is mediated by p38 mitogen-activated protein kinase, c-Jun N-terminal kinase, and nuclear factor-kappaB. Am J Respir Cell Mol Biol. 2005;33(2):186–94.
5. Gaffen SL. Structure and signalling in the IL-17 receptor family. Nat Rev Immunol. 2009;9(8):556–67.
6. Tang W, Smith SG, Beaudin S, Dua B, Howie K, Gauvreau G, et al. IL-25 and IL-25 receptor expression on eosinophils from subjects with allergic asthma. Int Arch Allergy Immunol. 2014;163(1):5–10.
7. Tang W, Smith SG, Salter B, Oliveria JP, Mitchell P, Nusca GM, Howie K, Gauvreau GM, O'Byrne PM, Sehmi R. Allergen-induced increases in interleukin-25 and interleukin-25 receptor expression in mature eosinophils from atopic asthmatics. Int Arch Allergy Immunol. 2016;170(4):234–42.
8. Salter BM, Sehmi R. Hematopoietic processes in eosinophilic asthma. Chest. 2017;152(2):410–6.
9. Cockcroft DW, Davis BE, Boulet LP, Deschesnes F, Gauvreau GM, O'Byrne PM, et al. The links between allergen skin test sensitivity, airway responsiveness and airway response to allergen. Allergy. 2005;60(1):56–9.
10. Smith SG, Gugilla A, Mukherjee M, Merim K, Irshad A, Tang W, et al. Thymic stromal lymphopoietin and IL-33 modulate migration of hematopoietic progenitor cells in patients with allergic asthma. J Allergy Clin Immunol. 2015;135(6):1594–602.
11. Johansson AK, Sergejeva SSjöstrand M, et al. Allergen-induced traffic of bone marrow eosinophils, neutrophils and lymphocytes to airways. Eur J Immunol. 2004;34:3135–45.
12. Radinger M, Johansson AK, Sitkauskiene B, et al. Eotaxin-2 regulates newly produced and $CD34^+$ airway eosinophils after allergen exposure. J Allergy Clin Immunol. 2004;113(6):1109–16.
13. Massoud AH, Charbonnier LM, Lopez D, et al. An asthma-associated IL4R variant exacerbates airway inflammation by promoting conversion of regulatory T cells to TH17-like cells. Nat Med. 2016;22(9):1013–22.
14. Chang SH, Dong C. Signaling of interleukin-17 family cytokines in immunity and inflammation. Cell Signal. 2011;23(7):1069–75.
15. Jung JS, Park BL, Cheong HS, Bae JS, Kim JH, Chang HS, et al. Association of IL-17RB gene polymorphism with asthma. Chest. 2009;135(5):1173–80.
16. Dorman SC, Babirad I, Post J, et al. Progenitor egress from the bone marrow after allergen challenge: role of stromal cell-derived factor 1alpha and eotaxin. J Allergy Clin Immunol. 2005;115(3):501–7.
17. Fort MM, Cheung J, Yen D, Li J, Zurawski SM, Lo S, et al. IL-25 induces IL-4, IL-5, and IL-13 and Th2-associated pathologies in vivo. Immunity. 2001;15(6):985–95.
18. Hurst SD, Muchamuel T, Gorman DM, Gilbert JM, Clifford T, Kwan S, et al. New IL-17 family members promote Th1 or Th2 responses in the lung: in vivo function of the novel cytokine IL-25. J Immunol. 2002;169(1):443–53.
19. Ballantyne SJ, Barlow JL, Jolin HE, Nath P, Williams AS, Chung KF, et al. Blocking IL-25 prevents airway hyperresponsiveness in allergic asthma. J Allergy Clin Immunol. 2007;120(6):1324–31.
20. Angkasekwinai P, Park H, Wang YH, Wang YH, Chang SH, Corry DB, et al. Interleukin 25 promotes the initiation of proallergic type 2 responses. J Exp Med. 2007;204(7):1509–17.
21. Suzukawa M, Morita H, Nambu A, et al. Epithelial cell-derived IL-25, but not Th17 cell-derived IL-17 or IL-17F, is crucial for murine asthma. J Immunol. 2012;189(7):3641–52.
22. Dorman SC, Efthimiadis A, Babirad I, Watson RM, Denburg JA, Hargreave FE, O'Byrne PM, Sehmi R. SputumCD34+IL-5Rα+ cells increase after allergen: evidence for in situ eosinophilopoieisis. Am J Respir Crit Care Med. 2004;169:573–7.
23. Southam DS, Widmer N, Ellis R, Hirota J, Inman MD, Sehmi R. Increased eosinophil-lineage committed progenitors in thelung of allergen challenged mice. J Allergy Clin Immunol. 2005;115:95–102.

3

Is fruit and vegetable intake associated with asthma or chronic rhino-sinusitis in European adults? Results from the Global Allergy and Asthma Network of Excellence (GA²LEN) Survey

Vanessa Garcia-Larsen[1,19]* ⓘ, Rhonda Arthur[2], James F. Potts[1], Peter H. Howarth[3], Matti Ahlström[4], Tari Haahtela[4], Carlos Loureiro[5], Ana Todo Bom[5], Grzegorz Brożek[6], Joanna Makowska[7], Marek L. Kowalski[7], Trine Thilsing[8], Thomas Keil[9,10], Paolo M. Matricardi[11], Kjell Torén[12], Thibaut van Zele[13], Claus Bachert[14], Barbara Rymarczyk[15], Christer Janson[16], Bertil Forsberg[17], Ewa Niżankowska-Mogilnicka[18] and Peter G. J. Burney[1]

Abstract

Background: Fruits and vegetables are rich in compounds with proposed antioxidant, anti-allergic and anti-inflammatory properties, which could contribute to reduce the prevalence of asthma and allergic diseases.

Objective: We investigated the association between asthma, and chronic rhino-sinusitis (CRS) with intake of fruits and vegetables in European adults.

Methods: A stratified random sample was drawn from the Global Allergy and Asthma Network of Excellence (GA²LEN) screening survey, in which 55,000 adults aged 15–75 answered a questionnaire on respiratory symptoms. Asthma score (derived from self-reported asthma symptoms) and CRS were the outcomes of interest. Dietary intake of 22 subgroups of fruits and vegetables was ascertained using the internationally validated GA²LEN Food Frequency Questionnaire. Adjusted associations were examined with negative binomial and multiple regressions. Simes procedure was used to control for multiple testing.

Results: A total of 3206 individuals had valid data on asthma and dietary exposures of interest. 22.8% reported having at least 1 asthma symptom (asthma score $\geq$1), whilst 19.5% had CRS. After adjustment for potential confounders, asthma score was negatively associated with intake of dried fruits (β-coefficient −2.34; 95% confidence interval [CI] −4.09, −0.59), whilst CRS was statistically negatively associated with total intake of fruits (OR 0.73; 95% CI 0.55, 0.97). Conversely, a positive association was observed between asthma score and *alliums* vegetables (adjusted β-coefficient 0.23; 95% CI 0.06, 0.40). None of these associations remained statistically significant after controlling for multiple testing.

Conclusion and clinical relevance: There was no consistent evidence for an association of asthma or CRS with fruit and vegetable intake in this representative sample of European adults.

Keywords: Fruits, Vegetables, Asthma, Chronic rhino-sinusitis, Adults, Europe, Meta-analysis, GA²LEN

*Correspondence: v.garcialarsen@imperial.ac.uk
[19] Respiratory Epidemiology, Occupational Medicine and Public Health Group, National Heart and Lung Institute, Imperial College London, Emmanuel Kaye Building, Manresa Road, London SW3 6LR, UK
Full list of author information is available at the end of the article

Background

Fruits and vegetables are rich sources of nutrients and compounds with antioxidant, anti-allergic and anti-inflammatory properties, which could modulate the expression of asthma and allergic diseases [1]. A recent systematic review suggested an overall reduced risk of wheeze or self-reported Dr diagnosed asthma in adults and children with higher intakes of fruits and vegetables [2]. Several observational studies in adults have shown a negative association between various asthma prevalence outcomes, and intake of apples [3], citrus fruits [4], tomatoes or leafy vegetables [4]. Smaller studies in asthmatic adults with a dietary pattern mainly comprised of fruits and vegetables have also been shown to have a lower risk of severe asthma [2]. The current evidence on a possible protective effect of fruits and vegetables on allergic diseases is mixed, with some studies showing a negative association between intake of vegetables [5] or food groups that contain them [6] and a lower asthma prevalence, whilst several population-based studies have reported no association between allergic symptoms and fruits or vegetables when measured individually [7, 8] or as part of a dietary pattern [9, 10].

Epidemiological studies use different operational definitions to assess asthma, as well as different instruments to ascertain usual dietary intake. These issues may make it more difficult to ascribe a consistent interpretation on their relationship. The current observational evidence in European adults is inconclusive, with very few multi-national studies examining in some standardised fashion, the association between asthma and diet [10]. Within the Global Allergy and Asthma Network of Excellence (GA^{2}LEN), we designed and piloted a single, common, food frequency questionnaire (FFQ) [11], which was used to estimate usual dietary intake of over 3500 adults from 10 European countries participating in the GA^{2}LEN Follow-up survey. In this analysis, we investigate the cross-sectional association between asthma and chronic rhino-sinusitis (CRS), with dietary intake of fruits and vegetables in these adults.

Methods

The GA^{2}LEN study—screening and clinical surveys

The core protocol for the GA^{2}LEN survey required 18 European participating centres to identify a random sample of at least 3000 adults aged 15–74 years from an available population-based sampling frame. A stratified random sample was drawn, in which 55,000 adults aged 15–75 answered a questionnaire on respiratory symptoms. The following countries (and cities) were included in this cross-sectional analysis: Belgium (Ghent), Denmark (Odense), Finland (Helsinki), Germany (Duisberg, Brandenburg), The Netherlands (Amsterdam), Poland (Krakow, Lodz, Katowice), Portugal (Coimbra), Sweden (Gothenburg, Stockholm, Umea, Uppsala), and the UK (Southampton, London). In 2008–2009, potential

participants were sent a short questionnaire by mail, and at least three attempts were made to elicit a response [12]. The questionnaire collected information on age, gender, smoking and the presence of symptoms of asthma (including age of onset), and CRS. Four sub-samples were selected to define cases and controls: (1) those with self-reported asthma and at least one respiratory symptom reported in the last 12 months ('asthma'), (2) those having chronic sinusitis (defined following the EP^{3}OS criteria, that is, the presence of at least two of the following symptoms for at least 12 weeks in the past year: (i) nasal blockage, (ii) nasal discharge, (iii) facial pain or pressure or (iv) reduction in sense of smell with at least one of the symptoms being nasal blockage or nasal discharge), (3) those who had both 'asthma' and 'chronic sinusitis', and those who had none of these conditions. [13] Five questions on symptoms in the last 12 months (breathless when wheezing, woken with tightness in chest, shortness of breath while at rest, shortness of breath after exercise, woken by shortness of breath) were used to construct an asthma symptom score on a five-point scale [14].

Dietary intake

The GA^{2}LEN food frequency questionnaire (FFQ) was designed to assess usual dietary intake across countries, using a single, common, and standardised instrument. The FFQ was validated in a random sample of adults from 5 participant centres in GA^{2}LEN, namely Finland, Portugal, Germany, Greece, and Poland, each representing a different European Region [11]. All centres adhered to the same standard operational procedure (SOP) to translate the questionnaires and the same procedure was used to translate and standardise all other questionnaires in the GA^{2}LEN survey. The GA^{2}LEN FFQ has been translated into more than 25 languages for use in several single and multi-national epidemiological studies [15]. To facilitate international food comparisons, the FFQ was organised into 32 sections of food groups [16]. The FFQ collected data on a wide range of foods, including 43 vegetables and 25 fruits (Table 1). Total energy intake (TEI) was calculated using the latest available food composition estimates from the British Food Composition Table [17].

Statistical analyses

Sampling probability weights were used to standardise prevalences by gender and age to a European Standard Population.

Multivariable logistic regression was used to assess the relationship between food consumption and CRS within each country, controlling for education, employment, smoking status (never, ex-smoker, current smoker), BMI, age, gender, supplement use and TEI. The country level logistic analyses were weighted to take into account

Table 1 Fruit and vegetable subgroup classification in the GA²LEN Follow-up study

Food group	Food items included
Vegetables	
Leafy vegetables	Lettuce, spinach, chard, fenugreek, wild greens
Fruit vegetables	Capers, tomatoes, aubergine, courgette, sweet peppers, pumpkin, artichoke, okra, mushroom
Cucurbitacea	Cucumber, melon, watermelon, bitter melon
Apiaceae	Celery, carrot, herbs (coriander, parsley, chervil, dill), parsnip
Other root vegetables	Turnip or swede, radish, beetroot, ginger, taro
Maiz/Corn	Sweet corn
Alliums	Onion, garlic, leek
Brassicaceae	Brussels sprouts, broccoli, cabbage, cauliflower, coleslaw
Potatoes	Mashed potatoes, baked/roasted/casserole potatoes, chips/french fries, potatoes in salad, potato dumping/bread dumpling/gnocchi, potato tortilla
Pickled vegetables	Cucumber, radish, cabbage
All vegetables	Average intake of all above
Fruits	
Hard fruits	Apple, pear
Citrus fruits	Lemon, orange, mandarin/tangerine, grape-fruit, kiwi
Oily fruits	Olives, avocado
Fruit juice	Freshly squeezed fruits
Berries	Blueberries, strawberries, raspberries ('forest berries')
Nectarines	Nectarine, apricot, peach
Dried fruits	Raisin, prune
Tropical fruits	Mango, pineapple (banana assessed individually)
Canned fruits	Any canned fruits
Dark pigmented fruit	Cherries, rhubarb, grape, fig, plum
All fruits	Average intake of all above

the case–control sampling selection. Negative binomial regression was used to assess the relationship between food consumption and asthma score within each country. This analysis controlled for the same variables and used the same sampling weights as in the logistic regression described above. There was only weak collinearity between the variables when we tested this in each of the multivariable models. The regression coefficients from the country level analyses were meta-analysed to give an overall coefficient. The I^2 statistic was used to assess heterogeneity between countries. Simes procedure was used to correct statistical estimates derived from multiple testing [18].

All analyses were run using Stata 13.1 (StataCorp, 4905 Lakeway Drive, College Station, Texas 77845 USA).

Results

The main characteristics of the 3202 participants with valid data on diet and asthma score are summarised in Table 2. Of these, 22.8% reported having at least 1 symptom of asthma (asthma score = 1) whereas 9.3% had 3 or more symptoms. CRS was reported by 23.4% of individuals. Over half of all participants reported eating fruits or vegetables 5 times a week, with Portugal and Poland having the highest intake of these food groups.

The association between asthma score and fruit and vegetable intake is illustrated in Table 3. After controlling for potential confounders, a statistically significant negative association was observed between having an increasing asthma score and eating dried fruits (β-coefficient −2.34; 95% CI −4.09, −0.59; P value = 0.009). No other fruit groups were associated with asthma. Intake of fruity vegetables (which included capers, tomatoes, aubergine, courgette, sweet peppers, pumpkin, artichoke, okra, and mushroom) was positively associated with asthma score (β-coefficient 0.17; 95% CI 0.04, 0.30). Similarly, a higher asthma score was related to intake of alliums vegetables (onion, garlic, leek) (β-coefficient 0.23; 95% CI 0.06, 0.40). Figure 1 illustrates the per-country associations between asthma score and total fruit intake and fruity vegetables. There was no heterogeneity across countries ($I^2 = 0\%$).

Table 4 shows the associations found between CRS and fruit and vegetable intake. A 27% lower risk of disease was observed in those with a total intake of fruit ≥ 5 versus those who ate fruit below this cut-off point (OR 0.23; 95% CI 0.55, 0.97). As illustrated in Fig. 2, there was no evidence of heterogeneity between the estimates across countries ($I^2 = 0.0\%$; P value = 0.62).

After applying Simes procedure, the statistical significance of the association between asthma score and dried fruits was attenuated (P value = 0.05), and all the other associations were no longer statistically significant (>0.15).

Discussion

In this multi-national study of adults participating in the GA²LEN Follow-up survey, asthma symptom score and CRS were negatively associated with dietary intake of dried fruits and total fruit intake, respectively. Asthma symptom score was also positively associated with a higher intake of fruity vegetables and alliums. These associations were observed after adjusting for several potential confounders, which included socio-economic, smoking, and lifestyle-related variables (including BMI, TEI, and nutritional supplement use). After controlling for multiple comparisons, the statistical significance of these associations was lost.

To our knowledge, this is the first multi-national population-based study to examine the association between

Table 2 General characteristics of the study population (based on individuals with complete data on dietary exposures and asthma score)

Variables	Countries					
	Denmark	Finland	Sweden	United Kingdom	Germany	The Netherlands
	Odense (359)	Helsinki (160)	Total (1261)	Total (173)	Total (376)	Amsterdam (215)
Age, years; mean (SD)	48.1 (14.5)	46.8 (15.1)	45.7 (15.1)	51.6 (13.2)	48.8 (15.6)	52.6 (13.9)
Males, n (%)	162 (45.1)	62 (38.8)	556 (44.1)	70 (40.5)	152 (403)	111 (51.6)
BMI (kg/m^2)	27.4 (14.8)	26.5 (4.6)	25.9 (7.2)	27.1 (5.6)	26.3 (4.8)	25.7 (3.7)
Age at completing full-time education; years (SD)	23.4 (5.5)	23.5 (5.5)	24.5 (7.7)	18.1 (3.6)	20.6 (5.2)	20.2 (4.6)
Employment status						
Employed	188 (52.7)	94 (58.9)	737 (58.5)	85 (49.7)	196 (52.0)	103 (47.9)
Retired	82 (23.0)	32 (20.0)	199 (15.8)	39 (22.8)	88 (23.3)	56 (21.1)
Unemployed	11 (3.1)	3 (1.9)	38 (3.0)	4 (2.3)	12 (3.2)	5 (2.3)
Other	76 (21.5)	31 (19.4)	286 (22.7)	43 (25.1)	81 (21.5)	51 (23.7)
Smoking						
Never smokers	155 (43.4)	83 (51.9)	672 (53.3)	77 (44.5)	183 (48.4)	84 (39.1)
Ex-smokers	102 (28.6)	37 (23.1)	428 (33.9)	70 (40.5)	131 (34.7)	88 (40.9)
Current smokers	100 (28.0)	40 (25.0)	162 (12.8)	26 (15.0)	64 (16.9)	43 (20.0)
Asthma score; N (%)						
0	145 (40.4)	96 (59.6)	583 (46.2)	66 (38.2)	161 (42.6)	100 (41.0)
1	85 (23.7)	31 (19.3)	276 (21.9)	37 (21.4)	107 (28.3)	40 (18.6)
2	50 (13.9)	15 (9.3)	195 (15.5)	22 (12.7)	47 (12.4)	37 (17.2)
3	47 (13.1)	10 (6.2)	114 (9.0)	17 (11.5)	35 (9.3)	23 (10.7)
4	24 (6.7)	7 (4.4)	61 (4.8)	26 (15.0)	16 (4.2)	12 (5.6)
5	8 (2.2)	2 (1.2)	33 (2.6)	5 (2.9)	12 (3.2)	3 (1.4)
Chronic rhino-sinusitis; n (%)	63 (17.6)	29 (17.8)	234 (18.3)	22 (12.6)	62 (16.2)	52 (23.9)
Asthma ever (n; %)	115 (32.0)	44 (27.0)	510 (39.8)	80 (45.7)	83 (21.7)	44 (20.2)
CRS only (n; %)	42 (11.7)	17 (10.4)	102 (8.0)	10 (5.7)	38 (9.9)	40 (18.4)
Both asthma ever and CRS (n; %)	21 (5.9)	12 (7.4)	132 (10.3)	12 (6.9)	23 (6.0)	12 (5.5)
Total Energy Intake (TEI)	2577 (761)	3197 (1140)	3110 (978)	2833 (889.6)	2821 (1049)	2817 (827)
Use of nutritional supplements, n (%)	143 (40.4)	70 (43.5)	325 (26.0)	58 (33.7)	102 (27.1)	88 (41.0)
% people eating fruits (all types) ≥5 times/week	202 (56.4)	93 (57.1)	717 (56.0)	101 (57.7)	213 (55.8)	114 (52.3)
% people eating total vegetables (all types) ≥5 times/week	224 (62.4)	128 (78.5)	906 (70.7)	92 (52.6)	194 (50.7)	78 (35.8)

Variables	Countries			
	Portugal	Belgium	Poland	Total
	Coimbra (266)	Ghent (148)	Total (244)	3202
Age, years; mean (SD)	47.1 (15.0)	45.7 (15.1)	49.7 (15.7)	47.6 (15.1)
Males, n (%)	93 (35.0)	71 (48.0)	104 (42.6)	1381 (43.1)
BMI, kg/m^2 (SD)	25.9 (5.1)	24.9 (4.4)	27.4 (5.2)	26.3 (5.2)
Age at completing full-time education; years (SD)	20.1 (4.6)	20.6 (6.6)	20.4 (3.4)	22.4 (6.6)
Employment status				
Employed	140 (52.6)	75 (51.0)	89 (38.0)	1707 (53.6)
Retired	56 (26.5)	26 (17.7)	86 (36.8)	664 (20.8)
Unemployed	11 (4.1)	3 (2.0)	12 (5.1)	99 (3.1)
Other	59 (22.2)	30 (22.4)	47 (20.0)	717 (22.5)
Smoking				
Never smokers	172 (64.7)	75 (50.7)	111 (45.7)	1612 (50.4)
Ex-smokers	56 (21.1)	45 (30.4)	78 (32.1)	1035 (32.2)

Table 2 continued

Variables	Countries			
	Portugal	Belgium	Poland	Total
	Coimbra (266)	Ghent (148)	Total (244)	3202
Current smokers	38 (14.3)	28 (18.9)	54 (22.2)	555 (17.3)
Asthma score				
0	109 (41.0)	57 (38.5)	78 (32.0)	1395 (43.5)
1	49 (18.4)	34 (23.0)	73 (29.9)	732 (22.8)
2	41 (15.4)	22 (14.9)	34 (13.9)	463 (14.4)
3	27 (910.2)	17 (11.5)	28 (11.5)	318 (9.9)
4	23 (8.7)	12 (8.1)	17 (7.0)	198 (6.2)
5	17 (6.4)	6 (4.1)	14 (5.7)	100 (3.1)
Chronic rhino-sinusitis; n (%)	78 (29.2)	43 (29.1)	50 (20.2)	633 (19.5)
Asthma ever (n; %)	59 (22.1)	23 (15.5)	37 (15.0)	995 (30.7)
CRS only (n; %)	44 (16.5)	28 (18.9)	39 (15.8)	360 (11.1)
Both asthma ever and CRS (n; %)	34 (12.7)	15 (10.1)	11 (4.5)	272 (8.4)
Total Energy Intake (TEI); mean (SD)	3195 (1296)	2937 (885)	3211 (1661)	2993 (1072)
Use of nutritional supplements, n (%)	16 (6.0)	50 (33.8)	53 (22.0)	905 (28.4)
% people eating fruits (all types) ≥5 times/week	189 (70.8)	80 (54.1)	158 (64.0)	1867 (57.6)
% people eating total vegetables (all types) ≥5 times/week	206 (77.2)	77 (52.0)	182 (73.7)	2087 (64.4)

Table 3 Association between severity of asthma (asthma score) and fruit and vegetable intake in adults from GA[2]LEN

Fruit and vegetable groups	Asthma score Effect size (β-coefficient (95% confidence intervals))	
	Unadjusted (n = 3206)	Adjusted (n = 2945)
Fruits		
Hard fruits	0.01 (−0.11, 0.14) n = 3196	−0.02 (0.15, 0.11) n = 2940
Bananas	0.03 (−0.14, 0.21) n = 3187	0.04 (−0.19, 0.27) n = 2934
Citrus fruits	−0.05 (−0.19, 0.09) n = 3196	−0.03 (−0.18, 0.12) n = 2938
Oily fruits	0.25 (0.02, 0.48) n = 3196	0.24 (0.01, 0.46) n = 2942
Freshly squeezed fruit	0.16 (−0.03, 0.36) n = 3184	0.18 (−0.01, 0.38) n = 2930
Berries	−0.07 (−0.32, 0.19) n = 3159	−0.12 (−0.37, 0.13) n = 2907
Nectarines	0.26 (−0.10, 0.62) n = 3197	0.16 (−0.33, 0.65) n = 2942
Dried fruits	*−1.89 (−3.36, −0.42) n = 3190*	*−2.34 (−4.09, −0.59) n = 2937*
Tropical fruits	0.13 (−0.31, 0.56) n = 3194	0.21 (−0.15, 0.55) n = 2940
Canned fruits	−4.62 (−6.50, −2.74) n = 3181	−5.66 (−11.4, 0.07) n = 2930
Dark pigmented fruits	−0.11 (−0.41, 0.19) n = 3201	−0.09 (−0.37, 0.19) n = 2944
All fruits	−0.03 (−0.16, 0.10) n = 3203	0.04 (−0.09, 0.17) n = 2944
Nuts	0.21 (−0.12, 0.54) n = 3192	0.20 (−0.21, 0.61) n = 2935
Vegetables		
Leafy vegetables	0.11 (−0.04, 0.26) n = 3195	0.03 (−0.15, 0.22) n = 2937
Fruity vegetables	*0.16 (0.04, 0.28) n = 3202*	*0.17 (0.04, 0.30) n = 2942*
Cucurbitacea	0.07 (−0.10, 0.24) n = 3202	−0.02 (−0.22, 0.18) n = 2943
Apiaceae	0.05 (−0.12, 0.21) n = 3204	0.05 (−0.09, 0.19) n = 2943
Other root vegetables	0.13 (−0.08, 0.33) n = 3200	0.12 (−0.13, 0.37) n = 2942
Maize/corn	0.41 (−0.12, 0.93) n = 3189	0.47 (−0.04, 0.98) n = 2936
Alliums	*0.27 (0.15, 0.39) n = 3203*	*0.23 (0.06, 0.40) n = 2944*
Brassicaceae	0.30 (0.01. 0.59) n = 3202	0.20 (−0.02, 0.41) n = 2943
Potatoes	0.09 (−0.21, 0.38) n = 3194	0.002 (−0.24, 0.24) n = 2937
Pickled vegetables	−2.32 (−4.17, −0.47) n = 3175	−1.90 (−3.94, 0.14) n = 2924
Legumes	*−2.10 (−3.65, −0.45) n = 3196*	−1.98 (−4.13, 0.18) n = 2939
All vegetables	0.12 (−0.001, 0.25) n = 3206	0.11 (−0.03, 0.25) n = 2945

Italics indicate a statistically significant effect size

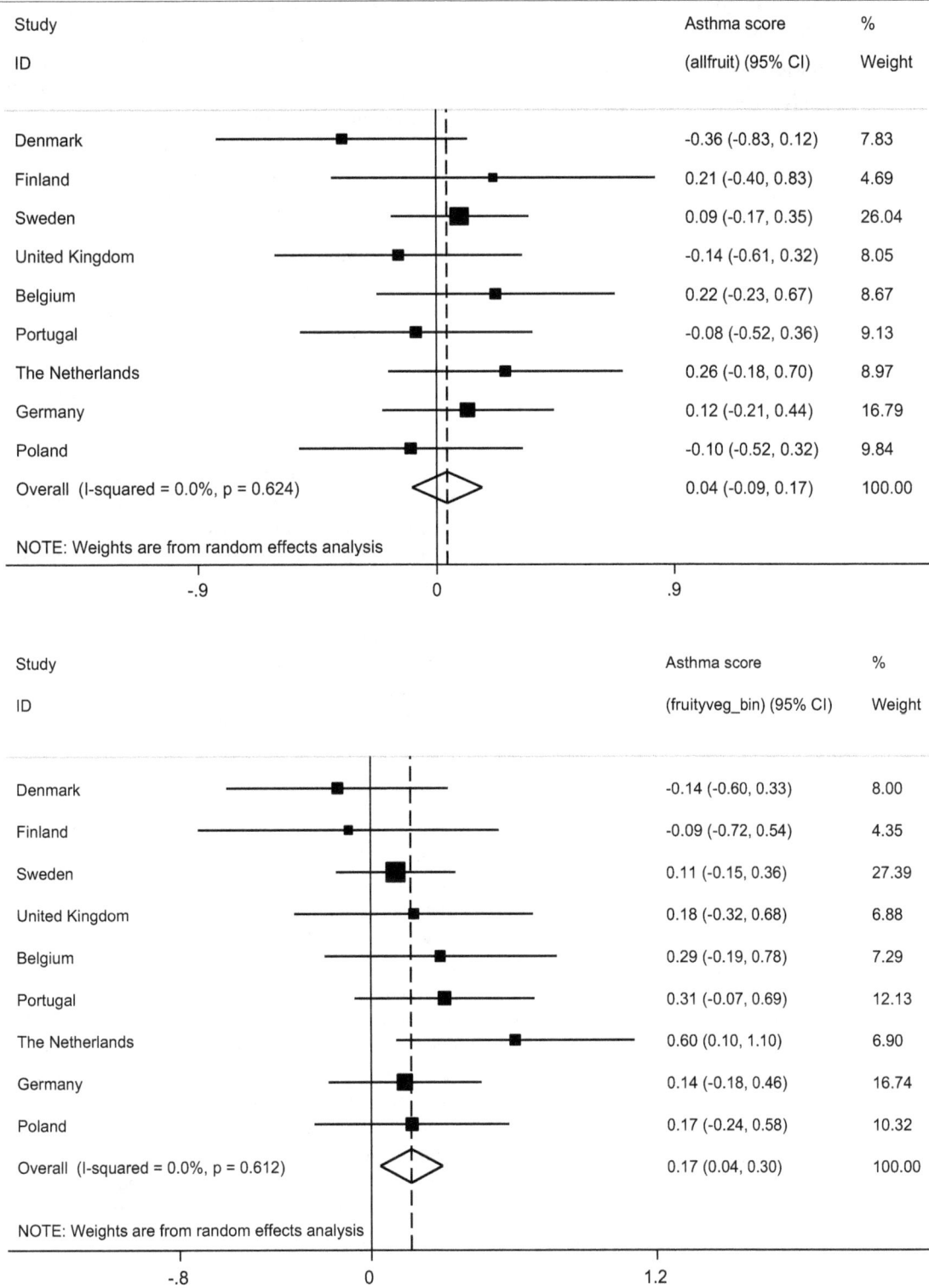

Fig. 1 Weighted adjusted negative binomial regressions of asthma score association with total intake of fruits (*top*) and fruity vegetables (*below*) (per centre, and meta-analysis of pooled results)

Table 4 Association between CRS and fruit and vegetable intake in adults from GA²LEN

Fruit and vegetable groups	Effect size (odds ratio (95% confidence intervals)	
	Unadjusted (n = 3242)	Adjusted (2970)
Fruit group		
Hard fruit	0.83 (0.64–1.06) n = 3232	0.82 (0.62–1.09) n = 2965
Bananas	1.04 (0.78–1.40) n = 3223	0.99 (0.68–1.44) n = 2959
Citrus fruit	0.78 (0.48–1.26) n = 3232	0.87 (0.52–1.46) n = 2963
Oily fruits	1.40 (0.91–2.16) n = 3232	1.67 (0.91–3.06) n = 2967
Freshly squeezed fruit	0.73 (0.44–1.20) n = 3219	0.74 (0.44–1.24) n = 2954
Berries	1.08 (0.61–1.94) n = n = 3195	1.23 (0.55–2.76) n = 2932
Nectarines	1.42 (0.84–2.41) n = 3233	1.57 (0.79–3.11) n = 2967
Dried fruits	0.95 (0.42–2.14) n = 3226	0.98 (0.42–2.32) n = 2962
Tropical fruits	2.14 (1.10–4.16) n = 3230	2.50 (0.91–6.92) n = 2965
Canned fruits[a]	–	–
Dark pigmented fruits	1.01 (0.71–1.45) n = 3237	1.11 (0.75–1.64) n = 2969
All fruits	*0.75 (0.58–0.96) n = 3239*	*0.73 (0.55–0.97) n = 2969*
Nuts	0.47 (0.21–1.06) n = 3227	0.64 (0.23–1.80) n = 2960
Vegetables		
Leafy vegetables	1.15 (0.86–1.53) n = 3229	1.22 (0.86–1.71) n = 2961
Fruity vegetables	1.16 (0.87–1.53) n = 3237	1.22 (0.81–1.85) n = 2967
Cucurbitacea	1.15 (0.85–1.56) n = 3238	1.03 (0.73–1.44) n = 2968
Apiaceae	1.22 (0.93–1.62) n = 3239	1.22 (0.90–1.64) n = 2968
Other root vegetables	1.63 (0.98–2.70) n = 3235	1.77 (0.89–3.53) n = 2967
Maize/corn	1.64 (0.55–4.87) n = 3224	1.74 (0.42–7.22) n = 2961
Alliums	1.19 (0.91–1.55) n = 3238	0.99 (0.68–1.42) n = 2969
Brassicaceae	1.09 (0.73–1.62) n = 3237	1.05 (0.67–1.65) n = 2968
Potatoes	*2.27 (1.47–3.52) n = 3229*	*1.82 (1.03–3.23) n = 2962*
Pickled vegetables	1.73 (0.88–3.4) n = 3210	1.61 (0.72–3.59) n = 2949
All vegetables	1.11 (0.80–1.54) n = 3242	1.09 (0.67–1.77) n = 2970
Legumes	1.54 (0.51–4.64) n = 3231	1.24 (0.30–5.10) n = 2964

Italics indicate a statistically significant effect size

[a] Not enough people with data on this exposure to carry out analyses

asthma, CRS and allergic rhinitis, with fruit and vegetable intake, using a standardised method to ascertain both respiratory outcomes and dietary exposures. The results of this study were weighted to make results generalizable to the European adult population. We used an asthma score to ascertain individuals with a variety of symptoms, for its good predictability to ascertain outcomes related to asthma [14, 19]. Asthma is characterised for its clinical phenotypic heterogeneity and temporal phenotypic variability. Being a multi-categorical measure, the score provides more power to detect risk factors for asthma [19].

The GA²LEN FFQ was translated into each of the participant countries' languages following international guidelines, and was previously piloted and validated in a subsample of 5 participating countries [11]. The FFQ uses a semi-quantitative approach to enquiring about the frequency of intake of 250 food items, which includes staple foods representative of each nation, but also foods that are commonly consumed in all these countries. The GA²LEN FFQ is being used in several other multinational countries and appears to be a functional and accurate tool to ascertain usual dietary intake [15]. Given the large number of dietary exposure studied, we used Simes procedure to adjust the P values for multiple testing. This method has more power to identify true associations and its use is helpful when there are several highly correlated variables, as it is the case of dietary exposures [18].

The absence of robust evidence suggesting an association between dietary intake of fruits and vegetables with respiratory outcomes in this study has been confirmed in other population-based observational studies. Several authors have reported no association between asthma risk and intake of citrus fruits. As reported in other studies, we did not observe an association between the outcomes studies and citrus fruits [3, 20–22] nor with vitamin C, for which observational studies show mixed evidence of a beneficial effect [23].

We did find a negative association between dried fruit intake and asthma score, which remained statistically significant after controlling for multiple comparisons. Recent experimental evidence has demonstrated in an asthma-induced model in rats, that administering *V. vinifera* dried fruits inhibited the recruitment of inflammatory cytokines (IL)-4, IL-5, IL-1β, tumour necrosis factor, as well as IgE levels, and circulating levels of eosinophils in blood/serum and broncho-alveolar fluid [24]. Treatment with raisin extract also normalised lung function and histamine levels compared to control animals. Although no experimental evidence has demonstrated that prunes might exert similar effects, it has been proposed that the potential beneficial role of prunes on asthma might be mediated through their role in maintaining the gut microbiota balance [25]. Our findings of a negative association between dried fruits (raisins and prunes) might be explained at least partly by these biological mechanisms.

Several other studies have used a more integrative approach to elucidate the association between asthma and dietary exposures using dietary patterns, derived from Principal Component or Factor analysis, or through other indexes. However, dietary patterns that include fruits and vegetables as main food contributors have so far been unrelated to prevalence [9] or risk of adult

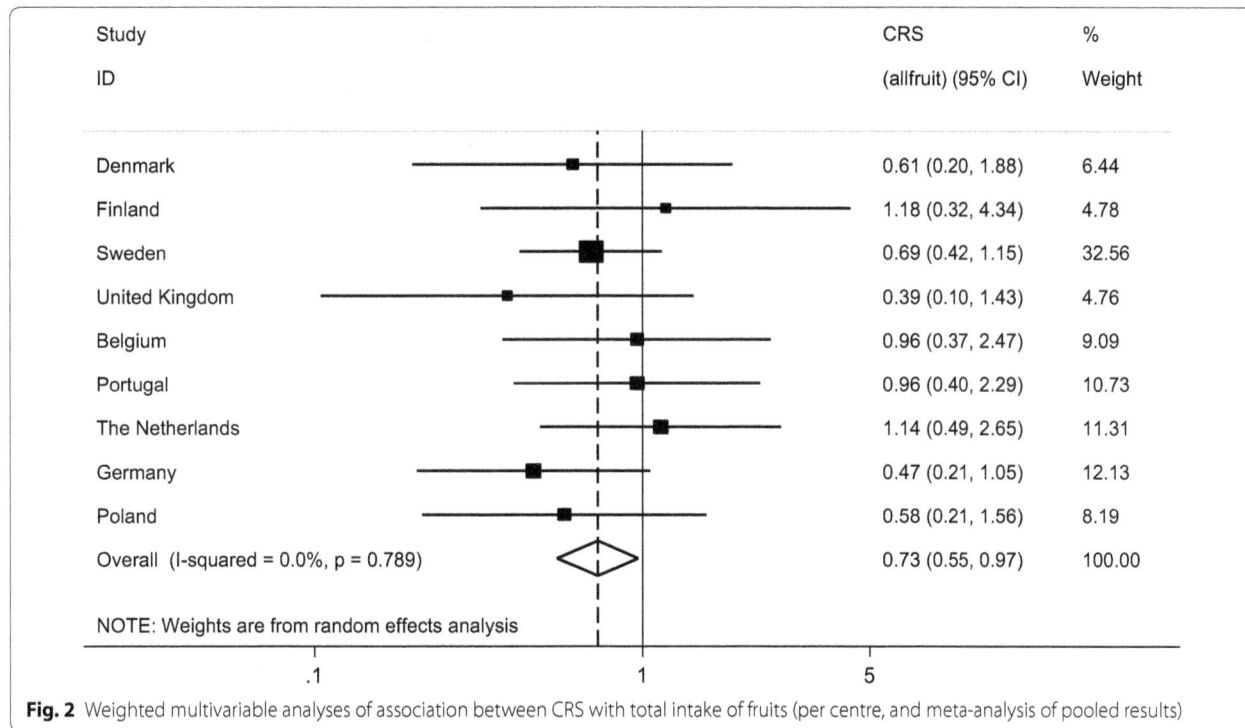

Fig. 2 Weighted multivariable analyses of association between CRS with total intake of fruits (per centre, and meta-analysis of pooled results)

asthma [26]. The uniformity of the associations observed per country in our study, and the absence of heterogeneity observed in most analyses, would lend further support to the notion that in general intakes of fruits and vegetables are not strongly associated with adult asthma.

Fruits and vegetables are also rich in various subclasses of flavonoids, for which strong anti-oxidant, anti-inflammatory and anti-allergic properties have been demonstrated in experimental studies of induced asthma [27]. These results have been echoed in some observational studies in adults showing a reduced risk of BHR [7] or asthma incidence [28], though others have reported no association with current asthma or allergic symptoms [29]. This is partly explained by the differences in the subclasses studied. In our study, we found some evidence that a lower risk of CRS was associated with a higher intake of fruits, which could partly be explained by the high content of vitamin C and flavonoids in them. We err on the cautious side though as this association was no longer statistically significant after controlling for multiple testing.

Due to the cross-sectional nature of our analysis, we cannot ascribe causality (or lack of) in the association between asthma, CRS, and allergic rhinitis with dietary intake of fruits and vegetables. Although we adjusted for several important potential confounders, there are likely to be other unmeasured confounders involved in the complex association between asthma and diet.

In conclusion, we found no consistent evidence for an association of asthma and allergic rhino-sinusitis with fruit and vegetable intake. The overall effect size observed for CRS and total fruit intake is suggestive of a protective effect, but this needs to be taken with caution given the multiple comparisons carried out in the study.

Abbreviations
GA[2]LEN: The Global Asthma and Allergy Network of Excellence; FFQ: food frequency questionnaire; CRS: chronic rhino-sinusitis; TEI: total energy intake; BMI: body mass index.

Authors' contributions
VGL and PGB conceived the hypothesis for this analysis. VGL wrote the first draft of manuscript. VGL designed the GA[2]LEN FFQ which was used to collect data on dietary intake in the GA[2]LEN participants. PGB led the research efforts to make possible the international validation of the GA[2]LEN FFQ. RA and JFP contributed with statistical analyses. RA helped to interpret and classify the nutritional variables used in the study. All co-authors listed in the manuscript contributed to and approved the final version of the manuscript and led the research efforts to assess dietary intake in their centres. All authors read and approved the final manuscript.

Author details
[1] Population Health and Occupational Medicine Group, National Heart and Lung Institute, Imperial College London, London, UK. [2] Department of Nutrition, King's College London, London, UK. [3] Faculty of Medicine, University of Southampton, London, UK. [4] Skin and Allergy Hospital, Helsinki University Hospital, Southampton, Finland. [5] Immuno-allergology Department, Coimbra University Hospital, Helsinki, Portugal. [6] Department of Epidemiology, College of Medicine, Medical University of Silesia, Katowice, Poland. [7] Department of Immunology, Rheumatology and Allergy, Medical University of Lodz, Coimbra, Poland. [8] Research Unit for Occupational and Environmental Medicine, Institute of Clinical Research, University of Southern Denmark,

Coimbra, Denmark. [9] Institute of Social Medicine, Epidemiology and Health Economics, Charité - Universitätsmedizin Berlin, Lodz, Germany. [10] Institute of Clinical Epidemiology and Biometry, Würzburg University, Würzburg, Germany. [11] Deptartment of Pediatrics, Charité – Universitätsmedizin Berlin, Berlin, Germany. [12] Section of Occupational and Environmental Medicine, University of Gothenburg, Odense, Sweden. [13] Upper Airway Research Laboratory, Ghent University, Ghent, Belgium. [14] Division of ENT Diseases, Karolinska Institute, Stockholm, Sweden. [15] Clinical Department of Internal Diseases, Allergology and Clinical Immunology, Medical University of Silesia, Katowice, Poland. [16] Department of Medical Sciences, Respiratory, Allergy and Sleep Research, Uppsala University, Ghent, Sweden. [17] Division of Occupational and Environmental Medicine, Department of Public Health and Clinical Medicine, Umeå University, Chorzów, Sweden. [18] Jagiellonian University School of Medicine, Krakow, Poland. [19] Respiratory Epidemiology, Occupational Medicine and Public Health Group, National Heart and Lung Institute, Imperial College London, Emmanuel Kaye Building, Manresa Road, London SW3 6LR, UK.

Acknowledgements
We are indebted to the participants of the GA[2]LEN Follow-up survey across Europe.

Competing interests
The authors declare that they have no competing interests.

Funding
The GA[2]LEN study was supported by EU Framework programme for research; contract no. FOOD-CT-2004-506378.

References
1. Julia V, Macia L, Dombrowicz D. The impact of diet on asthma and allergic diseases. Nat Rev Immunol. 2015;15:308–22.
2. Seyedrezazadeh E, Moghaddam MP, Ansarin K, Vafa MR, Sharma S, Kolahdooz F. Fruit and vegetable intake and risk of wheezing and asthma: a systematic review and meta-analysis. Nutr Rev. 2014;72:411–28.
3. Shaheen SO, Sterne JA, Thompson RL, Songhurst CE, Margetts BM, Burney PG. Dietary antioxidants and asthma in adults: population-based case–control study. Am J Respir Crit Care Med. 2001;164:1823–8.
4. Patel BD, Welch AA, Bingham SA, Luben RN, Day NE, Khaw KT, Lomas DA, Wareham NJ. Dietary antioxidants and asthma in adults. Thorax. 2006;61:388–93.
5. Romieu I, Varraso R, Avenel V, Leynaert B, Kauffmann F, Clavel-Chapelon F. Fruit and vegetable intakes and asthma in the E3N study. Thorax. 2006;61:209–15.
6. Barros R, Moreira A, Padrão P, Teixeira VH, Carvalho P, Delgado L, Lopes C, Severo M, Moreira P. Dietary patterns and asthma prevalence, incidence and control. Clin Exp Allergy. 2015;45:1673–80.
7. Garcia-Larsen V, Chinn S, Arts IC, Amigo H, Rona RJ. Atopy, wheeze and bronchial responsiveness in young Chilean adults. Do dietary antioxidants matter? Allergy. 2007;62:714–5.
8. Liang W, Chikritzhs T, Lee AH. Lifestyle of young Australian adults with asthma. Asia Pac J Public Health. 2015;27:NP248–54.
9. Lv N, Xiao L, Ma J. Dietary pattern and asthma: a systematic review and meta-analysis. J Asthma Allergy. 2014;7:105–21.
10. Hooper R, Heinrich J, Omenaas E, Sausenthaler S, Garcia-Larsen V, Bakolis I, Burney P. Dietary patterns and risk of asthma: results from three countries in European Community Respiratory Health Survey-II. Br J Nutr. 2010;103:1354–65.
11. Garcia-Larsen V, Luczynska M, Kowalski ML, et al. Use of a common food frequency questionnaire (FFQ) to assess dietary patterns and their relation to allergy and asthma in Europe: pilot study of the GA2LEN FFQ. Eur J Clin Nutr. 2011;65:750–6.
12. Bousquet J, et al. GA2LEN (Global Allergy and Asthma European Network) addresses the allergy and asthma 'epidemic'. Allergy. 2009;64:969–77.
13. Tomassen P, Newson RB, Hoffmans R, et al. Reliability of EP3OS symptom criteria and nasal endoscopy in the assessment of chronic rhinosinusitis: a GA[2]LEN study. Allergy. 2011;66:556–61.
14. Sunyer J, Pekkanen J, Garcia-Esteban R, Svanes C, Künzli N, Janson C, de Marco R, Antó JM, Burney P. Asthma score: predictive ability and risk factors. Allergy. 2007;62:142–8.
15. Palmer SC, Ruospo M, Campbell KL, et al. DIET-HD Study investigators. Nutrition and dietary intake and their association with mortality and hospitalisation in adults with chronic kidney disease treated with haemodialysis: protocol for DIET-HD, a prospective multinational cohort study. BMJ Open. 2015;5:e006897.
16. Ireland J, van Erp-Baart AM, Charrondière UR, Møller A, Smithers G. Trichopoulou A; EFCOSUM Group. Selection of a food classification system and a food composition database for future food consumption surveys. Eur J Clin Nutr. 2002;56:S33–45.
17. FSA (Food Standards Agency). McCance and widdowson's the composition of foods. Seventh Summary edn. Royal Society of Chemistry: Cambridge; 2002.
18. Simes RJ. An improved Bonferroni procedure for multiple tests of significance. Biometrika. 1986;73:751–4.
19. Pekkanen J, Sunyer J, Anto JM, Burney P, European Community Respiratory Survey. Operational definitions of asthma in studies on its aetiology. Eur Respir J. 2005;26:28–35.
20. Kelly Y, Sacker A, Marmot M. Nutrition and respiratory health in adults: findings from the health survey for Scotland. Eur Respir J. 2003;21:664–71.
21. Troisi RJ, Willett WC, Weiss ST, et al. A prospective study of diet and adult-onset asthma. Am J Respir Crit Care Med. 1995;151:1401–8.
22. Soutar A, Seaton A, Brown K. Bronchial reactivity and dietary antioxidants. Thorax. 1997;52:166–70.
23. Moreno-Macias H, Romieu I. Effects of antioxidant supplements and nutrients on patients with asthma and allergies. J Allergy Clin Immunol. 2014;133:1237–44.
24. Arora P, Ansari SH, Najmi AK, et al. Investigation of anti-asthmatic potential of dried fruits of Vitis vinifera L. in animal model of bronchial asthma. Allergy Asthma Clin Immunol. 2016;12:42.
25. Anhê FF, Varin TV, Le Barz M, et al. Gut microbiota dysbiosis in obesity-linked metabolic diseases and prebiotic potential of polyphenol-rich extracts. Curr Obes Rep. 2015;4:389–400.
26. Bédard A, Garcia-Aymerich J, Sanchez M, et al. Confirmatory factor analysis compared with principal component analysis to derive dietary patterns: a longitudinal study in adult women. J Nutr. 2015;145:1559–68.
27. Tanaka T, Takahashi R. Flavonoids and asthma. Nutrients. 2013;5:2128–43.
28. Garcia V, Arts IC, Sterne JA, et al. Dietary intake of flavonoids and asthma in adults. Eur Respir J. 2005;26:449–52.
29. Knekt P, Kumpulainen J, Jarvinen R, et al. Flavonoid intake and risk of chronic diseases. Am J Clin Nutr. 2002;76:560–8.

4

Allergen immunotherapy for allergic asthma: a systematic overview of systematic reviews

Felix Asamoah[1,2,3†], Artemisia Kakourou[4†], Sangeeta Dhami[5*] , Susanne Lau[6], Ioana Agache[7], Antonella Muraro[8], Graham Roberts[9,10,11], Cezmi Akdis[12], Matteo Bonini[13], Ozlem Cavkaytar[14], Breda Flood[15], Kenji Izuhara[16], Marek Jutel[17], Ömer Kalayci[18], Oliver Pfaar[19,20] and Aziz Sheikh[21]

Abstract

Background: There is clinical uncertainty about the effectiveness and safety of allergen immunotherapy (AIT) for the treatment of allergic asthma.

Objectives: To undertake a systematic overview of the effectiveness, cost-effectiveness and safety of AIT for the treatment of allergic asthma.

Methods: We searched nine electronic databases from inception to October 31, 2015. Systematic reviews were independently screened by two reviewers against pre-defined eligibility criteria and critically appraised using the Critical Appraisal Skills Programme quality assessment tool for systematic reviews. Data were descriptively and thematically synthesized.

Results: We identified nine eligible systematic reviews; these focused on delivery of AIT through the following routes: subcutaneous (SCIT; n = 3); sublingual (SLIT; n = 4); and both SCIT and SLIT (n = 2). This evidence found that AIT delivered by SCIT and SLIT can improve medication and symptom scores and measures of bronchial hyper-reactivity. The impact on measures of lung function or asthma control was however less clear. We found no systematic review level evidence on the cost-effectiveness of SCIT or SLIT. SLIT had a favorable safety profile when compared to SCIT, particularly in relation to the risk of systemic reactions.

Conclusions: AIT has the potential to achieve reductions in symptom and medication scores, but there is no clear or consistent evidence that measures of lung function can be improved. Bearing in mind the limitations of synthesizing evidence from systematic reviews and the fact that these reviews include mainly dated studies, a systematic review of current primary studies is now needed to update this evidence base, estimate the effectiveness of AIT on asthma outcomes and to investigate the relative effectiveness, cost-effectiveness and safety of SCIT and SLIT.

Introduction

Asthma is a major public health problem affecting over 300 million people worldwide [1]. Its prevalence and impact are particularly on the rise in urbanized regions. With a projected surge in the world's urban population it is estimated that by 2025 an additional 100 million people may develop asthma [2]. Asthma is therefore set to become one of the world's most prevalent chronic diseases.

Patho-physiologically, asthma is a chronic inflammatory disorder of the airways leading to airflow limitation and remodelling [3]. The resulting signs and symptoms are dyspnea, cough, chest discomfort and wheezing. Based on clinical and laboratory findings, different asthma phenotypes have been described [4]. This review focuses on allergic asthma. Allergic asthma is one of the best described asthma phenotypes.

*Correspondence: SangeetaDhami@hotmail.com
†Artemisia Kakourou and Felix Asamoah contributed equally to this work.
5 Evidence-Based Health Care Ltd, Edinburgh, UK
Full list of author information is available at the end of the article

Allergic sensitization is a strong risk factor for asthma inception and severity in children and in adults [5]. Currently, there is no cure for asthma, but symptomatic control can be achieved in the majority of patients through a combination of short-acting bronchodilators and inhaled corticosteroids with minimal, if any, side-effects. Long-acting beta-2 agonists, anti-leukotrienes, anticholinergics, theophylline, anti-IgE antibodies and other biologic agents can be added to achieve asthma control in more severe cases [6].

Allergen immunotherapy (AIT) is the only class of treatment for respiratory allergy that has the potential to change the course of the disease. Its immunological mechanisms of action involve induction of allergen-specific immune tolerance. AIT for allergic asthma is therefore a potential therapeutic option in appropriately selected patients with allergic asthma.

The European Academy of Allergy and Clinical Immunology (EAACI) is in the process of developing the *EAACI Guidelines on Allergen Immunotherapy for Allergic Asthma*. Guideline recommendations will be informed by formal evidence syntheses of the literature. This article is an overarching synthesis of the systematic review evidence on the effectiveness, cost-effectiveness and safety of AIT in the management of allergic asthma. It will be followed by a review of the primary studies.

Methods

A detailed description of our methods is available in the published systematic review protocol [7]. We therefore confine ourselves here to a summary of our methods.

Search strategy

Electronic literature searches were conducted to retrieve systematic reviews that have been conducted in relation to AIT for allergic asthma from the following electronic databases: Medline, Embase, Cochrane Library, HTA, EED, CINAHL, ISI Web of Science, TRIP, Current controlled trials and Australian and New Zealand Clinical Trials registry.

A highly sensitive search strategy was developed, and validated study design filters were applied to retrieve articles pertaining to the use of AIT for allergic asthma from electronic bibliographic databases ("Appendix"). We used the systematic review filter developed at McMaster University Health Information Research Unit (HIRU) (http://hiru.mcmaster.ca/hiru/HIRU_Hedges_MEDLINE_Strategies.aspx#Reviews). Based on further abstract and full paper screening, all systematic reviews were identified and screened for inclusion. The searches were for articles published from inception of the databases up to 31st October 2015. No language restrictions were applied. All titles were uploaded into the systematic review software Distiller SR (Evidence Partners, Ottawa, Canada).

Eligibility criteria

We were interested in systematic reviews of randomized controlled trials (RCTs) in which AIT for different allergens (e.g. pollens, mites, animal dander and cockroach) were administered through the subcutaneous (SCIT) or sublingual (SLIT) routes compared with placebo or any active comparator.

Participants of interest were patients of any age with a physician confirmed diagnosis of allergic asthma, plus evidence of clinically relevant allergic sensitization as assessed by an objective biomarker (e.g. skin prick test or specific-IgE), in combination with a history of asthma symptoms due to allergen exposure. Reviews that investigated participants with both asthma and rhinitis/rhinoconjuctivitis, but presented separate outcomes for the two conditions were also included.

The primary outcome of interest was the effectiveness—both short-term and long-term, where long-term was defined as persistence of benefit after discontinuation of treatment—of AIT as assessed by symptoms and/or medication scores.

Secondary outcomes of interest included asthma control, asthma specific quality of life, exacerbations, lung function, environmental exposure chamber or bronchial allergen challenge, cost-effectiveness and safety as assessed by local and systemic reactions.

Selection procedures

Title and abstract screening was conducted independently by two reviewers (SD and FS) and for those that appeared to meet the inclusion criteria full-texts were independently retrieved and screened (AK and FA). Any disagreements were resolved through discussion or, if necessary, arbitration by a third reviewer (SD).

Data extraction

Data were extracted independently in Distiller SR by two reviewers (FA and AK) using pre-defined criteria. Disagreements were resolved by discussion between the reviewers and where agreement could not be reached by arbitration with a third reviewer (SD).

Quality assessment

Independent quality assessment of all systematic reviews was undertaken by two reviewers (FA and AK) using the Critical Appraisal Skills Programme (CASP) tool for systematic reviews [8]. Disagreements were resolved through discussion; if agreement could not be reached a third reviewer (SD) arbitrated.

Synthesis of evidence

Abstracted data were included into descriptive tables that included information on search strategy, population characteristics, study design, quality assessment, exposure, outcomes and subgroup analyses. Because of multiple outcomes of this overview and since there is no consensus whether and how meta-analysis should be performed from systematic reviews, we did not undertake meta-analysis.

Results

Characteristics of included systematic review

Our searches retrieved nine systematic reviews, five of which included meta-analyses (see Fig. 1). The key features of these systematic reviews are summarized in Table 1.

The nine systematic reviews included 272 individual RCTs studying over 13,000 patients with asthma. Eight of the systematic reviews studied both children and adults [9–16]; whilst one focused on children only [17]. Two systematic reviews evaluated AIT for a single-allergen (i.e. house dust mite) [13, 17]. The remaining seven studied AIT for multiple allergens, these including animal dander, mold natural, pollens, modified allergens and latex [10–12, 14–16, 18]. Three systematic reviews evaluated SCIT [10, 14, 17], four evaluated SLIT [11, 13, 15, 16], and two examined a combination of SCIT and SLIT [12, 18].

The majority of the systematic reviews had primary outcomes which focused on asthma symptoms, medication usage, allergen-specific bronchial hyper-reactivity (BHR) and exacerbations with secondary outcomes of safety and disease specific quality of life (Table 1).

Quality assessment

Two reviews by Abramson et al. and Normansell et al. were judged to be at low risk of bias [10, 15]. The remaining reviews were classified as being at moderate risk of bias (Table 2) [11–14, 16, 17].

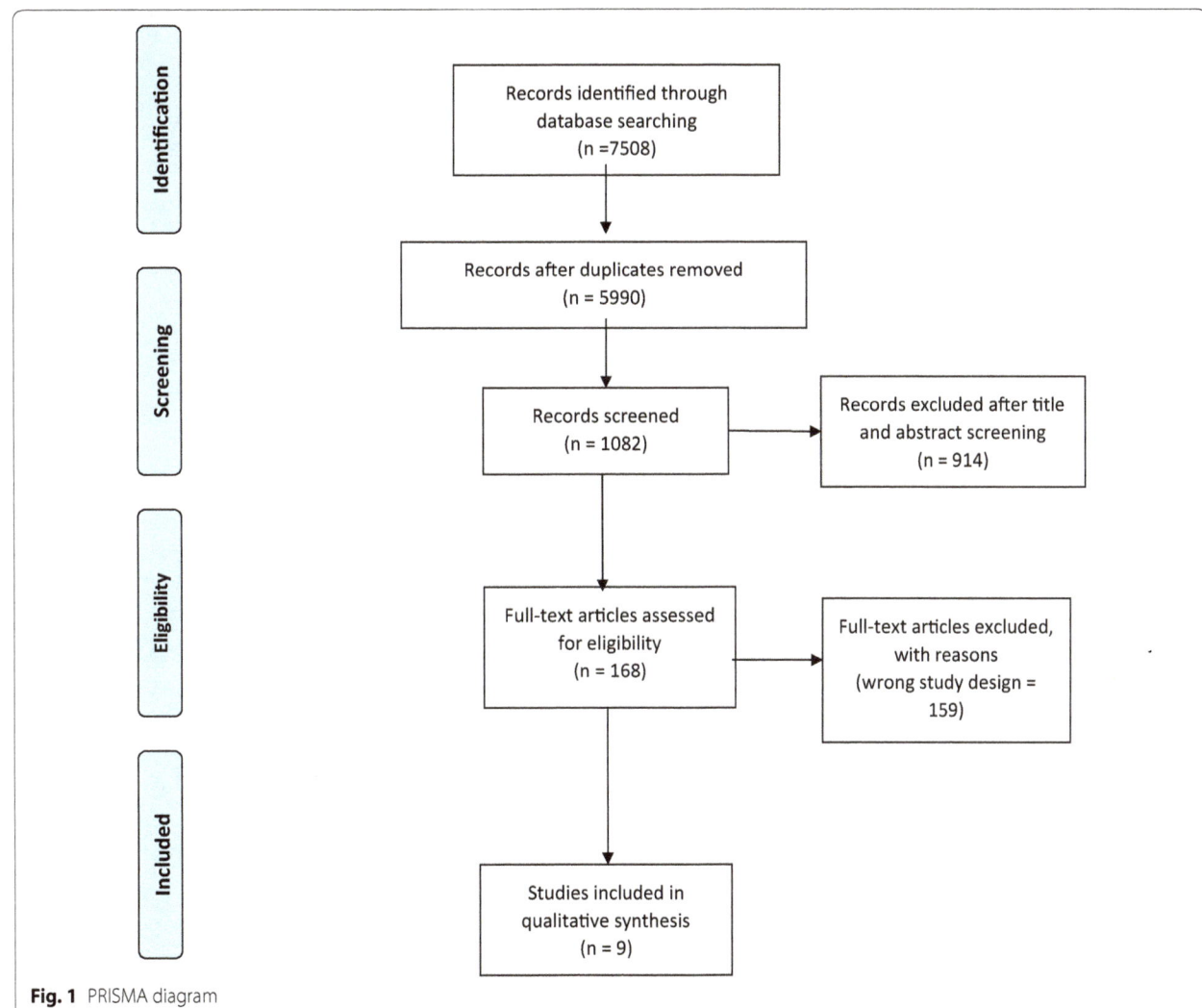

Fig. 1 PRISMA diagram

Table 1 Main characteristics of included studies

Author, Year (Country)	Databases searched	Search period	No of studies relevant to this SR (No of participants)	Population	Intervention relevant to this SR	Allrgens	Outcomes relevant to this SR	Subgroup analyses relevant to this SR
Abramson, 2010 (Australia)	CENTRAL, MEDLINE, EMBASE, CINAHL, AMED, PsycINFO, and handsearching of journals and meeting abstracts	1950–2005	88 RCTs (3459)	adults and children with allergic asthma	SCIT vs placebo SCIT vs inhaled steroid	HDM, pollens, animal dander, moulds, chemically modified allergoids, antigen–antibody complexes	Effectiveness, lung function, non-specific BHR, allergen-specific BHR, safety	NR
Calamita, 2006 (Brazil)	MEDLINE, EMBASE, LILACS and the Cochrane Library	1966–2005	25 RCTS (1706)	adults and children with allergic asthma	SLIT vs placebo	Mites, pollens, mould, dander, latex	Effectiveness, lung function, non-specific BHR, safety	Age, treatment duration (no details)
Chelladurai, 2013 (USA)	MEDLINE, Embase, LILACS and the Cochrane Central Register of Controlled Trials	Up to December 21, 2012	4 RCTs (NR)	adults and children with allergic asthma	SCIT vs SLIT	Mites, pollens	Effectiveness, safety	NR
Compalati, 2009 (Italy)	MEDLINE, EMBASE, LILACS, SCOPUS	Up to March 31, 2008	9 DBRCTs (452)	adults and children with allergic asthma	SLIT vs placebo	HDM	Effectiveness	Age (children vs adults)
Erekosima, 2014 (USA)	MEDLINE, Embase, LILACS, and the Cochrane Central Register of Controlled Trials	1947-May 21, 2012	38 RCTs (NR)	adults and children with allergic asthma ± rhinitis/rhino corjunctivitis	SCIT vs any comparator	Mites, pollen, dander, mould	Effectiveness, lung function, allergen-specific BHR, quality of life, safety	NR
Kim, 2013 (USA)	Medline, Embase, LILACS, CENTRAL, and the Cochrane Central Register of Controlled Trials	Up to May 2012	27 RCTs (NR)	Children w th allergic asthma ± rhinoconjuctivitis	SCIT vs any comparator SLIT vs any comparator SCIT vs SLIT	Dust mite, Rye, Cladosporium, Alternaria, Tree mix	Effectiveness, quality of life, safety	NR
Normansell, 2015 (UK)	CENTRAL, MEDLINE, EMBASE, CINAHL, AMED, PsycINFO, Clinical Trials.gov, WHO and handsearching of journals and meeting abstracts	Up to March 25, 2015	52 RCTs (5256)	adults and children with allergic asthma	SLIT vs placebo SLIT vs conventional pharmacotherapy	HDM, grass pollen, birch pollen, cockroach, cat dander, Alternaria, Parietaria, olive pollen, Artemisia, HDM + Parietaria (combination)	Effectiveness, Exacerbations, Quality of life, safety, BHR	Age (children vs adults)
Polzehl, 2006 (Germany)	MEDLINE and EMBASE	1970–2001	13 DBRCTs (442)	adults and children with allergic asthma	SCIT vs. placebo	HDM (D. pteronyssinus, D. farinae)	Effectiveness, safety, lung function, bronchial provocation	NR
Tao, 2013 (China)	PubMed, EMBASE and the Cochrane Central Register of Controlled Trials	Up to March 2012	16 DBRCTs (794)	adults and children with allergic asthma	SLIT vs placebo	Mite, pollen	Effectiveness, lung function, safety	Age (children vs adults)

Table 2 Quality assessment of included studies

Author, year	Focused question	Inclusion of appropriate studies	Inclusion of eligible studies	Quality assessment of studies	Appropriateness of synthesis	Overall results of review	Accuracy of results	Applicability to local populations	Considering all relevant outcomes	Benefits vs harms/costs	Overall risk of bias
Abramson	✓	✓	✓	✓	✓	✓	✓	n/a	✓	✓	Low
Calamita	✓	✓	Unclear	✓	✓	✓	✓	n/a	✓	Unclear	Unclear
Chelladurai	✓	✓	X	✓	✓	✓	✓	n/a	✓	✓	Unclear
Compalati	✓	✓	X	✓	✓	✓	✓	n/a	✓	✓	Unclear
Erekosima	✓	✓	X	✓	n/a	✓	✓	n/a	✓	✓	Unclear
Kim	✓	✓	X	✓	✓	✓	✓	n/a	✓	✓	Unclear
Normansell	✓	✓	✓	✓	✓	✓	✓	n/a	✓	✓	Low
Polzehl	✓	✓	✓	Unclear	✓	✓	✓	n/a	✓	✓	Unclear
Tao	✓	✓	X	✓	✓	✓	✓	n/a	✓	✓	Unclear

SCIT focused reviews

Asthma symptom scores

The strongest evidence for asthma symptom reduction was provided by the meta-analysis by Abramson et al., which included 88 RCTs of moderate quality randomizing a total of 3459 asthma patients [10]. Meta-analysis demonstrated a significant improvement in asthma symptoms scores based on data from thirty-five trials: the estimated standardised mean difference (SMD) for all allergens combined was −0.59 (95% CI −0.83 to −0.35) for AIT versus placebo, but there was high heterogeneity between studies (I^2 = 73%). The authors concluded that it would have been necessary to treat three patients (NNT = 3; 95% CI 3–5) to avoid one person's asthma symptoms deteriorating. Significant improvement of symptoms was most likely with AIT to pollen (NNT = 3; 95% CI 2–16); animal dander (NNT = 3; 95% CI 2–18) and other allergens such as molds, chemically modified allergoids or antigen–antibody complexes (NNT = 3; 95% CI 3–4). A smaller improvement was observed following HDM immunotherapy where six patients would need to be treated to avoid one deteriorating (NNT = 6; 95% CI 4–16). Only one trial directly compared AIT to inhaled corticosteroids and this found that symptoms improved more rapidly on inhaled steroids than AIT [18].

A further three reviews undertook a qualitative synthesis of the impact of AIT on asthma symptom scores. Erekosima et al. [14] reported on 10 studies [19–28], including 628 participants, that evaluated SCIT for control of asthma symptoms (eight compared SCIT to placebo, one compared SCIT to pharmacotherapy, and one compared SCIT to no SCIT); 90% of these studies reported a greater improvement in the SCIT arm than in the comparator arm. All of these trials used a single allergen: six were for HDM, one *Cladosporitum*, one timothy grass, one ragweed and one cat allergens. The review by Polzehl et al., which focused on the efficacy of SCIT with HDM extracts (*Dermatophagides pteronyssinus or farina*) in 442 adolescents and adults, reported that seven out of 12 studies showed a significant improvement in asthma symptom scores when compared to placebo [17].

Kim et al., using a narrative synthesis, reported evidence to demonstrate that SCIT improved asthma symptoms compared with placebo or pharmacotherapy [18]. This was only true however when using a single allergen; when multiple allergens were used, this was not the case. This evidence was from moderate to high quality studies.

Asthma medication scores

The review by Abramson et al. pooled evidence from 21 studies to show that AIT significantly decreased medication usage with an SMD for all allergens combined versus placebo of −0.53 (95% CI −0.80 to −0.27) with moderate between study heterogeneity (I^2 = 67%) [10]. Overall, it would have been necessary to treat four patients (NNT = 4; 95% CI 4–7) with AIT to avoid one patient requiring an increase in medication.

In Erekosima et al. [14], eight studies [18–22, 25, 29, 30], all using single allergen AIT, including 592 patients, reported on medication scores [18]. Five out of eight studies demonstrated a greater reduction in medication use in the SCIT group than in the comparator arm and two of the studies did not report the direction of change. Polzehl et al. [17] reported on asthma medication use in 10 studies: five of these showed a significant decrease in medication requirement after therapy whereas the remaining five studies showed no significant effect. Interestingly, no improvement was seen in four trials, which included patients with moderate-to-severe asthma.

Kim et al. presented results from four studies using single allergens which demonstrated that the SCIT group had a reduction in medication score greater than the control group [18]. A further study however reported the same scores for the treatment and placebo group.

Asthma control and exacerbations

No results were available for these outcomes.

Disease specific quality of life

Kim et al. reported quality of life outcomes in two SCIT studies [18]. Of these, a study of 50 patients with moderate risk of bias showed a significant improvement in quality of life in both patients and their parents and the other, a study of 300 patients with high risk of bias, showed no difference in SCIT and control groups.

Lung function

In Abramson et al., of the 88 included studies 20 provided results for lung function [10]. Data for peak expiratory flow (PEF) and forced expiratory volume in one second (FEV1) were meta-analyzed. The overall results were inconclusive regarding the impact of AIT on lung function when compared to placebo: SMD for PEF 0.14 (95% CI −0.33 to 0.61) and SMD for FEV1 −0.32 (95% CI −0.96 to 0.31).with high between study heterogeneity (I^2 = 81% for PEF; and I^2 = 61% for FEV1) In seven studies reporting on lung function deterioration (simply as improved, worsened or the same), there was an overall trend implying lung function improvement after immunotherapy, but this did not reach statistical significance (RR 0.89; 95% CI 0.73–1.10).

In Erekosima et al., 11 studies enrolling 873 participants reported that the impact on lung function was 'variable and inconsistent across studies' (no further details provided) [14]. Polzehl et al., from nine studies, found no significant changes in lung function between SCIT and placebo [17].

Environmental exposure chamber or bronchial allergen challenge

Three systematic reviews reported on bronchial allergen challenge . Meta-analysis results of 18 studies from Abramson et al. [10] showed that AIT reduced non-specific BHR following challenges when compared to placebo: overall SMD of −0.35 (95% CI −0.59 to −0.11). These effects were significant for methacholine: SMD of −0.25 (95% CI −0.51 to 0.00) and acetylcholine: SMD −1.29 (95% CI −2.28 to −0.31), but not for histamine: SMD −0.55 (95% CI −1.37 to 0.28) or cold air: SMD −0.52 (95% CI −1.31 to 0.26). Non-specific BHR was reported as increased, reduced or unchanged in five studies with an estimated RR for increased non-specific BHR of 0.48 (95% CI 0.33–0.72) favoring AIT.

In Erekosima et al., 13 studies reported on non-specific bronchial provocation tests on 568 participants in total [14]. Five out of 13 studies demonstrated greater improvement in the AIT group than the comparator. In Polzehl et al., two out of three studies showed significant improvement to methacholine challenge after 12–18 months [17].

Meta-analysis of 19 trials in the systematic review by Abramson et al. showed a significant reduction in allergen specific BHR following immunotherapy compared to placebo: mite SMD −0.98 (95% CI −1.39 to −0.58), pollen SMD −0.55 (95% CI −0.84 to −0.27), animal dander SMD −0.61 (95% CI −0.95 to −0.27), other allergens SMD −0.18 (95% CI −0.70 to 0.33) and overall SMD −0.61 (95% CI −0.79 to −0.43) [10]. Allergen specific BHR was reported as increased, reduced or unchanged in 16 studies with an estimated RR for increased allergen specific BHR of 0.51 (95% CI 0.41–0.63) favoring AIT.

In Erekosima et al., eight out of 11 studies demonstrated statistically significant improvement in the SCIT group that the comparator [14]. Finally, in Polzehl et al., three out of three studies showed significant improvement in the immunotherapy group [17].

Safety

Abramson and colleagues in their systematic review reported on both local and systemic adverse reactions [10]. The pooled relative risk for local adverse reactions, as it was reported in ten studies, was 1.4 (95% CI 0.97–2.02) and homogenous (I² = 0.0%). So, if sixteen patients were treated with immunotherapy, one would be expected to develop a local reaction. Systemic adverse reactions defined as anaphylaxis, asthma, rhinitis, urticaria or any combination of these were reported by 32 studies. The pooled relative risk for systemic reactions of

any severity was 2.45 (95% CI 1.91–3.13) and relatively homogenous (I² = 27%). They concluded that if nine patients were treated with immunotherapy, one would be expected to develop a systemic reaction.

Erekosima et al. reported data on safety from 35 trials [14]. Local reactions were reported in 11 studies, these showing that 71/346 (20.5%) patients in the SCIT arm experienced local reactions compared to 1/7 (14.3%) in the comparator arm. General reactions were reported in 14 studies, according to which 190/624 (30.4%) in the SCIT arm experienced general reactions, compared to 52/217 (24.0%) in the comparator arm. Finally anaphylactic reactions were reported in four studies and all events were concerning patients on immunotherapy (13/205 (6.3%) patients).The other study that reported on this outcome was Polzehl et al., which found that seven out of the thirteen studies showed no severe adverse events [17]. Four studies however, reported systemic adverse effects.

Kim et al. reported from 10 SCIT studies local reactions occurring at the injection site in both the treatment and placebo groups [18]. In terms of systemic reactions, bronchospasm occurred in 1–30% of patients and general systemic reactions in 3–34% of patients.

SLIT focused reviews
Asthma symptom scores

Evidence from the meta-analysis by Calamita et al. [11] which included 25 RCTs (19 double-blind and six open) showed a non-significant reduction in asthma symptoms in the SLIT arm compared to placebo: the SMD from meta-analysis of nine studies (enrolling 303 patients) t was −0.38 (95% CI −0.79 to 0.03).

The systematic review by Compalati et al., which included nine double-blind placebo controlled RCTs, found a significant reduction in symptom scores: SMD −0.95 (95% CI −1.74 to −0.15) compared to the placebo group; there was high heterogeneity (I² = 92%) [13].

Normansell et al. found symptom scores in 42 studies, but only 17 presented these in a numerical fashion [15]. Of these studies, five showed no statistical significant difference between groups, nine studies reported statistically significant reductions in the SLIT group compared with the placebo group; two studies showed a small improvement and one study reported a marked reduction in symptoms during cat exposure for the SLIT group.

Tao et al. [16] which included 16 double-blind placebo controlled RCTs demonstrated that there was a significant reduction in patients symptom scores in the SLIT group compared to the placebo group: pooled SMD of −0.74 (95% CI −1.26 to −0.22), with significant between study heterogeneity (I² = 91%). Subgroup analysis according to age showed that SMD was −0.87 (95% CI −1.54 to −0.21) in children and −0.40 (95% CI −1.36 to −0.25) in adults. Subgroup analysis by allergen showed a beneficial effect in the context of mite immunotherapy: SMD −0.97 (95% CI −1.69 to −0.25), but not pollen immunotherapy: SMD −0.29 (95% CI −0.96 to 0.38). Finally, subgroup analysis according to treatment duration showed that SMD was −0.96 (95% CI −1.69 to −0.22) for treatment less than 12 months whereas SMD was −0.60 (95% CI −1.30 to 0.10) for greater than 12 months of treatment.

Kim et al. using a narrative synthesis indicated that there was evidence to demonstrate that SLIT improved asthma symptoms compared with placebo or pharmacotherapy [18].

Asthma medications scores

Meta-analysis results of six studies (with 254 patients) from Calamita et al. showed that there was a tendency towards improved medication scores favored by SLIT, but this was not conclusively shown: SMD of −0.91 (95% CI −1.94 to 0.12) with significant between studies heterogeneity ($I^2 = 91.8\%$) [11]. The results from Compalati et al., from seven studies enrolling 220 patients looking at dust mite allergen, however presented a significant (P = 0.02) reduction in rescue medication use: SMD −1.48 (95% CI −2.70 to −0.26) but significant heterogeneity ($I^2 = 96\%$). Subgroup analysis according to age, showed a significant reduction in children (SMD −1.86; 95% CI −3.34 to −0.38) but not in adults (SMD 0.23; 95% CI −0.33 to 0.78) [13]. Normansell et al. reported this outcome numerically in twelve studies, five of which reported favorably for the SLIT group and seven of which showed no statistically significant difference between groups [15]. Results from Tao et al., indicated that medication score was significantly (P = 0.02) reduced in the SLIT group compared to their comparators (SMD of −0.78; 95% CI −1.45 to −0.11), but there was significant heterogeneity ($I^2 = 93\%$) [16]. They also looked at children and adults separately and found that whereas in children there was a statistically significant reduction in medication score with SLIT (SMD −1.1; 95% CI −2.06 to −0.14, P = 0.03) this was not the case for adults (SMD −0.00; 95% CI −0.36 to 0.36; P = 0.99). They also indicated that prolonged duration of treatment did not have any additive beneficial effect: SMD for less than 12 month treatment was −0.98 (95% CI −2.14 to 0.19) and SMD for more than 12 months of treatment was −0.51 (95% CI −1.17 to 0.16).

Kim et al. included nine studies which reported on this outcome in relation to asthma: seven for HDM showed a significant improvement compared to placebo [18].

Asthma control

Calamita et al. found that seven studies had reported on general asthma control, combining asthmatic symptoms, need for symptom relief medication, respiratory function test and lung hyper-reactivity, and found a significant improvement for AIT over placebo: RD −0.27 (95% CI −0.33 to −0.21) and RR 0.48 (95% CI 0.4–0.57). There was little heterogeneity between these studies ($I^2 = 36.3\%$) [11].

Tao et al. reported that two studies looked at 'global improvement', considering symptom remission, medication use and lung function, but they failed to identify any significant improvement (RR 3.31; 95% CI 0.25–44.44) [16].

Kim et al. reported two studies which looked at general asthma control [18]. One study found that after six months of SLIT to HDM compared to placebo, classification of asthma in the treatment group changed from 'mild-moderate persistent to mild intermittent'. The second study however concluded that after three years of SLIT treatment there was no difference in the number of children with mild intermittent asthma when compared to the placebo group.

Exacerbations

Normansell et al. reported on this outcome with data from one small study, enrolling 43 patients, which was assessed to be at high risk of bias [15]. It reported no exacerbations requiring emergency department attendance or hospital admission during the (four week) treatment period or the follow up period (5–6 weeks) in either the SLIT or placebo arms.

Disease specific quality of life

Normansell et al. reported data on this outcome from five of the included studies, but no meta-analysis could be performed [15]. Results from these five studies were variable, this possibly in part because a number of tools had been used not all of which were specific to asthma. Overall, two studies found no significant difference in disease specific quality of life scores, two found a significant improvement, and the fifth was equivocal.

Kim et al. reported quality of life outcomes in only two SLIT studies, both showed no improvement in quality of life [18].

Lung function

Calamita et al. indicated that treatment by SLIT failed to show a significant improvement in FEV1%: SMD of 1.48 (95% CI 0.13–2.82) among 144 patient in four of the studies that investigated this outcome. FEF 25–75% also did not achieve statistical significance: SMD 1.06 (95% CI 0.40–1.72) among 42 patients in two studies [11]. Similarly, Tao et al. found, from five studies, no improvement in FEV1% pooled SMD of 0.49 (95% CI −0.36 to 1.34; P = 0.26) in the SLIT group [16].

Environmental exposure chamber or bronchial allergen challenge

Calamata et al. reported that there was no significant improvement in bronchial provocation tests in the SLIT group, but no data were presented [11]. Normansell et al. found 11 studies which used the methacholine provocation test. Data from four of these trials were pooled; meta-analysis failed to show any evidence of benefit: SMD 0.69, 95% CI −0.04 to 1.43, with a high level of heterogeneity ($I^2 = 76\%$) [15].

Safety

Calamita et al. reported adverse effects reported in 20 studies enrolling 1501 patients. Only mild adverse events were seen, the majority resolving without the need for treatment [11]. The relative risk of adverse effects was 1.83 (95% CI 1.40–2.40) and RD was 0.07 (95% CI 0.04–0.10) with a number needed to harm (NNH) for AIT of 14.3.

Normansell et al., from 22 RCTs, reported that serious adverse events were uncommon, occurring in 1 in 100 patients using SLIT (RD 0.001, 95% CI −0.008 to 0.010; moderate-quality evidence) [15]. When they looked at all AEs, however, they showed an increase of AEs in the SLIT group compared to the placebo with an OR of 1.70 (95% CI 1.21–2.38). Most of these AEs were however mild.

Tao et al., also concluded that the AEs were mild such as mouth and throat itchiness, redness and swelling [16]. Pooled data analysis through meta-analysis resulted in a significant risk in a RR 2.23 (95% CI 1.17–4.2; P = 0.01) with high level of heterogeneity ($I^2 = 75\%$). Kim et al. found in 12 SLIT studies a rate of local reactions from 0.2–50% in the treatment group but 6–25% in the placebo group [18]. Systemic reactions were common, but not life threatening and occurred in both treatment and placebo groups.

Reviews including both SCIT and SLIT studies

Two systematic reviews examined the effect of SLIT versus SCIT on asthma. Kim et al. looked solely at children and included 27 trials: 12 SLIT and 12 SCIT, the results of which have been discussed above under the appropriate headings; there were a further three trials comparing the two treatment routes [18]. Chelladurai et al. looked at a head-to-head comparison of the two routes of administration [12].

Asthma symptom score

Kim et al., using a narrative synthesis, found that in the studies that looked at SLIT versus SCIT there was no conclusive evidence to favor one route of administration over the other in terms of symptom scores [18].

A comparison between SCIT and SLIT was undertaken in the review by Chelladurai et al., which included four studies of asthma patients all using HDM immunotherapy [12]. They demonstrated a greater reduction in asthma symptoms from three studies with SCIT compared to SLIT, whereas one study showed greater reduction in symptoms with SLIT. All of these studies were judged to be of moderate quality.

Asthma medication score

Kim et al. presented results from three studies of HDM immunotherapy directly comparing SLIT with SCIT, but there was no conclusive evidence to favor one route of administration over the other in terms of reducing medication scores. Two studies were described as favoring SCIT over SLIT for improving medication use, whereas one study favored SLIT.

Chelladurai et al., found that when comparing the HDM studies two studies favored SCIT in reducing medications usage while two favored SLIT [12].

Asthma control

No results were available for this outcome.

Disease specific quality of life

No results were available for these outcomes.

Lung function and environmental exposure chamber or bronchial allergen challenge

No results were available for these outcomes.

Safety

In Kim et al. among the three studies (including 135 children) that examined SCIT versus SLIT, local reactions were reported in three patients receiving SLIT and in three patients receiving SCIT. No systemic reactions were reported in patients receiving SLIT. Among the patients that received SCIT, four experienced systemic reactions, including one anaphylaxis event (anaphylaxis was defined as flushing, wheezing and dyspnea requiring adrenaline) [18].

In the comparison between SCIT and SLIT, Chelladurai et al. indicated that eight studies reported on AEs, however due to the heterogeneity data could not be pooled [12]. Local reactions occurred both in SCIT and SLIT with no fatalities; however SLIT was associated with an increased frequency of local reactions (7–56%) compared with SCIT (20%). The only episode of anaphylaxis was reported in one study in a child treated with SCIT.

Health economic outcomes

No results were available for this outcome.

Discussion

Statement of principal findings

We found clear evidence that AIT administered by the SCIT route is effective in improving medication and symptom scores. The evidence in relation to the effectiveness of SLIT for these outcomes was more mixed. It is interesting to note however, that the review by Compalati et al. [12] which looked only at HDM AIT shows significant reductions in both symptom and medication scores for asthma compared to the review by Calamita et al. [11] which looks at a number of allergens which shows no significant reduction when considering the same outcomes. In terms of lung function no positive result could be concluded for either SCIT or SLIT. With regards to BHR, some of the studies showed an improvement in the SCIT group, but no clear conclusions could be drawn and no improvement in the SLIT group could be demonstrated for this outcome. There was considerable variation in results dependent upon which allergen was used and whether multiple or single allergens were administered with single allergen AIT faring more favorably. The two systematic reviews by Kim et al. [18] and Chelladurai et al. [12] which compared the two routes of administration could not conclusively show any difference between the effectiveness of SLIT and SCIT. Furthermore, it was difficult to compare results from these two reviews due to the heterogeneity between them including the fact that one was focused on the pediatric population only whilst the other looked at both adults and children. Furthermore, although they both looked at AIT for HDM, they also looked at different allergens with one concentrating on tree mix and the other pollens. Across all of the reviews, there was considerable variation in results dependent upon which allergen was used and whether multiple or single allergens were administered.

Safety is a prime concern with any treatment and the safety profile of SLIT compares more favorably to SCIT particularly in relation to the risk of systemic reactions. However, no fatalities were reported with either route of administration.

There were very few studies which considered and reported on disease specific quality of life as a study outcome. As a result due to the paucity of data present no conclusions can be drawn. This is therefore clearly an area that warrants further enquiry. Studies that considered this outcome used many different tools to assess quality of life some of which were not disease specific. This is another area where uniformity of reporting is urgently required.

Strengths and limitations

We believe this is the first such synthesis of data from systematic reviews on AIT that has been undertaken. We used standard systematic overview techniques, which will have helped to minimize the risk of bias.

There are nonetheless some limitations of systematic overviews which should be considered when interpreting the results. First is in relation to the quality of studies that were included in the individual systematic reviews, many of which were at moderate or high risk of bias. Second is the wide variety of studies included within these systematic reviews, the majority of which are dated. They included patients with varying severities of asthma, allergies and treatment with single or multiple allergens and with treatment regimens of varying length and follow-up. Furthermore, there was no standardization of outcomes measured and even when outcomes overlapped there was still no standardization of measurements taken. This heterogeneity of studies may in part account for the varied results that were seen. Finally, meta-analysis was mainly confined in the studies that investigated SLIT rather than SCIT.

Conclusions

This systematic overview has identified a substantial evidence base investigating the effectiveness and safety of AIT for allergic asthma, this showing that overall this treatment modality has the potential to improve medication and symptom scores. There was some indirect evidence to suggest that the effectiveness of SCIT may be superior to SLIT, but that the safety profile of SLIT is superior in relation to systemic AEs. We found no evidence in relation to cost-effectiveness considerations and equivocal and little or no evidence in relation to many of our secondary effectiveness outcomes of interest. A follow-on, more up-to-date evidence synthesis of primary studies may help to provide further clarity on the effectiveness, safety and cost-effectiveness of AIT.

Authors' contributions

This review was drafted by Felix Asamoah, Artemisia Karakou and Sangeeta Dhami. It was revised following critical review initially by Aziz Sheikh, Ioana Agache and Susanne Lau, and then by all the co-authors All authors read and approved the final manuscript.

Author details

[1] Centre for Environmental and Preventive Medicine, Wolfson Institute of Preventive Medicine, London, UK. [2] Barts and the London School of Medicine and Dentistry, Queen Mary University of London, London, UK. [3] Neonatal Unit, Homerton University Hospital NHS Foundation Trust, London, UK. [4] Department of Hygiene and Epidemiology, University of Ioannina School of Medicine, Ioannina, Greece. [5] Evidence-Based Health Care Ltd, Edinburgh, UK. [6] Charite Medical University, Berlin, Germany. [7] Department of Allergy and Clinical Immunology, Faculty of Medicine, Transylvania University Brasov, Brasov, Romania. [8] Food Allergy Referral Centre Veneto Region, University Hospital of Padua, Padua, Italy. [9] The David Hide Asthma and Allergy Research Centre, St Mary's Hospital, Newport, Isle of Wight, UK. [10] NIHR Biomedical Research Centre, University Hospital Southampton NHS Foundation Trust and Faculty of Medicine, University of Southampton , Southampton, UK. [11] Faculty of Medicine, University of Southampton, Southampton, UK. [12] Swiss Institute for Allergy and Asthma Research, Davos, Switzerland. [13] Sapienza University Rome, Rome, Italy. [14] Department of Allergy and Clinical Immunology, Sami Ulus Maternity and Children Training and Research Hospital, Ankara,

Turkey. [15] European Federation of Allergy and Airways Diseases Patients Association, Brussels, Belgium. [16] Saga Medical School, Saga, Japan. [17] Wroclaw Medical University, Wrocław, Poland. [18] Hacettepe University, Ankara, Turkey. [19] Department of Otorhinolaryngology, Head and Neck Surgery, Universitätsmedizin Mannheim, Medical Faculty Mannheim, Heidelberg University, Mannheim, Germany. [20] Center for Rhinology and Allergology, Wiesbaden, Germany. [21] Asthma UK Centre for Applied Research, Usher Institute of Population Health Sciences and Informatics, The University of Edinburgh, Edinburgh, UK.

Acknowledgements
We would like to thank Z Sheikh for technical support. This study is part of the EAACI AIT guidelines project, chaired by Antonella Muraro and coordinated by Graham Roberts.

Competing interests
F Asamoah: reports payment from Evidence-Based Health Care Ltd during the conduct of the study; A Kakourou: has nothing to disclose; S Dhami: reports grants from EAACI to carry out the review, during the conduct of the study; S Lau: Allergopharma grant for SLIT grass pollen trial in children (AllerSLIT), Merck personal fees for Drug monitoring comittee (SLIT), Symbiopharm Herborn grant for prevention trail with ProSymbioflor, Boehringer grant for Tiotropiumbromid trial in children; I Agache: has nothing to disclose: A Muraro: reports personal fees from Novartis, personal fees from Meda Mylan, outside the submitted work; G Roberts: has a patent Use of sublingual immunotherapy to prevent the development of allergy in at risk infants issued and my University has received payments for activities I have undertaken giving expert advice to ALK, presenting at company symposia for ALK, Allergen Therapeutics and Meda plus as a member of an Independent Data Monitoring Committee for Merck; C Akdis: reports grants from Actellion, personal fees from Aventis, personal fees from Stallergenes, grants and personal fees from Allergopharma, personal fees from Circassia, grants from Novartis, grants from Christine Kuhne Center for Allergy Research and Education, outside the submitted work; M Bonini: has nothing to disclose; O Cavkaytar: has nothing to disclose; B Flood: has nothing to disclose; K Izuhara: reports grants and personal fees from Chugai Pharmaceutical Co. Ltd, grants from Shlno-test Co. Ltd, outside the submitted work; M Jutel: reports personal fees from ALLERGOPKARMA, personal fees from ANERGIS, personal fees from STALLERGEN, personal fees from ALK, personal fees from LETI, outside the submitted work; Ö Kalayci: none; O Pfaar: reports grants and personal fees from ALK-Abelló, grants and personal fees from Allergopharma, grants and personal fees from Stallergenes Greer, grants and personal fees from HAL Allergy Holding B.V./HAL Allergie GmbH, grants and personal fees from Bencard Allergie GmbH/Allergy Therapeutics, grants and personal fees from Lofarma, grants from Biomay, grants from Nuvo, grants from Circassia, grants and personal fees from Biotech Tools S.A., grants and personal fees from Laboratorios LETI/LETI Pharma, personal fees from Novartis Pharma, personal fees from MEDA Pharma, grants and personal fees from Anergis S.A., personal fees from Sanofi US Services, personal fees from Mobile Chamber Experts (a GA[2] Partner), personal fees from Pohl-Boskamp, outside the submitted work; A Sheikh: reports grants from EAACI, during the conduct of the study.

Funding
EAACI and BM4SIT project (grant number 601763) in the European Union's Seventh Framework Programme FP7. EU Grant: 601763.

Appendix
Search strategy 1
(MEDLINE, EMBASE)

1. exp asthma/
2. asthma.mp.
3. asthmatic children.mp.
4. acute asthmatic attack.mp.
5. asthma control.mp.
6. asthma exacerbations.mp.
7. wheez*.mp.
8. respiratory hypersensitivity/
9. bronchial disorder.mp.
10. hyper-responsiveness wheez*.mp.
11. lung function.mp.
12. ventilatory function.mp.
13. FEV.mp.
14. FEF.mp.
15. FVC.mp.
16. PEF.mp.
17. bronchial hyperreactivity.mp.
18. airway hyperreactivity.mp.
19. bronchial responsiveness.mp.
20. airway responsiveness.mp.
21. or/1-20
22. exp Desensitization, Immunologic/
23. exp Immunotherapy/
24. desensiti?ation.mp.
25. (immunotherapy or allergen immunotherapy or oral immunotherapy).mp.
26. subcutaneous immunotherapy.mp.
27. sublingual immunotherapy.mp.
28. specific immunotherapy.mp.
29. Or/22-28
30. exp Intervention Studies/
31. intervention studies.mp.
32. exp Clinical Trial/
33. (trial or clinical trial).mp.
34. Exp Randomized Controlled Trial/
35. randomi?ed controlled trial.mp.
36. exp Placebos/
37. placebos.mp.
38. exp Random allocation/
39. random allocation.mp.
40. random*.mp.
41. exp Double-blind method/
42. double-blind method.mp.
43. double-blind design.mp.
44. exp Single-blind method/
45. single-blind method.mp.
46. single-blind design.mp.
47. triple-blind method.mp.
48. search:.tw.
49. review.pt.
50. systematic review.tw.
51. meta analysis.mp,pt.
52. case series.mp.
53. (case$ and series).tw.
54. cost:.mp.
55. cost effective:.mp.
56. cost utility:.mp.

57. exp Health Care Costs/
58. (costs and costs analysis).mp.
59. economic evaluation*.mp.
60. ((cost effective* adj1 analys*) or cost minimi?ation analys* or cost benefit analys* or cost utility analys* or cost consequence analys* or finances).mp.
61. Or/30-60
62. 21 and 29 and 61

Search strategy 2
(Cochrane library, HTA, EED, CINAHL, ISI Web of Science, TRIP)

(Asthma or acute asthmatic attack or wheez* or respiratory hypersensitivity or bronchial disorder or hyper-responsiveness wheez* or lung function or ventilatory function or bronchial hyperreactivity or airway hyperreactivity or bronchial responsiveness or airway responsiveness)
AND
(Immunologic, desensiti* or immunotherapy or oral immunotherapy or allergen immunotherapy or specific immunotherapy or subcutaneous immunotherapy or sublingual immunotherapy)
AND
(Intervention stud* or experimental stud* or trial or clinical trial* or randomi* controlled trial or random allocation or single blind method or double blind method or triple blind method or random* or systematic review or meta-analysis or case series or economic evaluation* or cost effective* analys* or cost minimi?ation analys* or cost benefit analys* or cost utility analys* or cost consequence analys* or finances)

References

1. Report TGA. Global burden of disease due to Asthma. 2014; http://www.globalasthmareport.org/burden/burden.php.
2. Organization WH. Global surveillance, prevention and control of chronic respiratory diseases: a comprehensive approach; 2007.
3. Papadopoulos NG, Arakawa H, Carlsen K-H, Custovic A, Gern J, Lemanske R, et al. International consensus on (ICON) pediatric asthma. Allergy. 2012;67:976–97.
4. Haldar P, et al. Cluster analysis and clinical asthma phenotypes. Am J Respir Crit Care Med. 2008;178(3):218–24.
5. Gough H, Grabenhenrich L, Reich A, Eckers N, Nitsche O, Schramm D. Allergic multimorbidity of asthma, rhinitis and eczema over 20 years in the German birth cohort MAS. Pediatr Allergy Immunol. 2015;26(5):431–7.
6. SIGN BTS Asthma Guidelines 2012. https://www.brit-thoracic.org.uk/document-library/clinical-information/asthma/btssign-asthma-guideline-2014/. Last Accessed 23 Sept 2015.
7. Dhami S, et al. Allergen immunotherapy for allergic asthma: protocol for a systematic review. Clin Transl Allergy. 2015;6:5.
8. CASP checklist for systematic reviews. http://www.casp-uk.net/wp-content/uploads/2011/11/CASP_Systematic_Review_Appraisal_Checklist_14oct10.pdf. Last Accessed 3 Sept 2015.
9. Abramson MJ, Puy RM, Weiner JM. Injection allergen immunotherapy for asthma. Cochrane Database Syst Rev. 2010;8:CD001186.
10. Calamita Z, et al. Efficacy of sublingual immunotherapy in asthma: systematic review of randomized-clinical trials using the Cochrane Collaboration method. Allergy. 2006;61(10):1162–72.
11. Chelladurai Y, et al. Effectiveness of subcutaneous versus sublingual immunotherapy for the treatment of allergic rhinoconjunctivitis and asthma: a systematic review. J Allergy Clin Immunol Pract. 2013;1(4):361–9.
12. Compalati E, et al. The efficacy of sublingual immunotherapy for house dust mites respiratory allergy: results of a GA2LEN meta-analysis. Allergy. 2009;64(11):1570–9.
13. Erekosima N, et al. Effectiveness of subcutaneous immunotherapy for allergic rhinoconjunctivitis and asthma: a systematic review. Laryngoscope. 2014;124(3):616–27.
14. Normansell R, Kew KM, Bridgman AL. Sublingual immunotherapy for asthma. Cochrane Database Syst Rev. 2015;8:CD011293.
15. Tao L, et al. Efficacy of sublingual immunotherapy for allergic asthma: retrospective meta-analysis of randomized, double-blind and placebo-controlled trials. Clin Respir J. 2014;8(2):192–205.
16. Polzehl D, Keck T, Riechelmann H. Analysis of the efficacy of specific immunotherapy with house-dust mite extracts in adults with allergic rhinitis and/or asthma. Laryngorhinootologie. 2003;82(4):272–80.
17. Kim J, Lin S, Suarez-Cuervo C, Chelladurai Y, Ramanathan M, Segal J, Erekosima N. Allergen-specific immunotherapy for pediatric asthma and rhinoconjunctivitis: a systematic review PEDIATRICS, Vol 131, Number 6; 2013.
18. Shaikh WA. Immunotherapy vs inhaled budesonide in bronchial asthma: an open, parallel, comparative trial. Clin Exp Allergy. 1997;27(11):1279–84.
19. Maestrelli P, et al. Effect of specific immunotherapy added to pharmacologic treatment and allergen avoidance in asthmatic patients allergic to house dust mite. J Allergy Clin Immunol. 2004;113(4):643–9.
20. Olsen OT, et al. A 1-year, placebo-controlled, double-blind house-dust-mite immunotherapy study in asthmatic adults. Allergy. 1997;52(8):853–9.
21. Pichler CE, et al. Specific immunotherapy with *Dermatophagoides pteronyssinus* and *D. farinae* results in decreased bronchial hyperreactivity. Allergy. 1997;52(3):274–83.
22. Wang H, et al. A double-blind, placebo-controlled study of house dust mite immunotherapy in Chinese asthmatic patients. Allergy. 2006;61(2):191–7.
23. Bousquet J, et al. Specific immunotherapy with a standardized *Dermatophagoides pteronyssinus* extract. II. Prediction of efficacy of immunotherapy. J Allergy Clin Immunol. 1988;82(6):971–7.
24. Kohno Y, et al. Effect of rush immunotherapy on airway inflammation and airway hyperresponsiveness after bronchoprovocation with allergen in asthma. J Allergy Clin Immunol. 1998;102(6 Pt 1):927–34.
25. Nouri-Aria KT, et al. Grass pollen immunotherapy induces mucosal and peripheral IL-10 responses and blocking IgG activity. J Immunol. 2004;172(5):3252–9.
26. Creticos PS, et al. Ragweed immunotherapy in adult asthma. N Engl J Med. 1996;334(8):501–6.
27. Ohman JL Jr, Findlay SR, Leitermann KM. Immunotherapy in cat-induced asthma. Double-blind trial with evaluation of in vivo and in vitro responses. J Allergy Clin Immunol. 1984;74(3 Pt 1):230–9.
28. Malling HJ, Dreborg S, Weeke B. Diagnosis and immunotherapy of mould allergy. III. Diagnosis of Cladosporium allergy by means of symptom score, bronchial provocation test, skin prick test, RAST, CRIE and histamine release. Allergy. 1986;41(1):57–67.
29. Rak S, et al. A double-blinded, comparative study of the effects of short preseason specific immunotherapy and topical steroids in patients with allergic rhinoconjunctivitis and asthma. J Allergy Clin Immunol. 2001;108(6):921–8.
30. Malling HJ. Diagnosis and immunotherapy of mould allergy. IV. Relation between asthma symptoms, spore counts and diagnostic tests. Allergy. 1986;41(5):342–50.

5

Lung function in severe pediatric asthma: a longitudinal study in children and adolescents in Brazil

Mônica Versiani Nunes Pinheiro de Queiroz[1,4*], Cristina Gonçalves Alvim[2], Álvaro A. Cruz[3] and Laura Maria de Lima Belizário Facury Lasmar[2] [ID]

Abstract

Background: In severe asthma, high doses of inhaled corticosteroids (ICS) are used in order to achieve clinical and functional control. This study aimed to evaluate lung function in outpatients (children and adolescents) with severe asthma in Brazil, all of whom were treated with high doses of ICS. We evaluated all spirometry tests together and by ICS dose: 800 and > 800 µg/day.

Methods: This was a 3-year longitudinal study in which we analyzed 384 spirometry tests in 65 severe asthma patients (6–18 years of age), divided into two groups by the dose of ICS (budesonide or equivalent): 800 and > 800 µg/day.

Results: At baseline, the forced expiratory volume in one second (FEV_1) and the FEV_1/forced vital capacity (FVC) ratio were both < 80% of the predicted values in 50.8% of the patients. The median age of the patients was 10.4 years (interquartile range 7.8–13.6 years). In the sample as a whole, there were significant increases in FEV_1% and in the FEV_1/FVC% ratio ($p = 0.01$ and $p < 0.001$, respectively) over the course of the study. In the > 800 µg/day group, there were no statistical increases or decreases in FEV_1, the FEV_1/FVC ratio, or forced expiratory flow between 25 and 75% of the FVC ($FEF_{25-75\%}$), when calculated as percentages of the predicted values. However, the z-score for $FEF_{25-75\%}$ showed a statistically significant reduction, in the sample as a whole and in the > 800 µg/day group. Also in the > 800 µg/day group, there was a significant reduction in the post-bronchodilator FEV_1% ($p = 0.004$).

Conclusions: The fact that the spirometric parameters (as percentages of the predicted values) remained constant in the > 800 µg/day group, whereas there was a gain in lung function in the sample as a whole, suggests an early plateau phase in the > 800 µg/day group. However, there was some loss of lung function in the > 800 µg/day group, as evidenced by a decrease in the z-score for $FEF_{25-75\%}$, suggesting irreversible small airway impairment, and by a reduction in the post-bronchodilator FEV_1%, suggesting reduced reversibility of airway obstruction. Among children and adolescents with severe asthma, the use of ICS doses higher than those recommended for age does not appear to improve lung function.

Keywords: Asthma in childhood and adolescence, Spirometry, Forced expiratory flow, Longitudinal study, Adherence to treatment

*Correspondence: monicaversiani@medicina.ufop.br
[4] Departamento de Clínicas Pediátrica e do Adulto, Escola de Medicina, Universidade Federal de Ouro Preto, Rua Dois 697, Ouro Preto, MG 35400-000, Brazil
Full list of author information is available at the end of the article

Background

In most children with asthma, the disease is controlled with low to moderate doses of inhaled corticosteroids (ICS). However, approximately 5% of such children present with severe asthma that is uncontrolled or obtain asthma control only with the use of high doses of ICS, in combination with a long-acting β_2 agonist (LABA) or leukotriene receptor antagonist, and still require frequent or prolonged treatment with oral corticosteroids [1–3]. In that population of patients, there is an increased risk of adverse reactions to the medications used, chronic morbidity, severe exacerbations, and death [1]. Pediatric asthma patients are also more likely to have presented with impaired lung growth and lung function during childhood, together with an early onset of asthma, as well as a more rapid decline in lung function, which can be lower than that expected, in adult life [4].

The finding of an abnormal trajectory through monitoring of the forced expiratory volume in one second (FEV_1) can help identify pediatric patients at risk for abnormal lung function and irreversible airflow obstruction. Careful follow-up evaluation can identify the plateau phase and a subsequent decline [5].

The evolution of lung function in asthma patients, as determined by monitoring FEV_1, forced vital capacity (FVC), the FEV_1/FVC ratio, and forced expiratory flow between 25 and 75% of the vital capacity ($FEF_{25-75\%}$), has been described in longitudinal studies [5–8]. In a study conducted in the United States [5], children with mild to moderate asthma on budesonide treatment were found to show an abnormal pattern of lung growth, as determined by assessing FEV_1 as a percentage of the predicted value ($FEV_1\%$), which persisted into adult life. The authors also identified an early decline in lung function in 52% of the patients. Among children with moderate asthma in Europe [8], the use of 600 µg/day of budesonide resulted in a gain in lung function, as determined by measuring the post-bronchodilator parameters related to the central and intermediate airways. However, the authors also observed a loss of lung function in the distal airways. In a study in which 38.7% of the pediatric patients had severe asthma, functional alterations in the distal airways of those patients were associated with the persistence of asthma, as evidenced by a lower $FEF_{25-75\%}$ [6]. In children with uncontrolled asthma symptoms, $FEF_{25-75\%}$ can express airway obstruction better than can FEV_1 and the FEV_1/FVC ratio, both of which are often normal in children with asthma [7].

The scope of ICS treatment in preventing a loss of lung function in children and adolescents with asthma has also been a concern. In a study involving children with mild to moderate asthma in the United States, the use of budesonide was not found to increase the post-bronchodilator $FEV_1\%$. Because those patients entered treatment between 5 and 12 years of age, the authors suggested that an irreversible loss of lung function might have occurred prior to the initiation of treatment [9]. It has been demonstrated that deficits in the FEV_1/FVC ratio, FEV_1, and $FEF_{25-75\%}$ observed at 2 months of age persist at 22 years of age, suggesting that reduced lung function is a risk factor for early airway obstruction in adulthood [10]. In a study involving children and adolescents with severe refractory asthma treated with 1600 µg/day of budesonide in England [11], a gain in lung function, expressed as pre-bronchodilator FEV_1 %, was observed only in the first year of follow-up. That gain was not progressive, reaching a plateau, with a mean FEV_1 below 80% of the predicted value, that was maintained over the following 3 years [11]. In pediatric patients with poorly controlled severe asthma, increasing the dose of ICS is recommended, because it is believed that doses > 500 µg/day of fluticasone or equivalent can be beneficial [12].

There have been few longitudinal studies of lung function in pediatric patients with severe asthma. Therefore, the objective of the present prospective study was to analyze the evolution of lung function over a 3-year period in a cohort of children and adolescents with severe asthma treated using high doses of ICS, considering all of the spirometry tests together and by dose of ICS: 800 and > 800 µg/day.

Methods

Study design and participants

This was a prospective cohort study in which 384 spirometry tests of 65 patients with severe asthma, obtained over a period of 3 years, were referred by pediatric pulmonologists affiliated with the Wheezing Baby Program [13], which operates under the auspices of the *Centro Multidisciplinar de Asma de Difícil Controle* (CEMAD, Multidisciplinary Center for Difficult-to-Control Asthma), a university center in the city of Belo Horizonte, in southeastern Brazil. The methods of evaluation and therapeutic management of this cohort have previously been described [14]. We excluded 192 spirometry tests: 108 because the patients had experienced exacerbations in the last 3 weeks; 33 because the tests were carried out in the learning phase; and 51 because the tests were performed less than 15 days apart.

Severe asthma is defined as asthma which requires treatment with high doses of ICS, plus a second controller (with or without oral corticosteroids) to prevent it from becoming "uncontrolled", or which remains "uncontrolled" despite this therapy [1–3]. High doses of ICS (budesonide or equivalent) are defined as > 400 µg/day for individuals between 6 and 11 years of age and as > 800 µg/day for those over 12 years of age [3]. Because all of the patients in our cohort were being treated with a minimum of 800 µg/day of ICS (budesonide or equivalent), treatment with > 800 µg/day was classified as very-high-dose treatment.

Patients were recruited into the study between September 2010 and July 2015. At enrollment, all were in step 4 or 5 of the Global Initiative for Asthma (GINA) treatment plan and were using $\geq$ 800 µg/day of budesonide or equivalent [3]. All of the patients were between 6 and 18 years of age (median age, 10.4 years) and had been diagnosed with severe asthma. In all cases, the diagnosis had been confirmed after the factors associated with a lack of control (differential diagnosis, comorbidities, environmental factors, treatment adherence, and inhaler technique) had been reviewed and the treatment regimen had been adjusted according to the level of control [1–3].

The patients were evaluated periodically according to a standardized protocol that follows the recommendations of an expert panel convened by the World Health Organization to discuss severe asthma, in 2009 [1].

Evaluation of lung function
All spirometry tests were performed at the same place and time, with a spirometer (Spirobank II; Medical International Research, Rome, Italy). The tests were performed in accordance with the recommendations of the American Thoracic Society [15]. Before and after administration of a bronchodilator (400 µg albuterol by metered-dose inhaler), we measured FEV_1, FVC, the FEV_1/FVC ratio, and $FEF_{25-75\%}$. Increases of 200 mL or 12% were considered significant post-bronchodilator variations in FEV_1. The bronchodilator response was evaluated according to the proportional post-bronchodilator increase in FEV_1 in relation to the baseline value [15].

The parameters are expressed as percentages of the values predicted value for age, gender, and height [15], as well as in z-scores, according to the Global Lung Initiative reference values [16], because the latter have been deemed valid for expressing and describing the changes over time in growing individuals [7].

Measurement of the fraction of exhaled nitric oxide
In all patients, the fraction of exhaled nitric oxide (FeNO) was measured prior to spirometry and only when the patients were free of upper airway infections. Using a portable analyzer (NIOX MINO; Aerocrine AB, Solna, Sweden), we obtained the FeNO values at an expiratory flow rate of 50 ml/s [17].

Optimizing treatment
At each visit, the level of asthma control was evaluated on the basis of the following parameters: daytime and nighttime symptoms; the ability to perform physical activities; and the need for rescue medication [18]. We also used the Asthma Control Test (ACT), on which a score < 20 (out of a total of 25) indicates a lack of control [19]. At each visit, the treatment regimen and specific doses were adjusted according to the level of control [2, 3, 18].

All medications were provided free of charge to the patients by the pharmacies of secondary referral centers [13]. Over the course of the study, we monitored blood pressure, growth curves, body mass index, and the basal serum level of cortisol (measured annually), as well as monitoring clinical variables to identify any adverse effects of the medication prescribed. Annual evaluations were performed by ophthalmologists and by other specialists when indicated [2].

The patients were receiving one of two types of treatment: dry-powder inhalers delivering a combination of budesonide and formoterol—Symbicort (AstraZeneca, Lund, Sweden) or Alenia (Aché Laboratórios Farmacêuticos S.A., Guarulhos, Brazil); or dry-powder or metered-dose inhalers containing fluticasone, combined with salmeterol (Seretide; GlaxoSmithKline, Stevenage, England), montelukast (Montelair; Aché Laboratórios Farmacêuticos S.A.), oral prednisolone (generic), or omalizumab (Xolair; Novartis Biociências S.A., São Paulo, Brazil).

Inhaler technique
Every patient used a dry-powder inhaler or a metered-dose inhaler with a spacer fitted to the mouthpiece. The inhalation technique was evaluated at each visit, and the interventions proposed were reviewed at subsequent visits [1, 20].

Adherence rate
We determined the rate of adherence to the use of the ICS by calculating the proportion of doses used in relation to the expected number of doses for each time period, on the basis of the dose counters of the devices or counting the empty capsules (for the dry-powder inhalers) and the records of the dates on which the medicines were dispensed [1, 21].

Associated factors
In accordance with the criteria of the Allergic Rhinitis and its Impact on Asthma guidelines [22], the diagnosis of rhinitis was based on an adapted six-item clinical scale for rhinitis, each item scored from 0 to 3, corresponding to the best and worst scores, respectively [23]. Patients classified as having severe rhinitis were followed by specialists, underwent diagnostic assessments and received the necessary interventions.

We performed forearm skin prick tests using allergens obtained from ALK-Abelló (Hørsholm, Denmark), and positivity for allergic sensitization was defined as a wheal 3 mm larger than that observed for the negative control. The positive and negative controls were histamine and saline solution, respectively. We tested the following allergens [24]: *Dermatophagoides pteronyssinus, Dermatophagoides farinae, Blomia tropicalis, Alternaria alternata*, *Aspergillus fumigatus*, cat dander, dog dander, and cockroach allergens (from *Periplaneta americana* and *Blattella germanica*). We determined total immunoglobulin E by fluorescence enzyme immunoassay (ImmunoCAP, Phadia, Uppsala, Sweden), considering reference values by age group [25].

At each visit, we reviewed the level of environmental control in the home, considering reports of exposure to mold, passive smoking, household dust, and domestic animals, and the recommended interventions were reevaluated in subsequent visits [1, 20].

Patients with symptoms suggestive of gastroesophageal reflux disease were followed by specialists and underwent diagnostic assessment as necessary [26]. Patients for whom there were reports of emotional or behavioral disorders were referred to and monitored by specialists [18].

Statistical analysis

Descriptive analyses were performed by calculating frequencies, means, medians, and standard deviations. Because of the considerable variability observed in the individual profiles, we employed a mixed-effects linear regression model, with a random intercept and a random slope, in our evaluation of lung function over time. The inclusion of the random effects allowed us to estimate a specific intercept for each patient, and the random slope evaluated the estimated trend for individual patients to gain or lose lung function over time.

The graphics for the longitudinal profiles were then constructed, considering all of the spirometry tests together and by treatment group: 800 μg/day of ICS; and > 800 μg/day of ICS. To smooth the longitudinal profiles and determine the mean behavior among the groups, we adopted the locally weighted scatter-plot smoothing method.

Separate models were adjusted for the pre- and post-bronchodilator values of each of the response variables, calculated as percentages of the predicted values and as z-scores: FVC, FEV_1, $FEF_{25-75\%}$, and FEV_1/FVC ratio. The post-bronchodilator variation in FEV_1 was expressed in mL and in percentage. For each of these variables, we constructed two models. An initial model included only the length of follow-up (in months) and allowed us to infer the longitudinal trend (slope) for the sample as a whole. A second model was constructed in order to determine the influence that an ICS dose > 800 μg/day has on the mean behavior of lung function over time. To identify factors associated with pulmonary function, we also created a third model, which included the following covariates: gender; age at first spirometry; duration of illness; self-reported exposure to passive smoking; ACT score; occurrence of exacerbation since the previous consultation; FeNO; and length of follow-up. The models were initially adjusted for all of the covariates listed above. The covariates were selected manually: at each step, the least significant covariant (that with the highest *p* value) was removed, and the process was repeated until all non-significant covariates had been excluded. Covariates for which the estimated *p* value was less than 0.05 were considered significant. The suitability of the model was determined by visual inspection of residual plots, which did not indicate major deviations from the distributional assumptions. Data were analyzed with the program R (R Development Core Team—www.r-project.org). The level of significance was set at $p < 0.05$.

Results

Table 1 presents the general characteristics of the patients, at enrollment and over the course of the study. At enrollment, the mean age of the patients was 10.4 years (interquartile range, 7.8–13.6 years). All of the patients were referred from pediatric pulmonology clinics, after a median follow-up of 6.1 years, having been in GINA treatment step 4 or 5 at enrollment [3]. In the 12 months prior to enrollment in the study, 94.0% of the patients had experienced severe exacerbations, 20.0% had been admitted to an intensive care unit, and 12.3% had been under continuous treatment with oral corticosteroids, all of which indicate the severity of their asthma at enrollment. At the end of the follow-up period, only one patient was classified as obese.

The median FeNO was 22.5 ppb at enrollment and 13.5 ppb at the end of the follow-up period. The majority of the patients were allergic, *D. pteronyssinus*, *D. farinae*, and *B. tropicalis* being the most common aeroallergens to which they were sensitized.

During the study, we addressed the factors that influence asthma control, such as allergic rhinitis (the median score for which dropped from 9.5 at baseline to 6.0 at the end of the study) and exposure to secondhand smoke within the home, adopting measures for its elimination. The patients with gastroesophageal reflux disease were treated by specialists, and two of those patients underwent fundoplication. All patients were reminded of the importance of correct inhalation technique and treatment adherence, both of which showed improvement over the course of the study. During the study, the median dose of ICS increased from 800 to 876.1 μg/day and the maximum dose increased from 1600 to 2400 μg/day. At enrollment, all of the patients were using a LABA in combination with the ICS. During the study, the proportion of patients using leukotriene receptor antagonists increased from 16.9 to 61.5%, whereas there was a reduction in the proportion of patients on a regimen of continuous oral corticosteroid use. Omalizumab was started in 7.8% of the patients. During the follow-up

Table 1 Characteristics of children and adolescents with severe asthma ($N = 65$), at enrollment in the study and over the course of the follow-up period

Variable	At enrollment	At the end of follow-up
Female gender, n (%)	41 (63.0)	41 (63.0)
Age (years)[a]	10.4 (7.8; 13.6)	13.5 (8.7; 16.1)
BMI	0.31 (− 0.64; 0.88)	− 0.01 (− 0.65; 1.05)
Z-score > 3	0	1.0 (1.67)
Time followed by a pediatric pulmonologist (years)[a]	6.1 (4.3; 9.3)	–
Age of onset symptoms (years)	0.6 (1.3; 0.3)	–
Duration of disease (years)[a]	9.8 (6.1; 12.6)	–
Duration of ICS treatment (years)[a]	7.0 (4.6; 9.7)	–
Severe exacerbations in the last 12 months, n (%)	61 (94)	19 (29.2)
History of ICU admission due to asthma, n (%)	13 (20)	0
Asthma Control Test score[a]	15.5 (12.0; 20.0)	22.0 (19.0; 24.0)
Treatment adherence, %[a]	92.0 (75; 100)	93.2 (80; 100)
Inhaler technique, n (%)	49 (75.4)	52 (80.0)
Lung function, n (%)		
FEV_1 and FEV_1/FVC ratio $\geq$ 80% of predicted	32 (49.2)	52 (80.0)
FEV_1 and FEV_1/FVC ratio < 80% of predicted	33 (50.8)	13 (20.0)
$FEF_{25-75\%}$ < 70% of predicted	32 (49.2)	22 (44.4)
$FEF_{25-75\%}$ < 30% of predicted	1 (1.5)	1 (1.5)
Medication(s) used		
Dose of ICS (μg/day)[a,b]	800.0 (800.0; 1600.0)	876.1 (800.0; 2400.0)
Long-acting β_2 agonist, n (%)	65 (100)	65 (100.0)
Leukotriene receptor antagonist, n (%)	11 (16.9)	40 (61.5)
Oral corticosteroid (continuous use), n (%)	8 (12.3)	6 (9.2)
Omalizumab, n (%)	0	6 (7.8)
Comorbidities		
Allergic rhinitis, n (%)	62.0 (95.4)	62.0 (95.4)
Allergic rhinitis score[a]	9.5 (5.3; 12.8)	6.0 (3.0; 10.0)
Gastroesophageal reflux disease, n (%)	9.0 (13.9)	9.0 (13.9)
Psychosocial problems, n (%)	10.0 (15.4)	15.0 (23.4)
Reported passive smoking in the home, n (%)	26.0 (40.0)	0
Fraction of exhaled nitric oxide (ppb)	22.5 (10.0; 43.3)	13.5 (4.3; 36.5)
Serum IgE (IU/mL)[a]	821.0 (299.0; 1441.0)	–
Serum IgE of 30–1500 IU/mL, n (%)	10 (15.4)	–
Positive skin prick test result, n (%)	62 (95.4)	–
Dermatophagoides pteronyssinus, n (%)	51 (78.5)	–
Dermatophagoides farinae, n (%)	43 (66.2)	–
Blomia tropicalis, n (%)	49 (75.4)	–
Periplaneta americana, n (%)	13 (20.3)	–
Cat dander, n (%)	7 (10.8)	–
Blattella germanica, n (%)	12 (18.5)	–
Dog dander, n (%)	10 (15.4)	–
Interval between spirometry tests (months)[a]		
Cohort as a whole	–	3.03 (1.87; 3.97)
> 800 μg/day subgroup	–	2.57 (1.63; 4.20)

ICU intensive care unit

[a] Median (interquartile range)

[b] Budesonide or equivalent

period, there was improvement in the median ACT score (which increased from 15.5 at enrollment to 22.0 at the end of the study), a reduction in the frequency of severe exacerbations, and no intensive care unit admissions, showing that treatment optimization provided clinical improvement.

Table 2 shows the pre- and post-bronchodilator values for the 384 spirometry tests evaluated. The results were analyzed in the cohort as a whole, and, to understand the influence of dose, the subgroups of patients treated with 800 and > 800 µg/day of ICS were analyzed separately [3]. The mixed-effects linear regression model provided estimates of lung function parameters, with the intercepts and their respective 95% CIs, together with the slopes, indicating the monthly variation in response.

In the cohort as a whole, statistically significant increases were observed in the pre-bronchodilator FEV_1%, in the FEV_1/FVC ratio, and in $FEF_{25-75\%}$ (% predicted). In the > 800 µg/day subgroup, the intercept values were lower and no gain in lung function was observed for any of the parameters evaluated. However, we observed a significant reduction in the z-score for $FEF_{25-75\%}$. That phenomenon was observed in the cohort as a whole and in the > 800 µg/day subgroup.

In the longitudinal evaluation, the post-bronchodilator lung function parameters remained constant throughout the study in the cohort as a whole, with the exception of the z-score for the FEV_1/FVC ratio, which showed a statistically significant increase. In the > 800 µg/day subgroup, most of the parameters remained constant, with no gain or loss of function, although there was a reduction in the FEV_1%. Over the course of the study, there was a significant reduction in the FEV_1 response to bronchodilator administration in the cohort as a whole. In the > 800 µg/day subgroup, the post-bronchodilator variation in FEV_1 remained unchanged over the 3 years of follow-up.

Figure 1a, b depict the evolution of the pre- and post-bronchodilator spirometry parameters, expressed in z-scores, for the cohort as a whole and for the > 800 µg/day subgroup.

The evolution of the pre- and post-bronchodilator spirometry parameters, in z-scores, can be seen in Fig. 1. In the > 800 µg/day subgroup, there was a decline in lung function, especially in FEV_1 and $FEF_{25-75\%}$, for which the values were below the lower limit of the normal range at several points.

Table 2 Longitudinal evaluation of spirometry tests, including pre-and post-bronchodilator values

Variables	Cohort as a whole (65 patients; 384 spirometry tests) Intercept (95% CI)	Slope (95% CI)[a]	p	Subgroup of patients receiving > 800 µg/day of ICS (22 patients; 57 spirometry tests) Intercept (95% CI)	Slope (95% CI)[a]	p
Pre-bronchodilator						
FVC (% predicted)	90.87 (87.54; 94.20)	0.09 (−0.05; 0.22)	0.20	84.65 (76.69; 92.60)	0.15 (−0.30; 0.60)	0.50
FVC (z-score)	−0.73 (−1.01; −0.45)	0.00 (−0.01; 0.01)	0.70	−1.24 (−1.92; −0.55)	−0.01 (−0.05; 0.03)	0.60
FEV_1 (% predicted)	81.24 (77.35; 85.13)	0.20 (0.05; 0.34)	0.01	77.07 (67.92; 86.22)	−0.04 (−0.60; 0.51)	0.90
FEV_1 (z-score)	−1.22 (−1.58; −0.86)	0.01 (−0.01; 0.02)	0.40	−1.80 (−2.56; −1.03)	−0.01 (−0.04; 0.03)	0.80
FEV_1/FVC ratio	81.58 (79.31; 83.85)	0.12 (0.04; 0.20)	0.00	81.97 (75.49; 88.44)	−0.11(−0.39; 0.17)	0.50
FEV_1/FVC ratio (z-score)	−0.89 (−1.21; −0.57)	0.01 (0.00; 0.03)	0.03	−1.15 (−1.97; −0.32)	0.01 (−0.03; 0.05)	0.50
$FEF_{25-75\%}$ (% predicted)	71.53 (65.48; 77.58)	0.43 (0.20; 0.65)	0.00	72.75 (55.33; 90.18)	−0.24 (−1.25; 0.76)	0.60
$FEF_{25-75\%}$ (z-score)	−1.43 (−1.74; −1.11)	−0.02 (−0.02; −0.01)	0.00	−2.02 (−2.60; −1.44)	−0.02 (−0.04; 0.00)	0.03
Post-bronchodilator						
FVC (% predicted)	93.96 (90.96; 96.96)	−0.01 (−0.16; 0.13)	0.90	89.45 (81.62; 97.28)	−0.07 (−0.47; 0.33)	0.70
FVC (z-score)	−0.42 (−0.71; −0.13)	−0.01 (−0.02; 0.00)	0.10	−0.89 (−1.59; −0.19)	−0.02 (−0.04; 0.01)	0.30
FEV_1 (% predicted)	88.09 (84.61; 91.56)	0.06 (−0.06; 0.18)	0.30	89.58 (80.62; 98.50)	−0.48 (−0.93; −0.03)	0.04
FEV_1 (z-score)	−0.79 (−1.11; −0.46)	0.00 (−0.01; 0.01)	0.10	−1.38 (−2.20; −0.55)	−0.01 (−0.05; 0.03)	0.70
FEV_1/FVC ratio	93.31 (90.75; 95.87)	0.09 (−0.04; 0.23)	0.20	92.02 (85.11; 98.94)	0.04 (−0.21; 0.30)	0.70
FEV_1/FVC ratio (z-score)	−0.44 (−0.71; −0.15)	0.02 (0.00; 0.03)	0.02	−0.45 (−1.43; 0.52)	0.01 (−0.05; 0.07)	0.70
$FEF_{25-75\%}$ (% predicted)	90.60 (83.46; 97.75)	0.11 (−0.24; 0.46)	0.50	87.98 (69.48; 106.47)	−0.17 (−1.12; 0.78)	0.70
$FEF_{25-75\%}$ (z-score)	−0.51 (−0.87; −0.16)	0.01 (−0.01; 0.02)	0.30	−0.72 (−1.64; 0.20)	−0.01 (−0.05; 0.04)	0.80
Increase in FEV_1 (%)	9.48 (7.12; 11.84)	−0.18 (−0.32; −0.03)	0.02	12.07 (6.18; 17.97)	−0.28 (−0.67; 0.11)	0.20

[a] Monthly variation in response

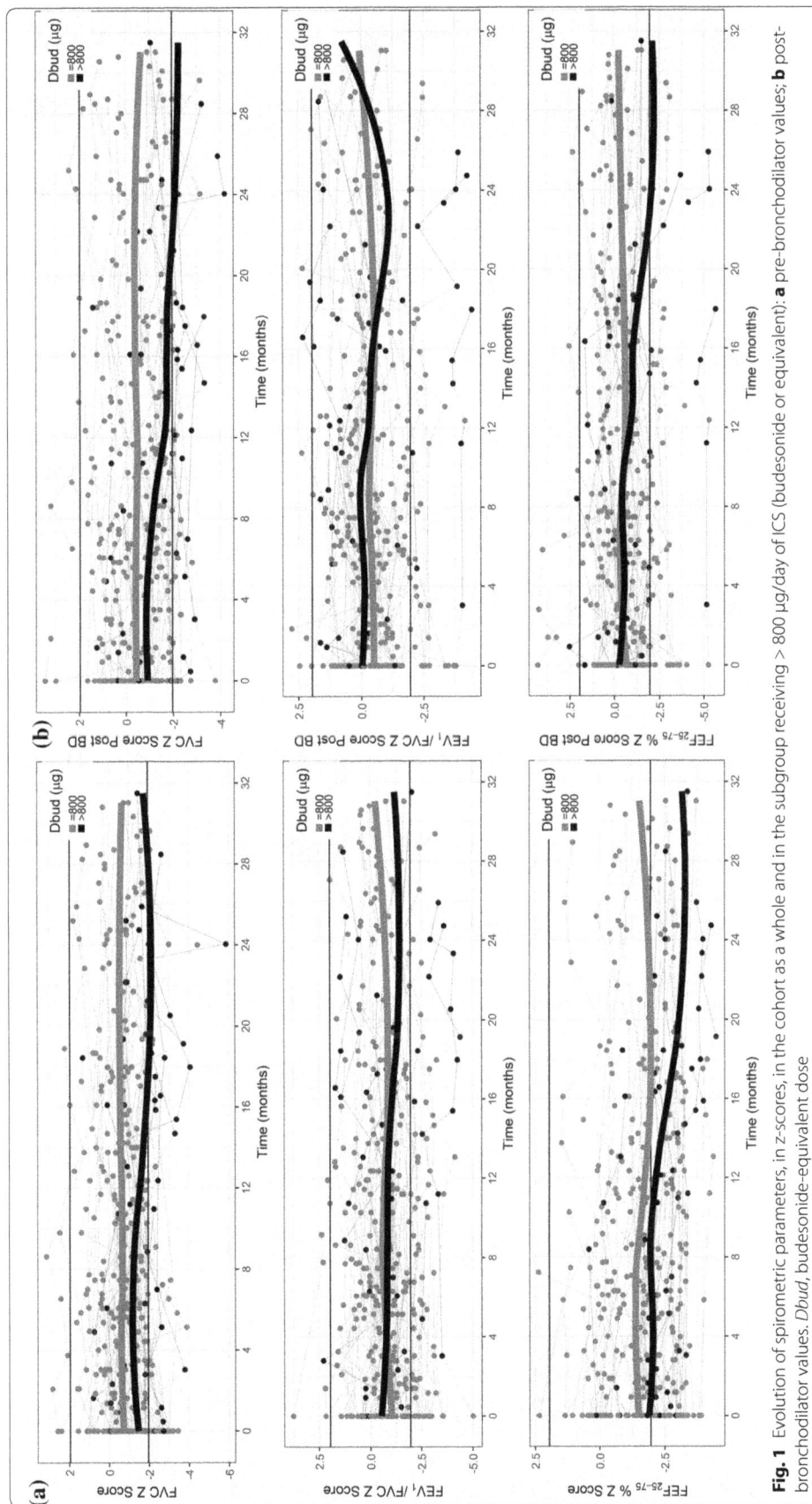

Fig. 1 Evolution of spirometric parameters, in z-scores, in the cohort as a whole and in the subgroup receiving > 800 μg/day of ICS (budesonide or equivalent): **a** pre-bronchodilator values; **b** post-bronchodilator values. *Dbud*, budesonide-equivalent dose

Table 3 **Variables associated with a decline in the z-score for FEF$_{25-75\%}$**

FEF$_{25-75\%}$ (z-score)	Slope (95% CI)[a]	p
(Intercept)	1.74 (0.97; 2.50)	0.000
Study follow-up (months)	− 0.02 (− 0.02; − 0.01)	0.000
Age at first spirometry	− 0.26 (− 0.33; − 0.20)	0.000
FeNO	− 0.01 (− 0.01; 0.00)	0.001

[a] Monthly variation in response

Table 3 shows the final multivariate model of the factors associated with a decrease in FEF$_{25-75\%}$. The covariates that remained in the final model were the length of the follow-up period ($p < 0.001$), age ($p < 0.001$), and the FeNO ($p = 0.001$).

Discussion

In individuals without lung disease, a normal pattern of growth and decline in lung function, based on the FEV$_1$%, has been shown to be characterized by a phase of elevation during childhood and adolescence, a plateau in young adulthood, and a subsequent decline after 30 years of age [27]. A pattern of reduced growth or early decline in lung function was demonstrated by the pre-bronchodilator FEV$_1$% in patients with mild to moderate asthma in a cohort studied in the United States [5]. The authors found that lower lung function in childhood was one of the predictors of abnormal evolution and an early decline in adult life.

During follow-up at our referral outpatient clinic, the patients in our cohort showed a statistically significant increase in lung function, as determined by measurements of FEV$_1$, the FEV$_1$/FVC ratio, and FEF$_{25-75\%}$ (% predicted). However, in the > 800 μg/day subgroup, FEV$_1$, the FEV$_1$/FVC ratio, and FEF$_{25-75\%}$ remained constant over time, a behavior that suggests an early plateau. At the end of the study, the median age of our patients was 13.5 years, when they would be expected to be in the FEV$_1$ gain phase.

In a four-year longitudinal study involving 47 children and adolescents (mean age, 11.2 years) with severe asthma that was refractory to treatment with 1600 μg/day of budesonide or equivalent, an early plateau phase was also observed [11]. The authors reported an annual gain in FEV$_1$ of 2.6% only in the first year, with a plateau in the following 3 years.

In the Tucson birth cohort [10], which comprised children with below-normal lung function, that pattern was maintained until the age of 22. In a long-term cohort study conducted in Australia, the authors found that adults who subsequently developed chronic obstructive pulmonary disease had not presented the expected increase in lung function during adolescence [28].

The interpretation of lung function in the transition from childhood to adolescence is complex and is influenced by the multitude of predictive equations of normal values and the differences among the various age groups. Unlike the majority of biological indices in medicine, such as plasma concentrations of chemical analytes or hormones, lung function varies with age, height, gender, and ethnicity. Few equations take into account the changing relationship between lung function and height during the adolescent growth spurt [7]. The percentage of predicted does not necessarily correspond to the z-score, and, in growing individuals, the Global Lung Initiative reference equations have been deemed adequate to express and describe the changes over time [7, 16]. The use of these two reference criteria in our study (% predicted and z-score) provided an expanded view of the evolution of lung function. Although some results were discordant, the main parameter used in the assessment of obstructive diseases, the FEV$_1$/FVC ratio, showed the same tendency in percentage of predicted and in z-score—an increase in the cohort as a whole and stability in the > 800 μg/day subgroup. In our study, the z-scores revealed a statistically significant reduction in the pre-bronchodilator FEF$_{25-75\%}$, in the cohort as a whole and in the > 800 μg/day subgroup.

A low FEF$_{25-75\%}$ is a sensitive indicator of small airways disease and has been shown to be useful in distinguishing patients with persistent symptoms from those with transient symptoms [7]. Small airway obstruction, evaluated by determining FEF$_{25-75\%}$, could function as a predictor of persistent asthma and of difficult-to-control asthma. Unlike FEV$_1$, FEF$_{25-75\%}$ is independent of abnormalities indicative of alterations in large airways [6]. Studies have indicated that low FEF$_{25-75\%}$ in childhood is predictive of asthma in adult life, whereas it is not necessarily the case for FEV$_1$ [29].

The use of FEF$_{25-75\%}$ as a diagnostic tool has limitations related to its reproducibility and interindividual variability, which are usually greater than those associated with FEV$_1$ and FVC. The coefficient of variation for FEF$_{25-75\%}$ is approximately 6%, which is high but acceptable [6]. It is possible that FEF$_{25-75\%}$ is more sensitive to detecting increased airway resistance because the growth of the pulmonary parenchyma can be disproportionate or because of "distal displacement" of the middle portion of the forced expiratory curve when there is lung deflation [28]. In our study, the variables associated with a decrease in FEF$_{25-75\%}$ were the length of follow-up, age, and FeNO. These findings are consistent with those of a study involving patients with severe asthma with a median age of 10 years (range, 6–17 years), in whom changes in the obstructive pulmonary function pattern and elevated FeNO persisted over time despite high doses of ICS.

This suggests that persistence of airway inflammation defines a subpopulation of pediatric patients with severe asthma [30]. The prolonged early wheezing and persistent wheezing phenotypes have been associated with the FEV_1/FVC ratio and $FEF_{25-75\%}$ both being lower at 14–15 years of age than at 8–9 years of age, whereas the persistent wheezing phenotype has been associated with higher ratios of FeNO at 14–15 years of age [31]. Children with severe asthma have been found to show persistent, progressive airflow limitation despite treatment with high doses of ICS and other asthma controller medications. That raises major questions about corticosteroid sensitivity, as well as about whether this decline in lung function represents a reduction in the rate of lung growth or the progression of airway remodeling [32].

In a 4-year, placebo-controlled study of the use of budesonide and nedocromil sodium in children with mild persistent asthma (mean age, 9.2 years), conducted by the Childhood Asthma Management Program Research Group [9], budesonide was found to provide no gain in pulmonary function, as determined by monitoring the post-bronchodilator $FEV_1\%$ over the course of the study, in comparison with the placebo and nedocromil sodium. The authors stated that, as a measure of lung function, post-bronchodilator $FEV_1\%$ presents less variability over time than do pre-bronchodilator values.

The use of pre- or post-bronchodilator spirometry values to determine the degree of airway obstruction is open to discussion. Although post-bronchodilator spirometry is recommended in patients with chronic obstructive pulmonary disease, its use in asthma patients, especially in younger patients, is more controversial [6]. A high degree of reversibility of airway obstruction is a recognized marker of a lack of asthma control [4].

Among the post-bronchodilator parameters evaluated in the present study, we observed a decrease in $FEV_1\%$ in the group of asthma patients that required even higher doses of ICS. In a study involving adults with severe asthma [33], there was a significant decline in post-bronchodilator $FEV_1\%$ over time ($p < 0.001$) and asthma severity was associated with a greater decline in lung function, supporting the concept that there is a specific endotype of progressive airway remodeling.

In a study involving children with moderate asthma in Europe [8], the group treated with ICS for approximately 2 years showed a significant, sustained increase in pre- and post-bronchodilator expiratory flows. However, the expiratory flows in the peripheral airways remained low, even after bronchodilator administration. The authors speculated that, even in asymptomatic individuals, residual lung function abnormalities persist, and that those abnormalities could be the result of irreversible changes

or peripheral deposition of budesonide that is insufficient to reduce the distal inflammatory process.

The post-bronchodilator FEV_1 response is a characteristic of asthma, and the magnitude of that response can decrease over the course of treatment [28]. In the present study, the z-scores for spirometry parameters remained below the lower limit of the normal range in the > 800 μg/day subgroup, even after administration of the bronchodilator. These data suggest persistent airflow limitation [34].

In one long-term study, the slopes for changes in the FEV_1/FVC ratio indicated that a reduction in lung function occurs in early childhood [35]. Among atopic children, that reduction can occur as early as 3 years of age [10].

The patients in our study used high doses of ICS, always in combination with a LABA. Other controllers, such as leukotriene receptor antagonists and oral corticosteroids, were prescribed as needed. Omalizumab was prescribed for patients over 6 years of age who had a serum immunoglobulin E level of 30–1500 IU/mL and in whom asthma was uncontrolled despite treatment with high doses of ICS and a LABA. Over the course of the study, the mean treatment adherence rate was 93.2%. The inhalation technique, reviewed at all visits, was found to be adequate. In addition, after initial efforts to educate the patients and their relatives, exposure to secondhand smoke in the home was reportedly eliminated and the comorbidities were addressed. All of our patients were treated within the public health care system, via the CEMAD and Wheezing Baby Program, which is the first of its kind in Brazil [13]. Since 1994, it has been offering specialized treatment with medications provided free of charge. Given these considerations, we believe that the loss of lung function observed in our cohort, as determined from the $FEF_{25-75\%}$ z-score and post-bronchodilator $FEV_1\%$, was not due to insufficient doses of ICS, lack of other controllers, or potentially modifiable factors.

The high treatment adherence rates observed in the present study were likely due to the fact that the CEMAD is a referral center structured for the treatment of asthma patients. A study involving adult patients with severe asthma in the city of Salvador, Brazil, also showed high treatment adherence rates, which the authors suggested was attributable to the fact that those patients were under treatment at specialized centers [36].

Our study has certain limitations. The results might have limited external validity, because the patients with severe asthma were recruited from among those who had been referred to our university center and had already been followed for a median of 6 years. Our patients, all of whom were referred by pediatric pulmonologists, had not achieved control despite being in GINA treatment step 4 or 5. Nevertheless, we believe that our sample was representative of this specific patient population.

It has been postulated that an irreversible loss of pulmonary function occurs early in life [10]. Our 3-year follow-up evaluation did not include the spirometry parameters during the first years of life. At patient enrollment, the mean duration of illness was 9.8 years and the mean time of ICS use was 7.0 years.

Our results indicate that the need for higher doses of medication is associated with greater asthma severity. Over the course of our study, we observed an improvement in asthma control, as evaluated by the ACT score, although functional alterations in the distal airways persisted, as did low post-bronchodilator FEV_1%. We observed an early plateau phase in an age group in which the majority of individuals should be gaining lung function. In the group of patients studied here, higher doses of ICS doses > 800 μg/day of budesonide or equivalent did not improve lung function parameters and the decrease in $FEF_{25-75\%}$ might reflect remodeling of the smaller airways.

Conclusions

In conclusion, among children and adolescents with severe asthma undergoing treatment in a referral outpatient clinic in Brazil, our longitudinal evaluation evidenced a gain in lung function, based on the majority of the spirometric variables evaluated. However, there was a decline in the z-scores for pre-bronchodilator $FEF_{25-75\%}$. Nevertheless, in the > 800 μg/day subgroup, there was also a significant reduction in the post-bronchodilator FEV_1%. The significant reduction in $FEF_{25-75\%}$ in the cohort as a whole and, more clearly, in the > 800 μg/ day subgroup, suggests small airway impairment that is unresponsive to ICS and to the other controllers used. It is possible that the $FEF_{25-75\%}$ z-score is a more sensitive measure of asthma obstruction. The behavior of lung function in the > 800 μg/day subgroup (no significant gain over the 3-year follow-up period) suggests an early plateau phase. The results of our study corroborate those of previous studies showing an abnormal pattern of growth or a decline in lung function among children with asthma, provide new evidence that treatment with ICS, even at very high doses, is insufficient to prevent the problem, and underscore the fact that low $FEF_{25-75\%}$ might be a sensitive biomarker of asthma severity, potentially indicating a subpopulation of pediatric patients with severe asthma.

Abbreviations

ICS: inhaled corticosteroids; FEV1: forced expiratory volume in one second; FVC: forced vital capacity; $FEF_{25-75\%}$: forced expiratory flow between 25 and 75% of the FVC; LABA: long-acting β2 agonist; CEMAD: Centro Multidisciplinar de Asma de Difícil Controle (Multidisciplinary Center for Difficult-to-Control Asthma); GINA: Global Initiative for Asthma; ACT: Asthma Control Test.

Authors' contributions

MVNPQ and LMLBFL designed the study, drafted, analyzed the data, interpreted the results, drafted, edited and revised the manuscript. CGA and AAC analyzed the data, interpreted the results, drafted, edited and revised the manuscript. All authors read and approved the final manuscript.

Author details

[1] Department of Pediatrics, School of Medicine, Federal University of Ouro Preto, Ouro Preto, Brazil. [2] Department of Pediatrics, School of Medicine, Federal University of Minas Gerais, Belo Horizonte, Brazil. [3] ProAR - Federal University of Bahia, Salvador, Brazil. [4] Departamento de Clínicas Pediátrica e do Adulto, Escola de Medicina, Universidade Federal de Ouro Preto, Rua Dois 697, Ouro Preto, MG 35400-000, Brazil.

Acknowledgements

Not applicable.

Competing interests

MVNPQ, CGA, and LMLBFL have no competing interests to declare. AAC has received institutional funding for research (investigator-initiated and industry trials) from the Brazilian *Conselho Nacional de Desenvolvimento Científico e Tecnológico* (CNPq, National Council for Scientific and Technological Development), GlaxoSmithKline, Novartis, MSD, Astrazeneca, and Sanofi, as well as personal honoraria from GSK, Boehringer Ingelheim, Roche, MEDA, CHIESI, Astrazeneca, Novartis, and Eurofarma.

Funding

Not applicable.

References

1. Bousquet J, Mantzouranis E, Cruz AA, Aït-Khaled N, Baena-Cagnani CE, Bleecker ER, et al. Uniform definition of asthma severity, control, and exacerbations: document presented for the World Health Organization Consultation on Severe Asthma. J Allergy Clin Immunol. 2010;126(5):926–38.
2. Chung KF, Wenzel SE, Brozek JL, Bush A, Castro M, Sterk PJ, et al. International ERS/ATS guidelines on definition, evaluation and treatment of severe asthma. Eur Respir J. 2014;43(2):343–73.
3. Global Strategy for Asthma Management and Prevention, Global Initiative for Asthma (GINA) 2012. http://www.ginasthma.org/.
4. Ulrik CS. Outcome of asthma: longitudinal changes in lung function. Eur Respir J. 1999;13(4):904–18.
5. McGeachie MJ, Yates KP, Zhou X, Guo F, Sternberg AL, Van Natta ML, et al. Patterns of growth and decline in lung function in persistent childhood asthma. N Engl J Med. 2016;374(19):1842–52.
6. Siroux V, Boudier A, Dolgopoloff M, Chanoine S, Bousquet J, Gormand F, et al. Forced midexpiratory flow between 25% and 75% of forced vital capacity is associated with long-term persistence of asthma and poor asthma outcomes. J Allergy Clin Immunol. 2015.
7. Piccioni P, Tassinari R, Carosso A, Carena C, Bugiani M, Bono R. Lung function changes from childhood to adolescence: a seven-year follow-up study. BMC Pulm Med. 2015;15:31.
8. Merkus PJ, van Pelt W, van Houwelingen JC, van Essen-Zandvliet LE, Duiverman EJ, Kerrebijn KF, et al. Inhaled corticosteroids and growth of airway function in asthmatic children. Eur Respir J. 2004;23(6):861–8.
9. Szefler S, Weiss S, Tonascia J, Adkinson NF, Bender B, Cherniack R, et al.

Long-term effects of budesonide or nedocromil in children with asthma. N Engl J Med. 2000;343(15):1054–63.

10. Stern DA, Morgan WJ, Wright AL, Guerra S, Martinez FD. Poor airway function in early infancy and lung function by age 22 years: a non-selective longitudinal cohort study. Lancet. 2007;370(9589):758–64.

11. Sharples J, Gupta A, Fleming L, Bossley CJ, Bracken-King M, Hall P, et al. Long-term effectiveness of a staged assessment for paediatric problematic severe asthma. Eur Respir J. 2012;40(1):264–7.

12. Bush A, Pedersen S, Hedlin G, Baraldi E, Barbato A, de Benedictis F, et al. Pharmacological treatment of severe, therapy-resistant asthma in children: what can we learn from where? Eur Respir J. 2011;38(4):947–58.

13. Lasmar L, Fontes MJ, Mohallen MT, Fonseca AC, Camargos P. Wheezy child program: the experience of the belo horizonte pediatric asthma management program. World Allergy Organ J. 2009;2(12):289–95.

14. de Andrade WC, Lasmar LM, Ricci CA, Camargos PA, Cruz Á. Phenotypes of severe asthma among children and adolescents in Brazil: a prospective study. BMC Pulm Med. 2015;15:36.

15. Miller MR, Hankinson J, Brusasco V, Burgos F, Casaburi R, Coates A, et al. Standardisation of spirometry. Eur Respir J. 2005;26(2):319–38.

16. Quanjer PH, Stanojevic S, Cole TJ, Baur X, Hall GL, Culver BH, et al. Multiethnic reference values for spirometry for the 3-95-yr age range: the global lung function 2012 equations. Eur Respir J. 2012;40(6):1324–43.

17. Society AT, Society ER. ATS/ERS recommendations for standardized procedures for the online and offline measurement of exhaled lower respiratory nitric oxide and nasal nitric oxide, 2005. Am J Respir Crit Care Med. 2005;171(8):912–30.

18. Program NAEaP. Expert Panel Report 3 (EPR-3). Guidelines for the diagnosis and management of asthma-summary report 2007. J Allergy Clin Immunol. 2007;120(5 Suppl):S94–138.

19. Roxo JP, Ponte EV, Ramos DC, Pimentel L, D'Oliveira Júnior A, Cruz AA. Portuguese-language version of the Asthma Control Test. J Bras Pneumol. 2010;36(2):159–66.

20. Bracken M, Fleming L, Hall P, Van Stiphout N, Bossley C, Biggart E, et al. The importance of nurse-led home visits in the assessment of children with problematic asthma. Arch Dis Child. 2009;94(10):780–4.

21. Lasmar L, Camargos P, Champs NS, Fonseca MT, Fontes MJ, Ibiapina C, et al. Adherence rate to inhaled corticosteroids and their impact on asthma control. Allergy. 2009;64(5):784–9.

22. Bousquet J, Reid J, van Weel C, Baena Cagnani C, Canonica GW, Demoly P, et al. Allergic rhinitis management pocket reference 2008. Allergy. 2008;63(8):990–6.

23. Wilson AM, Dempsey OJ, Sims EJ, Lipworth BJ. A comparison of topical budesonide and oral montelukast in seasonal allergic rhinitis and asthma. Clin Exp Allergy. 2001;31(4):616–24.

24. Bousquet J, Heinzerling L, Bachert C, Papadopoulos NG, Bousquet PJ, Burney PG, et al. Practical guide to skin prick tests in allergy to aeroallergens. Allergy. 2012;67(1):18–24.

25. Hamilton RG. Clinical laboratory assessment of immediate-type hypersensitivity. J Allergy Clin Immunol. 2010;125(2 Suppl 2):S284–96.

26. Gibson PG, Henry RL, Coughlan JL. Gastro-oesophageal reflux treatment for asthma in adults and children. Cochrane Database Syst Rev. 2003;(2):CD001496. http://doi.org/10.1002/14651858.CD001496

27. Speizer FE, Tager IB. Epidemiology of chronic mucus hypersecretion and obstructive airways disease. Epidemiol Rev. 1979;1:124–42.

28. Tai A, Tran H, Roberts M, Clarke N, Wilson J, Robertson CF. The association between childhood asthma and adult chronic obstructive pulmonary disease. Thorax. 2014;69(9):805–10.

29. Hamid Q, Song Y, Kotsimbos TC, Minshall E, Bai TR, Hegele RG, et al. Inflammation of small airways in asthma. J Allergy Clin Immunol. 1997;100(1):44–51.

30. Fitzpatrick AM, Gaston BM, Erzurum SC, Teague WG, National Institutes of Health/National Heart Ln, and Blood Institute Severe Asthma Research Program. Features of severe asthma in school-age children: atopy and increased exhaled nitric oxide. J Allergy Clin Immunol. 2006;118(6):1218–25.

31. Duijts L, Granell R, Sterne JA, Henderson AJ. Childhood wheezing phenotypes influence asthma, lung function and exhaled nitric oxide fraction in adolescence. Eur Respir J. 2016;47(2):510–9.

32. Fitzpatrick AM, Teague WG, National Institutes of Health/National Heart, Lung, and Blood Institute's Severe Asthma Research Program. Progressive airflow limitation is a feature of children with severe asthma. J Allergy Clin Immunol. 2011;127(1):282–4.

33. Witt CA, Sheshadri A, Carlstrom L, Tarsi J, Kozlowski J, Wilson B, et al. Longitudinal changes in airway remodeling and air trapping in severe asthma. Acad Radiol. 2014;21(8):986–93.

34. Lødrup Carlsen KC, Hedlin G, Bush A, Wennergren G, de Benedictis FM, De Jongste JC, et al. Assessment of problematic severe asthma in children. Eur Respir J. 2011;37(2):432–40.

35. Sears MR, Greene JM, Willan AR, Wiecek EM, Taylor DR, Flannery EM, et al. A longitudinal, population-based, cohort study of childhood asthma followed to adulthood. N Engl J Med. 2003;349(15):1414–22.

36. Souza-Machado A, Santos PM, Cruz AA. Adherence to treatment in severe asthma: predicting factors in a program for asthma control in Brazil. World Allergy Organ J. 2010;3(3):48–52.

6

Innate lymphocyte cells in asthma phenotypes

Leyla Pur Ozyigit[1*], Hideaki Morita[2,3] and Mubeccel Akdis[2,3]

Abstract

T helper type 2 (T_H2) cells were previously thought to be the main initiating effector cell type in asthma; however, exaggerated T_H2 cell activities alone were insufficient to explain all aspects of asthma. Asthma is a heterogeneous syndrome comprising different phenotypes that are characterized by their different clinical features, treatment responses, and inflammation patterns. The most-studied subgroups of asthma include T_H2-associated early-onset allergic asthma, late-onset persistent eosinophilic asthma, virus-induced asthma, obesity-related asthma, and neutrophilic asthma. The recent discovery of human innate lymphoid cells capable of rapidly producing large amounts of cytokines upon activation and the mouse data pointing to an essential role for these cells in asthma models have emphasized the important role of the innate immune system in asthma and have provided a new means of better understanding asthma mechanisms and differentiating its phenotypes.

Keywords: Asthma, Innate immunity, Airways, Phenotype, Cytokines

Introduction

The immune system is classically divided into two categories, innate and adaptive immunity, according to the speed and the duration of the response, and they collaborate with each other to target different agents and perform effector functions. Through recent advances in understanding the different subsets of immune system effector cells, Annunziato et al. have recently suggested a new classification [1]. They proposed that the innate and adaptive immune systems could also be generally classified into three major kinds of cell-mediated effector immunity: categorized as type 1, comprising T-bet[+] IFN-γ–producing helper cells, type 2, composed of GATA-3[+] lymphocytes producing interleukin-4 (IL-4), IL-5, and IL-13, and type 3, characterized by RORγt[+] lymphocytes that produce IL-17 alone or in combination with IL-22 as signature cytokines [1].

Innate immunity is known to respond quickly and without antigen specificity to signals derived from the environment or from other immune cells. Innate lymphoid cells (ILCs) are the newest described elements of the innate immune system and have received much attention over the last few years [2]. Early in the immune response, ILCs possess a lymphoid morphology, similar to adaptive B and T cells, and produce many different T helper (T_H) cell cytokines but lack the recombination-activating gene (RAG)-mediated antigen specific receptors; therefore, these cells are not antigen-specific. Because ILCs are very similar to the other effector cell phenotypes, it was proposed that ILCs could be classified in a similar manner to that of T_H cells. Type 1 immunity includes the IFN-γ-producing group 1 ILCs (ILC1s) that cope with intracellular pathogens through activation of mononuclear phagocytes. Group 2 ILCs (ILC2s), which secrete IL-4, IL-5, IL-9, and IL-13, are an example of Type 2 immunity. This type of immunity induces mast cell, basophil, and eosinophil activation leading to an increase in serum IgE levels and, therefore, fosters the eradication of helminthes and venoms. Group 3 ILCs (ILC3s), which are an example of type 3 immunity, produce IL-17 and/or IL-22, activate mononuclear phagocytes, recruit neutrophils, and induce epithelial antimicrobial responses, all of which help protect against extracellular fungal and bacterial infections [1]. This group includes lymphoid tissue inducer (LTi) cells that promote the formation of lymph nodes [3].

In general, ILCs constitute a distinct element of the innate immune system, providing an initial host response via specific cytokines after sensing external stimuli on the frontline. The initial priming of immune responses to pathogenic challenges is executed by ILCs with the capacity to rapidly secrete effector cytokines. All ILCs

---

* Correspondence: sozyigit@ku.edu.tr
[1]Department of Allergy and Immunology, Koç University, School of Medicine, Istanbul, Turkey
Full list of author information is available at the end of the article

are developmentally related, and they all require the expression of the transcriptional repressor inhibitor of DNA binding 2 (Id2) and the common IL-2 cytokine receptor (γ_c) chain. Moreover, they all possess the IL-7 receptor α-chain (CD-127) [4].

The ILC lineage incorporates the classic cytotoxic natural killer (NK) cells and the non-cytotoxic ILC family [5]. Natural killer cells are also capable of responding to invading pathogens and exterior threats without the need for prior sensitization, and they function in the absence of RAG-recombined antigen receptor recognition. Beside their ability to release a variety of cytokines, they also have the capacity to kill other cells. NK cells were initially categorized into ILC1s, but recently it has been shown that these cells are different from non-cytotoxic ILCs because they undergo different developmental pathways [6, 7].

Non-cytotoxic ILCs have the capacity to rapidly respond to the environment by producing various cytokines, and their goal is to maintain homeostasis with tissue repair and remodeling. They are involved in lymphoid organ development and in resistance to pathogenic and non-pathogenic microorganisms. Non-cytotoxic ILCs also interact with mast cells, natural killer T (NKT) cells, eosinophils, epithelial cells, and macrophages, and they may configure the optimal milieu for setting up an adaptive response [8, 5].

Asthma includes complex innate and adaptive immune responses to environmental factors. For decades, researchers investigating the immune responses in asthma have focused on adaptive immunity, mostly on memory responses to antigens. Therefore, asthma was previously considered to be the airway manifestation of a T_H2-driven response from adaptive immunity toward some specific triggers [9]. Today, advances in molecular technology and recent immunology studies have allowed us to understand much more about the impact of the innate immune system on the development of asthma and on its evolution. Negative results from the initial monoclonal treatment drug studies and cluster analysis have demonstrated that "asthma syndrome" covers distinct subgroups of a reversible obstructive lung disease with different clinical properties termed different "phenotypes" [10–12]. Although there is no consensus on a single phenotype classification for asthma, the most-studied subgroups include: T_H2-associated with early-onset allergic asthma, late-onset persistent eosinophilic asthma, virus-induced asthma, obesity-related asthma, and neutrophilic asthma. All of these subgroups can be distinguished from each other by clinical factors, such as the patient age at disease onset and the involvement of particular biological pathways.

Understanding new innate pathways will allow for more accurate asthma phenotyping and, subsequently, will help direct us to personalized care for our asthmatic patients. In this review, we provide an updated view on the emerging roles of non-cytotoxic ILCs in different asthma phenotypes.

Review

ILC1s and its possible role in asthma phenotypes

ILC1s, formerly known as conventional NK cells, are present in mucosal tissues, express the IL-7 receptor, and rapidly secrete IFN-γ upon stimulation with IL-12 and IL-18, which are produced by macrophages and other cells. ILC1s are involved in the antiviral response and have been shown to expand in the intestines of patients with Crohn's disease [13]. Although we now know that NK cells are developmentally different from ILC1s and that ILC1s lack cytotoxicity, these two cell types share some common properties [14]. Therefore, it is postulated that, like NK cells in a mouse model [15] and in human asthmatics [16], ILC1s might also have a role in the development of eosinophilic airway inflammation, which can be seen in most asthma phenotypes and even in the microbiota–immune interactions of asthma [17]. Intraepithelial ILC1s, another subset of ILC1s, have been found in human tonsillar tissue [18]. Unlike typical ILC1s, these cells are not stimulated with IL-12 and IL-18, but rather with IL-15.

ILC2s and early onset allergic asthma

For many years, early onset allergic asthma has been considered to be an adaptive immune response that develops after the prior sensitization phase to allergens. Airway epithelial cells are the frontline cells initially exposed to inhaled substances, and they actively collaborate with other immune cells, specifically pulmonary dendritic cells (DC) followed by M2 macrophages, to mount a T_H2 response through the production of epithelial cell-derived cytokines, such as IL-33, IL-25 and thymic stromal lymphopoietin (TSLP) [8].

After recent studies questioning the requirement for antigen-specific adaptive T_H cells in allergic asthma, the existence of a new class of the innate type-2 lymphocyte group, the ILC2s, has been described. ILC2s were first observed in the gut, emphasizing their physiological role against helminth infection [19–21]. Later, their presence was confirmed in various other tissues, including in the human lung [22]. ILC2s are also present in human peripheral blood, and their percentage is greater in asthma patients than it is in allergic rhinitis patients or in healthy controls [23, 24].

Following contact with certain microbial products, helminth infection, physical injury, or allergens in the airway, epithelial cells secrete TSLP, IL-25, and IL-33 [25, 26, 23, 19]. Afterwards the recruitment and activation of innate type 2 cells can initiate the immune response independently of adaptive immunity [27–29]. Lung ILC2s are an important source of IL-5, a growth and differentiation factor for eosinophils, and of IL-13, which can directly cause airway hyperreactivity (AHR). Cytokine production is followed by a progressive accumulation of eosinophils and mucus secretion. IL-13 is also crucial for the differentiation of T_H2 cells from naive CD4+ T cells (Fig. 1) [22, 21, 20, 30]. Mouse studies have demonstrated a role for ILC2s in OVA-, HDM-, papain protease-, and *Alternaria alternata*-induced airway inflammation [31, 29, 32, 22, 33, 34]. Some of these observations are from RAG-deficient animals, which are adaptive immunity-deficient mice. Although evidence supporting this in human asthma has not been found yet, we speculate that the activation of ILC2s in the absence of T cells and B cells is enough to induce asthma-like symptoms, and that ILC2s may play a role in early onset allergic asthma.

A papain-induced asthma model showed that even in the presence of T cells, ILC2s were the major source of type 2 cytokines [22]. Another mouse model with papain-induced airway inflammation revealed that lung

ILCs also produce IL-9, depending on the amount of IL-2 from the adaptive immune system, and IL-33 [35]. Moreover, a recent study showed that ILC2s in the lungs secrete arginase-1, a key enzyme in the pathophysiology of acute and chronic allergic asthma (Fig. 1) [36–38].

Being at the side that first contacts the environment, as well as the first source of type 2 cytokines, it is likely that ILC2s have a role in preparing a type 2 milieu for setting up the adaptive immune response [8]. Furthermore, major histocompatibility complex II (MHCII) is expressed on ILC2s, which provides them with the capacity for antigen presentation [39, 20]. ILC2s can promote the effector functions of CD4+ T cells via costimulatory molecules OX40L and IL-4 and by a contact-dependent mechanism favoring T_H2 polarization [40, 41]. Mutually-activated ILC2s also need IL-2, possibly derived from T cells, for activation and survival [21, 20].

ILC2s and late onset asthma with nasal polyposis

Asthma onset after 12 years of age and the presence of blood eosinophilia are two important parameters for differentiating the immunologically and pathologically

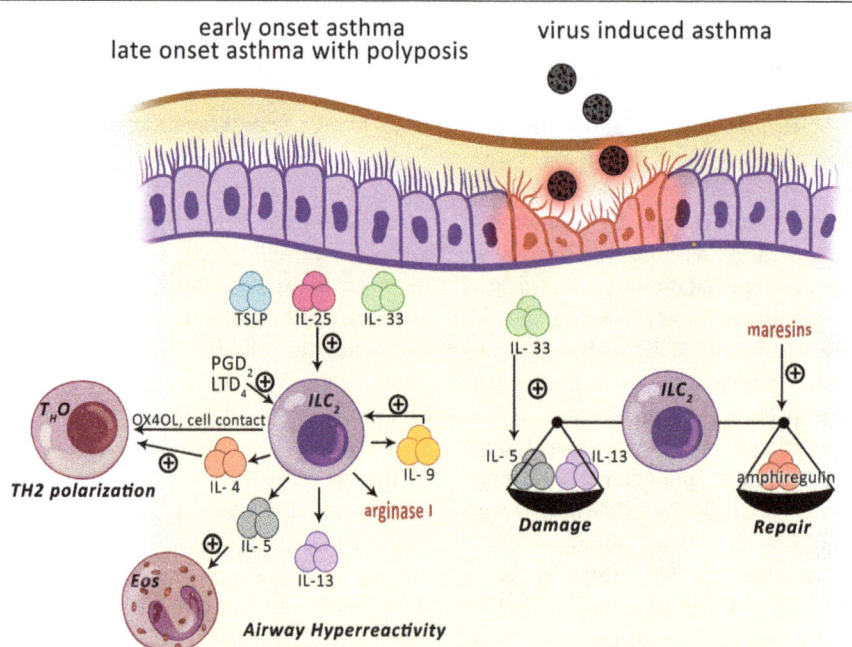

Fig. 1 Function and regulation of group 2 lymphoid cells in different asthma phenotypes. Innate lymphoid cells group 2 (ILC2s) of early onset asthma and late onset asthma with polyposis are regulated by several elements such as the epithelial cell derived thymic stromal lymphopoietin (TSLP), interleukin 25 (IL-25) and IL-33; arachidonic acid metabolites, like prostaglandin D_2 (PGD2) and leukotriene D_4 (LTD$_4$). Lung ILC2s produces IL-9 that also regulates their activation. ILC2s release IL-4, IL-5 and IL-13; then increase the airway hyperreactivity and eosinophilia. Lung ILC2s also secrete arginase 1. ILC2s can stimulate naive T cells (TH0) by IL-4, costimulatory molecules OX40L and a contact-dependent mechanism favoring T_H2 polarization. In the virus induced asthma phenotype, lungs ILC2s constitute a balance between tissue repair and tissue damage via amphiregulin and type 2-cytokine secretion. The damage is potentialized by IL-33 and the repairing capacity is enhanced by maresins. Eos, eosinophil

distinct asthma phenotype known as late onset asthma with nasal polyposis [42]. This phenotype is frequently associated with nasal polyposis and sometimes with aspirin-sensitivity [11]. Nevertheless, allergy skin test results are often positive in asthma patients with this phenotype, and even though these patients may rarely feel that their allergy symptoms were triggered by the allergens for which they tested positive [42].

Mjösberg et al. first identified ILC2s in nasal polyps of patients with rhinosinusitis (CRSwNP) [23]. Several studies have reported an increased percentage of ILC2s in the sinus mucosa of these patients compared with that in chronic rhinosinusitis patients without nasal polyps [43–45]. IL-25, IL-33, and eotaxin-3 levels, released from the sinus mucosa epithelium were also increased in CRSwNP [46]. Additionally, these patients had upregulated IL-5 and IL-13 mRNA levels [43]. The stimulation of ILC2s from human nasal polyps with TSLP has been shown to result in IL-4 release (Fig. 1) [47]. Another report found that ILC2s frequencies were associated with tissue and blood eosinophilia [45]. Additional studies focusing on the effects of ILC2s frequency on asthma control, the severity of this phenotype, and the association with the presence of aspirin sensitivity are needed.

ILC2s in virus-associated asthma and AHR

Viruses can pave the way for the development of asthma in susceptible individuals. After 2 years of age, viruses can be the trigger for a distinct phenotype of asthma known as "virus-induced asthma". Moreover, viruses frequently provoke asthma exacerbations [48–51].

In an experimental mouse model, researchers have shown that influenza A virus can rapidly induce AHR by inducing the activation of ILCs independently of the adaptive immune system [52]. During influenza virus infection, IL-33 is released from alveolar macrophages and NKT cells, which induces ILC2 activation and the subsequent production of type 2 cytokines, IL-13 and IL-5 [52, 53]. The presence of IL-5 enables the growth and the later persistence of eosinophils, even after viral clearance. IL-5 and IL-13 are mainly responsible for the clinical symptoms of AHR. Consequently, ILC2s can promote inflammation, but they also have an opposing role during virus-induced AHR- specifically the repair of wounded lung tissue after virus infection. This effect is attained through amphiregulin, an epidermal growth factor-like growth factor (Fig. 1) [4]. The balance between the damage and repair of airways constitutes the homeostatic function of ILC2s.

Regulation of ILC2s function during asthma

Recent work on ILC2s has provided new insights into T_H2-mediated asthma phenotypes, but additional questions remain. Future studies are needed to determine how this newly found source of type 2 cytokines could be regulated and how this knowledge will ameliorate our treatment options.

Role of TSLP, IL-25, and IL-33 in regulating ILC2s

Human ILC2s can be stimulated by TSLP, IL-25, and IL-33 [23, 44, 22]. Intranasal administration of IL-25 or IL-33 induces an increase in cytokine-releasing ILC2s in the lungs, bronchoalveolar lavage fluid, and mediastinal lymph nodes [31, 29, 54, 55].

- IL-25 has an essential role in allergic airway inflammation and also in remodeling [56]. Neutralizing antibodies against IL-25 may prevent airway hyperresponsiveness in allergic asthma [57].
- IL-33 can also activate mast cells and basophils through IgE receptors, and is a survival factor for eosinophils [58, 59]. Its effect on ILC2s is even faster and stronger than that of IL-25 [60]. These properties make IL-33 a possible target for future therapies. Like neutralizing antibodies to IL-25, neutralizing antibodies to IL-33 or to IL-33 receptor (ST2) has been shown to reduce AHR and to lessen the eosinophilic response [61].

Role of specialized pro-resolving mediators (SPM)

Asthma is an inflammatory lung disease with impaired resolution mechanisms, and understanding more about immune resolution could provide new treatments for this disease. SPM, which are essential fatty acids derived from regulating molecules, possess potent anti-inflammatory and pro-resolving capacities [62, 63]. They include lipoxins, resolvins, protectins, and maresins [64]. Investigating how ILC2s can be regulated through SPM will provide new insights into asthma pathobiology and could result in new therapeutic approaches [62].

- Lipoxins are the leading family of SPM [63]. Lipoxin A_4 might inhibit the stimulatory effects of PGD_2, IL-25, and IL-33 [16].
- Maresins are the most recently described SPM family. In a recent study, researchers demonstrated that maresins reduce lung inflammation and ILC2s expression of cytokines and increase the repairing capacity of ILC2s through amphiregulin (Fig. 1) [65]. Furthermore, regulatory T cells (Tregs) play a mandatory role in this interaction. Therefore, as potent regulators of Tregs and ILC2s, maresins may be promising therapeutic targets for asthma.

Role of leukotrienes and prostaglandins

Human ILC2s are stimulated by arachidonic acid metabolites, such as leukotrienes [32] and prostaglandins [16].

- Lung ILC2s express receptors for cysteinyl leukotrienes, including cysteinyl leukotriene receptor 1 (CysLT1R), the high-affinity receptor for leukotriene D_4 (LTD_4). Following stimulation by LTD_4, ILC2s produce IL-4, IL-5, and IL-13. Montelukast, a CysLT1R antagonist, can prevent the IL-5 production stimulated by leukotriene C_4 and LTD_4 [32].
- Prostaglandin D_2 (PGD2) is a positive regulator of ILC2s, inducing ILC2s migration and production of type 2 cytokines [16, 66]. PGD2 binds to its recently characterized receptor, Chemokine receptor, a homologous molecule expressed on T helper type 2 cells (CRTH2), which is a receptor expressed on ILC2s that is similar to a T_H2 receptor [67].

Recently, a study evaluating the effect of subcutaneous grass pollen immunotherapy (SCIT) on peripheral ILC2s demonstrated that the percentage of ILC2s in untreated allergic rhinitis patients increased during pollen season, and that this percentage is correlated with the patient's symptom scores. In contrast, the percentage of peripheral ILC2s in allergic rhinitis patients who were treated with SCIT and in control patients did not increase during pollen season [68]. An evaluation of whether this same effect occurs in allergic asthma patients remains to be conducted.

ILC3s in non-allergic asthma

Non-T_H2 asthma is poorly defined and is less well understood than allergic asthma phenotypes, even though it represents a large proportion of total asthma cases [11]. This group of asthma phenotypes includes obesity-associated asthma and neutrophilic asthma.

Although the role in non-allergic asthma of type 3 immunity and IL-17, which is believed to be a T_H2-released cytokine, have only recently become an area of interest, a combination of bench and bedside approaches should improve our understanding of these phenotypes [11]. Recent studies have emphasized the role of IL-17 on steroid-resistant AHR [69, 70].

ILC3s are mainly found in gut-associated lymphoid tissue (GALT) [71], but their presence in the lung has also been demonstrated [72]. They express MHC class II and are able to regulate the adaptive immune system by presenting antigens [73]. IL-23 and IL-1β rapidly stimulate ILC3s to produce IL-22, which plays a protective role through lung epithelial cells during T_H2 asthma (Fig. 2) [74]. ILC3s may also produce IL-17A, which is a potent neutrophil chemotactic agent. The presence of IL-22 and IL-17A in the sputum or peripheral blood is positively correlated with the severity of asthma [75–79]. However, further studies are needed to show the role of these cytokines in non-T_H2 asthma.

Obesity-associated asthma

This asthma phenotype is difficult to control because of comorbidities and a lack of responsiveness to classic asthma treatments [11, 80]. In a mouse model of obesity-induced AHR, researchers showed a crucial role in AHR for IL-17A, which is secreted mainly from ILC3s in the

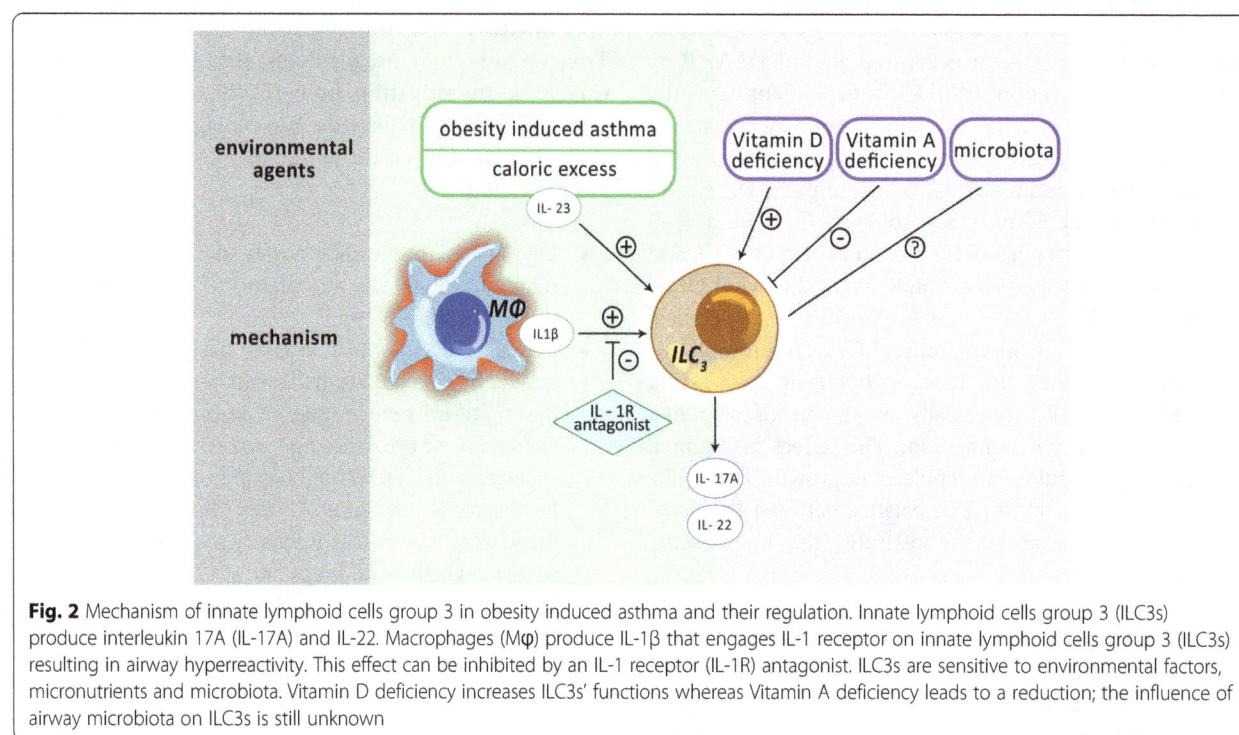

Fig. 2 Mechanism of innate lymphoid cells group 3 in obesity induced asthma and their regulation. Innate lymphoid cells group 3 (ILC3s) produce interleukin 17A (IL-17A) and IL-22. Macrophages (Mφ) produce IL-1β that engages IL-1 receptor on innate lymphoid cells group 3 (ILC3s) resulting in airway hyperreactivity. This effect can be inhibited by an IL-1 receptor (IL-1R) antagonist. ILC3s are sensitive to environmental factors, micronutrients and microbiota. Vitamin D deficiency increases ILC3s' functions whereas Vitamin A deficiency leads to a reduction; the influence of airway microbiota on ILC3s is still unknown

absence of adaptive immunity. The same study was the first to report the presence of ILC3s in the bronchoalveolar lavage fluid of patients with lung diseases. The researchers also reported that patients with severe asthma had a higher percentage of lung IL-17-producing ILC3s, than patients with mild or no asthma. Surprisingly, a protective role for ILC2s, in which they maintain the metabolic homeostasis in obesity, has been recently demonstrated [81, 82]. This unexpected finding suggests that the role of ILC2s in obesity-associated asthma should be studied further.

Regulation of ILC3s function and asthma

Although ILC3s are typically stimulated by IL-23 and IL-1β, they are also sensitive to environmental signals, such as caloric excess, micronutrients, and microbiota. A vitamin A deficit in mice resulted in greatly decreased numbers of ILC3s in the intestine, which increased the susceptibility of these mice to bacterial infections. Subsequently, treatment with vitamin A restored the number of ILC3s to normal levels; however, this treatment reduced the percentage of ILC2s [83]. In another study, vitamin D deficiency improved ILC3s responses (Fig. 2) [84]. ILCs are influenced by the ability of macrophages to sense microbial signals and produce IL-1β [85]. Interestingly, a study demonstrated that the AHR in obese mice was completely resolved with an IL-1 receptor antagonist, anakinra. The researchers also reported a decrease in the number of IL-17-producing lung ILC3s [72]. The microbiota possessed by asthmatic individuals in their airways is believed to have a higher potential to be pathogenic than that of non-asthmatic individuals [86]. How ILC3s contribute to and/or are impacted by the roles of these vitamins and the influence of this crosstalk with microbiota has not yet been evaluated.

Conclusion

Knowledge gained from recently recognized ILCs will help us to fill in the missing gaps of innate molecular pathways regarding asthma immunopathology. The lung ILCs on the frontier, sensitive to environmental factors including toxic and non-toxic substances, pathogenic and nonpathogenic microorganisms, and allergens, maintain homeostasis with tissue repair and remodeling. They can initiate AHR and appropriately set up the milieu for adaptive immunity by producing various cytokines, generally previously described in other contexts, and by interacting with different immune cells. ILCs represent one of the very first mediators for the different phenotypes of asthma 'syndrome' [10]. However, it is still unclear whether additional subsets of ILCs exist, and their role in innate immune memory has yet to be determined. We need further studies investigating their interaction with other immune cells,

exogenous factors, and other micronutrients. A better understanding of their pathogenesis in asthma will be important for a better understanding of asthma phenotypes and for developing better strategies for preventive and therapeutic interventions.

Competing interests
The authors declare that they have no competing interests.

Authors' contributions
LPO drafted the manuscript. HM and MA reviewed and finalized the manuscript. All authors read and approved the final manuscript.

Acknowledgements
The authors wish to thank the European Academy of Allergy and Clinical Immunology, and its Junior Members and Affiliates for supporting the mentorship program and encouraging the authors to write this review. The authors also thank the artist, Merve Evren, for her work in creating the illustrations for this review.

Author details
[1]Department of Allergy and Immunology, Koç University, School of Medicine, Istanbul, Turkey. [2]Swiss Institute of Allergy and Asthma Research, University of Zurich, Zurich, Switzerland. [3]Christine Kühne-Center for Allergy Research and Education, Davos, Switzerland.

References
1. Annunziato F, Romagnani C, Romagnani S. The 3 major types of innate and adaptive cell-mediated effector immunity. J Allergy and Clinical Immunology. 2014. doi:10.1016/j.jaci.2014.11.001
2. Mjosberg J, Eidsmo L. Update on innate lymphoid cells in atopic and non-atopic inflammation in the airways and skin. Clin Exp Allergy. 2014;44(8):1033–43. doi:10.1111/cea.12353.
3. Mebius RE, Rennert P, Weissman IL. Developing lymph nodes collect CD4 + CD3- LTbeta + cells that can differentiate to APC, NK cells, and follicular cells but not T or B cells. Immunity. 1997;7(4):493–504.
4. Monticelli LA, Sonnenberg GF, Abt MC, Alenghat T, Ziegler CG, Doering TA, et al. Innate lymphoid cells promote lung-tissue homeostasis after infection with influenza virus. Nat Immunol. 2011;12(11):1045–54. doi:10.1031/ni.2131.
5. Artis D, Spits H. The biology of innate lymphoid cells. Nature. 2015;517(7534):293–301. doi:10.1038/nature14189.
6. Klose CS, Flach M, Mohle L, Rogell L, Hoyler T, Ebert K, et al. Differentiation of type 1 ILCs from a common progenitor to all helper-like innate lymphoid cell lineages. Cell. 2014;157(2):340–56. doi:10.1016/j.cell.2014.03.030.
7. Daussy C, Faure F, Mayol K, Viel S, Gasteiger G, Charrier E, et al. T-bet and Eomes instruct the development of two distinct natural killer cell lineages in the liver and in the bone marrow. J Exp Med. 2014;211(3):563–77. doi:10.1084/jem.20131560.
8. Pulendran B, Artis D. New paradigms in type 2 immunity. Science. 2012;337(6093):431–5. doi:10.1126/science.1221064.
9. Robinson DS, Hamid Q, Ying S, Tsicopoulos A, Barkans J, Bentley AM, et al. Predominant TH2-like bronchoalveolar T-lymphocyte population in atopic asthma. N Engl J Med. 1992;326(5):298–304. doi:10.1056/nejm199201303260504.
10. Lotvall J, Akdis CA, Bacharier LB, Bjermer L, Casale TB, Custovic A, et al. Asthma endotypes: a new approach to classification of disease entities within the asthma syndrome. J Allergy Clin Immunol. 2011;127(2):355–60. doi:10.1016/j.jaci.2010.11.037.
11. Wenzel SE. Asthma phenotypes: the evolution from clinical to molecular approaches. Nat Med. 2012;18(5):716–25. doi:10.1038/nm.2678.
12. Agache I, Akdis C, Jutel M, Virchow JC. Untangling asthma phenotypes and endotypes. Allergy. 2012;67(7):835–46. doi:10.1111/j.1398-9995.2012.02832.x.
13. Bernink JH, Peters CP, Munneke M, te Velde AA, Meijer SL, Weijer K, et al. Human type 1 innate lymphoid cells accumulate in inflamed mucosal tissues. Nat Immunol. 2013;14(3):221–9. doi:10.1038/ni.2534.
14. Cella M, Miller H, Song C. Beyond NK cells: the expanding universe of innate lymphoid cells. Front Immunol. 2014;5:282. doi:10.3389/fimmu.2014.00282.

15. Korsgren M, Persson CG, Sundler F, Bjerke T, Hansson T, Chambers BJ, et al. Natural killer cells determine development of allergen-induced eosinophilic airway inflammation in mice. J Exp Med. 1999;189(3):553–62.

16. Barnig C, Cernadas M, Dutile S, Liu X, Perrella MA, Kazani S, et al. Lipoxin A4 regulates natural killer cell and type 2 innate lymphoid cell activation in asthma. Sci Transl Med. 2013;5(174):174ra26. doi:10.1126/scitranslmed.3004812.

17. Huang YJ. The respiratory microbiome and innate immunity in asthma. Curr Opin Pulm Med. 2015;21(1):27–32. doi:10.1097/MCP.0000000000000124.

18. Fuchs A, Vermi W, Lee JS, Lonardi S, Gilfillan S, Newberry RD, et al. Intraepithelial type 1 innate lymphoid cells are a unique subset of IL-12- and IL-15-responsive IFN-gamma-producing cells. Immunity. 2013;38(4):769–81. doi:10.1016/j.immuni.2013.02.010.

19. Saenz SA, Siracusa MC, Monticelli LA, Ziegler CG, Kim BS, Brestoff JR, et al. IL-25 simultaneously elicits distinct populations of innate lymphoid cells and multipotent progenitor type 2 (MPPtype2) cells. J Exp Med. 2013;210(9):1823–37. doi:10.1084/jem.20122332.

20. Neill DR, Wong SH, Bellosi A, Flynn RJ, Daly M, Langford TK, et al. Nuocytes represent a new innate effector leukocyte that mediates type-2 immunity. Nature. 2010;464(7293):1367–70. doi:10.1038/nature08900.

21. Moro K, Yamada T, Tanabe M, Takeuchi T, Ikawa T, Kawamoto H, et al. Innate production of T(H)2 cytokines by adipose tissue-associated c-Kit(+)Sca-1(+) lymphoid cells. Nature. 2010;463(7280):540–4. doi:10.1038/nature08636.

22. Halim TY, Krauss RH, Sun AC, Takei F. Lung natural helper cells are a critical source of Th2 cell-type cytokines in protease allergen-induced airway inflammation. Immunity. 2012;36(3):451–63. doi:10.1016/j.immuni.2011.12.020.

23. Mjosberg JM, Trifari S, Crellin NK, Peters CP, van Drunen CM, Piet B, et al. Human IL-25- and IL-33-responsive type 2 innate lymphoid cells are defined by expression of CRTH2 and CD161. Nat Immunol. 2011;12(11):1055–62. doi:10.1038/ni.2104.

24. Bartemes KR, Kephart GM, Fox SJ, Kita H. Enhanced innate type 2 immune response in peripheral blood from patients with asthma. J Allergy Clin Immunol. 2014;134(3):671–8. doi:10.1016/j.jaci.2014.06.024.

25. Allakhverdi Z, Comeau MR, Jessup HK, Yoon BR, Brewer A, Chartier S, et al. Thymic stromal lymphopoietin is released by human epithelial cells in response to microbes, trauma, or inflammation and potently activates mast cells. J Exp Med. 2007;204(2):253–8. doi:10.1084/jem.20062211.

26. Angkasekwinai P, Park H, Wang YH, Wang YH, Chang SH, Corry DB, et al. Interleukin 25 promotes the initiation of proallergic type 2 responses. J Exp Med. 2007;204(7):1509–17. doi:10.1084/jem.20061675.

27. Oliphant CJ, Barlow JL, McKenzie AN. Insights into the initiation of type 2 immune responses. Immunology. 2011;134(4):378–85. doi:10.1111/j.1365-2567.2011.03499.x.

28. Kondo Y, Yoshimoto T, Yasuda K, Futatsugi-Yumikura S, Morimoto M, Hayashi N, et al. Administration of IL-33 induces airway hyperresponsiveness and goblet cell hyperplasia in the lungs in the absence of adaptive immune system. Int Immunol. 2008;20(6):791–800. doi:10.1093/intimm/dxn037.

29. Bartemes KR, Iijima K, Kobayashi T, Kephart GM, McKenzie AN, Kita H. IL-33-responsive lineage- CD25+ CD44(hi) lymphoid cells mediate innate type 2 immunity and allergic inflammation in the lungs. J Immunol. 2012;188(3):1503–13. doi:10.4049/jimmunol.1102832.

30. Price AE, Liang HE, Sullivan BM, Reinhardt RL, Eisley CJ, Erle DJ, et al. Systemically dispersed innate IL-13-expressing cells in type 2 immunity. Proc Natl Acad Sci U S A. 2010;107(25):11489–94. doi:10.1073/pnas.1003988107.

31. Barlow JL, Bellosi A, Hardman CS, Drynan LF, Wong SH, Cruickshank JP, et al. Innate IL-13-producing nuocytes arise during allergic lung inflammation and contribute to airways hyperreactivity. J Allergy Clin Immunol. 2012;129(1):191–8 e1-4. 10.1016/j.jaci.2011.09.041.

32. Doherty TA, Khorram N, Lund S, Mehta AK, Croft M, Broide DH. Lung type 2 innate lymphoid cells express cysteinyl leukotriene receptor 1, which regulates TH2 cytokine production. J Allergy Clin Immunol. 2013;132(1):205–13. doi:10.1016/j.jaci.2013.03.048.

33. Kim HY, Chang YJ, Subramanian S, Lee HH, Albacker LA, Matangkasombut P, et al. Innate lymphoid cells responding to IL-33 mediate airway hyperreactivity independently of adaptive immunity. J Allergy Clin Immunol. 2012;129(1):216–27 e1-6. doi:10.1016/j.jaci.2011.10.036.

34. Klein Wolterink RG, Kleinjan A, van Nimwegen M, Bergen I, de Bruijn M, Levani Y, et al. Pulmonary innate lymphoid cells are major producers of IL-5 and IL-13 in murine models of allergic asthma. Eur J Immunol. 2012;42(5):1106–16. doi:10.1002/eji.201142018.

35. Wilhelm C, Hirota K, Stieglitz B, Van Snick J, Tolaini M, Lahl K, et al. An IL-9 fate reporter demonstrates the induction of an innate IL-9 response in lung inflammation. Nat Immunol. 2011;12(11):1071–7. doi:10.1038/ni.2133.

36. Bando JK, Nussbaum JC, Liang HE, Locksley RM. Type 2 innate lymphoid cells constitutively express arginase-I in the naive and inflamed lung. J Leukoc Biol. 2013;94(5):877–84. doi:10.1189/jlb.0213084.

37. Maarsingh H, Dekkers BG, Zuidhof AB, Bos IS, Menzen MH, Klein T, et al. Increased arginase activity contributes to airway remodelling in chronic allergic asthma. Eur Respir J. 2011;38(2):318–28. doi:10.1183/09031936.00057710.

38. Maarsingh H, Zaagsma J, Meurs H. Arginase: a key enzyme in the pathophysiology of allergic asthma opening novel therapeutic perspectives. Br J Pharmacol. 2009;158(3):652–64. doi:10.1111/j.1476-5381.2009.00374.x.

39. Oliphant CJ, Hwang YY, Walker JA, Salimi M, Wong SH, Brewer JM, et al. MHCII-mediated dialog between group 2 innate lymphoid cells and CD4(+) T cells potentiates type 2 immunity and promotes parasitic helminth expulsion. Immunity. 2014;41(2):283–95. doi:10.1016/j.immuni.2014.06.016.

40. Drake LY, Iijima K, Kita H. Group 2 innate lymphoid cells and CD4+ T cells cooperate to mediate type 2 immune response in mice. Allergy. 2014;69(10):1300–7. doi:10.1111/all.12446.

41. Mirchandani AS, Besnard AG, Yip E, Scott C, Bain CC, Cerovic V, et al. Type 2 innate lymphoid cells drive CD4+ Th2 cell responses. J Immunol. 2014;192(5):2442–8. doi:10.4049/jimmunol.1300974.

42. Miranda C, Busacker A, Balzar S, Trudeau J, Wenzel SE. Distinguishing severe asthma phenotypes: role of age at onset and eosinophilic inflammation. J Allergy Clin Immunol. 2004;113(1):101–8. doi:10.1016/j.jaci.2003.10.041.

43. Miljkovic D, Bassiouni A, Cooksley C, Ou J, Hauben E, Wormald PJ, et al. Association between group 2 innate lymphoid cells enrichment, nasal polyps and allergy in chronic rhinosinusitis. Allergy. 2014;69(9):1154–61. doi:10.1111/all.12440.

44. Shaw JL, Fakhri S, Citardi MJ, Porter PC, Corry DB, Kheradmand F, et al. IL-33-responsive innate lymphoid cells are an important source of IL-13 in chronic rhinosinusitis with nasal polyps. Am J Respir Crit Care Med. 2013;188(4):432–9. doi:10.1164/rccm.201212-2227OC.

45. Ho J, Bailey M, Zaunders J, Mrad N, Sacks R, Sewell W, et al. Group 2 innate lymphoid cells (ILC2s) are increased in chronic rhinosinusitis with nasal polyps or eosinophilia. Clinical and experimental allergy : journal of the British Society for Allergy and Clinical Immunology. 2015;45(2):394–403. doi:10.1111/cea.12462.

46. Lam M, Hull L, McLachlan R, Snidvongs K, Chin D, Pratt E, et al. Clinical severity and epithelial endotypes in chronic rhinosinusitis. International forum of allergy & rhinology. 2013;3(2):121–8. doi:10.1002/alr.21082.

47. Mjosberg J, Bernink J, Golebski K, Karrich JJ, Peters CP, Blom B, et al. The transcription factor GATA3 is essential for the function of human type 2 innate lymphoid cells. Immunity. 2012;37(4):649–59. doi:10.1016/j.immuni.2012.08.015.

48. Singh AM, Moore PE, Gern JE, Lemanske Jr RF, Hartert TV. Bronchiolitis to asthma: a review and call for studies of gene-virus interactions in asthma causation. Am J Respir Crit Care Med. 2007;175(2):108–19. doi:10.1164/rccm.200603-435PP.

49. Bacharier LB, Boner A, Carlsen KH, Eigenmann PA, Frischer T, Gotz M, et al. Diagnosis and treatment of asthma in childhood: a PRACTALL consensus report. Allergy. 2008;63(1):5–34. doi:10.1111/j.1398-9995.2007.01586.x.

50. Gern JE. The ABCs of rhinoviruses, wheezing, and asthma. J Virol. 2010;84(15):7418–26. doi:10.1128/JVI.02290-09.

51. Jackson DJ, Evans MD, Gangnon RE, Tisler CJ, Pappas TE, Lee WM, et al. Evidence for a causal relationship between allergic sensitization and rhinovirus wheezing in early life. Am J Respir Crit Care Med. 2012;185(3):281–5. doi:10.1164/rccm.201104-0660OC.

52. Chang YJ, Kim HY, Albacker LA, Baumgarth N, McKenzie AN, Smith DE, et al. Innate lymphoid cells mediate influenza-induced airway hyper-reactivity independently of adaptive immunity. Nat Immunol. 2011;12(7):631–8. doi:10.1038/ni.2045.

53. Gorski SA, Hahn YS, Braciale TJ. Group 2 innate lymphoid cell production of IL-5 is regulated by NKT cells during influenza virus infection. PLoS Pathog. 2013;9(9), e1003615. doi:10.1371/journal.ppat.1003615.

54. Hurst SD, Muchamuel T, Gorman DM, Gilbert JM, Clifford T, Kwan S, et al. New IL-17 family members promote Th1 or Th2 responses in the lung: in vivo function of the novel cytokine IL-25. J Immunol. 2002;169(1):443–53.

55. Schmitz J, Owyang A, Oldham E, Song Y, Murphy E, McClanahan TK, et al. IL-33, an interleukin-1-like cytokine that signals via the IL-1 receptor-related protein ST2 and induces T helper type 2-associated cytokines. Immunity. 2005;23(5):479–90. doi:10.1016/j.immuni.2005.09.015.

56. Gregory LG, Jones CP, Walker SA, Sawant D, Gowers KH, Campbell GA, et al. IL-25 drives remodelling in allergic airways disease induced by house dust mite. Thorax. 2013;68(1):82–90. doi:10.1136/thoraxjnl-2012-202003.

57. Ballantyne SJ, Barlow JL, Jolin HE, Nath P, Williams AS, Chung KF, et al. Blocking IL-25 prevents airway hyperresponsiveness in allergic asthma. J Allergy Clin Immunol. 2007;120(6):1324–31. doi:10.1016/j.jaci.2007.07.051.

58. Cherry WB, Yoon J, Bartemes KR, Iijima K, Kita H. A novel IL-1 family cytokine, IL-33, potently activates human eosinophils. J Allergy Clin Immunol. 2008;121(6):1484–90. doi:10.1016/j.jaci.2008.04.005.

59. Silver MR, Margulis A, Wood N, Goldman SJ, Kasaian M, Chaudhary D. IL-33 synergizes with IgE-dependent and IgE-independent agents to promote mast cell and basophil activation. Inflamm Res. 2010;59(3):207–18. doi:10.1007/s00011-009-0088-5.

60. Barlow JL, Peel S, Fox J, Panova V, Hardman CS, Camelo A, et al. IL-33 is more potent than IL-25 in provoking IL-13-producing nuocytes (type 2 innate lymphoid cells) and airway contraction. J Allergy Clin Immunol. 2013;132(4):933–41. doi:10.1016/j.jaci.2013.05.012.

61. Liu X, Li M, Wu Y, Zhou Y, Zeng L, Huang T. Anti-IL-33 antibody treatment inhibits airway inflammation in a murine model of allergic asthma. Biochem Biophys Res Commun. 2009;386(1):181–5. doi:10.1016/j.bbrc.2009.06.008.

62. Levy BD, Serhan CN. Resolution of acute inflammation in the lung. Annu Rev Physiol. 2014;76:467–92. doi:10.1146/annurev-physiol-021113-170408.

63. Serhan CN, Chiang N, Van Dyke TE. Resolving inflammation: dual anti-inflammatory and pro-resolution lipid mediators. Nat Rev Immunol. 2008;8(5):349–61. doi:10.1038/nri2294.

64. Serhan CN, Yang R, Martinod K, Kasuga K, Pillai PS, Porter TF, et al. Maresins: novel macrophage mediators with potent antiinflammatory and proresolving actions. J Exp Med. 2009;206(1):15–23. doi:10.1084/jem.20081880.

65. Krishnamoorthy N, Burkett PR, Dalli J, Abdulnour RE, Colas R, Ramon S, et al. Cutting edge: maresin-1 engages regulatory T cells to limit type 2 innate lymphoid cell activation and promote resolution of lung inflammation. J Immunol. 2015;194(3):863–7. doi:10.4049/jimmunol.1402534.

66. Xue L, Salimi M, Panse I, Mjosberg JM, McKenzie AN, Spits H, et al. Prostaglandin D2 activates group 2 innate lymphoid cells through chemoattractant receptor-homologous molecule expressed on TH2 cells. J Allergy Clin Immunol. 2014;133(4):1184–94. doi:10.1016/j.jaci.2013.10.056.

67. Pettipher R, Hansel TT, Armer R. Antagonism of the prostaglandin D2 receptors DP1 and CRTH2 as an approach to treat allergic diseases. Nat Rev Drug Discov. 2007;6(4):313–25. doi:10.1038/nrd2266.

68. Lao-Araya M, Steveling E, Scadding GW, Durham SR, Shamji MH. Seasonal increases in peripheral innate lymphoid type 2 cells are inhibited by subcutaneous grass pollen immunotherapy. J Allergy Clin Immunol. 2014;134(5):1193–5. doi:10.1016/j.jaci.2014.07.029. 5.

69. Kudo M, Melton AC, Chen C, Engler MB, Huang KE, Ren X, et al. IL-17A produced by alphabeta T cells drives airway hyper-responsiveness in mice and enhances mouse and human airway smooth muscle contraction. Nat Med. 2012;18(4):547–54. doi:10.1038/nm.2684.

70. McKinley L, Alcorn JF, Peterson A, Dupont RB, Kapadia S, Logar A, et al. TH17 cells mediate steroid-resistant airway inflammation and airway hyperresponsiveness in mice. J Immunol. 2008;181(6):4089–97.

71. Geremia A, Arancibia-Carcamo CV, Fleming MP, Rust N, Singh B, Mortensen NJ, et al. IL-23-responsive innate lymphoid cells are increased in inflammatory bowel disease. J Exp Med. 2011;208(6):1127–33. doi:10.1084/jem.20101712.

72. Kim HY, Lee HJ, Chang YJ, Pichavant M, Shore SA, Fitzgerald KA, et al. Interleukin-17-producing innate lymphoid cells and the NLRP3 inflammasome facilitate obesity-associated airway hyperreactivity. Nat Med. 2014;20(1):54–61. doi:10.1038/nm.3423.

73. Hepworth MR, Monticelli LA, Fung TC, Ziegler CG, Grunberg S, Sinha R, et al. Innate lymphoid cells regulate CD4+ T-cell responses to intestinal commensal bacteria. Nature. 2013;498(7452):113–7. doi:10.1038/nature12240.

74. Taube C, Tertilt C, Gyulveszi G, Dehzad N, Kreymborg K, Schneeweiss K, et al. IL-22 is produced by innate lymphoid cells and limits inflammation in allergic airway disease. PLoS One. 2011;6(7):e21799. doi:10.1371/journal.pone.0021799.

75. Buonocore S, Ahern PP, Uhlig HH, Ivanov II, Littman DR, Maloy KJ, et al. Innate lymphoid cells drive interleukin-23-dependent innate intestinal pathology. Nature. 2010;464(7293):1371–5. doi:10.1038/nature08949.

76. Sun YC, Zhou QT, Yao WZ. Sputum interleukin-17 is increased and associated with airway neutrophilia in patients with severe asthma. Chin Med J (Engl). 2005;118(11):953–6.

77. Agache I, Ciobanu C, Agache C, Anghel M. Increased serum IL-17 is an independent risk factor for severe asthma. Respir Med. 2010;104(8):1131–7. doi:10.1016/j.rmed.2010.02.018.

78. Zhao Y, Yang J, Gao YD, Guo W. Th17 immunity in patients with allergic asthma. Int Arch Allergy Immunol. 2010;151(4):297–307. doi:10.1159/000250438.

79. Sherkat R, Yazdani R, Ganjalikhani Hakemi M, Homayouni V, Farahani R, Hosseini M, et al. Innate lymphoid cells and cytokines of the novel subtypes of helper T cells in asthma. Asia Pacific allergy. 2014;4(4):212–21. doi:10.5415/apallergy.2014.4.4.212.

80. Gibeon D, Batuwita K, Osmond M, Heaney LG, Brightling CE, Niven R, et al. Obesity-associated severe asthma represents a distinct clinical phenotype: analysis of the British Thoracic Society Difficult Asthma Registry Patient cohort according to BMI. Chest. 2013;143(2):406–14. doi:10.1378/chest.12-0872.

81. Brestoff JR, Kim BS, Saenz SA, Stine RR, Monticelli LA, Sonnenberg GF, et al. Group 2 innate lymphoid cells promote beiging of white adipose tissue and limit obesity. Nature. 2014. doi:10.1038/nature14115.

82. Lee MW, Odegaard JI, Mukundan L, Qiu Y, Molofsky AB, Nussbaum JC, et al. Activated type 2 innate lymphoid cells regulate beige fat biogenesis. Cell. 2015;160(1–2):74–87. doi:10.1016/j.cell.2014.12.011.

83. Spencer SP, Wilhelm C, Yang Q, Hall JA, Bouladoux N, Boyd A, et al. Adaptation of innate lymphoid cells to a micronutrient deficiency promotes type 2 barrier immunity. Science. 2014;343(6169):432–7. doi:10.1126/science.1247606.

84. Chen J, Waddell A, Lin YD, Cantorna MT. Dysbiosis caused by vitamin D receptor deficiency confers colonization resistance to Citrobacter rodentium through modulation of innate lymphoid cells. Mucosal immunology. 2014. doi:10.1038/mi.2014.94.

85. Mortha A, Chudnovskiy A, Hashimoto D, Bogunovic M, Spencer SP, Belkaid Y, et al. Microbiota-dependent crosstalk between macrophages and ILC3 promotes intestinal homeostasis. Science. 2014;343(6178):1249288. doi:10.1126/science.1249288.

86. Hilty M, Burke C, Pedro H, Cardenas P, Bush A, Bossley C, et al. Disordered microbial communities in asthmatic airways. PLoS One. 2010;5(1):e8578. doi:10.1371/journal.pone.0008578.

7

On-demand intermittent beclomethasone is effective for mild asthma in Brazil

Paulo Camargos[1]*[iD], Alessandra Affonso[2], Geralda Calazans[2], Lidiana Ramalho[2], Marisa L. Ribeiro[2], Nulma Jentzsch[2], Simone Senna[2] and Renato T. Stein[3]

Abstract

Background: Daily inhaled corticosteroids are widely recommended for mild persistent asthma. This study aimed to assess the efficacy of the intermittent use of beclomethasone as an alternative treatment for mild persistent asthma.

Methods: In this 16-week trial, children aged 6–18 years were evaluated. Subjects in the continuous treatment arm of the study received 500 µg/day of beclomethasone, whereas the intermittent ones were given 1000 µg/day (250 µg every 6 h) in combination with albuterol for 7 days upon exacerbations or worsening of symptoms. Primary outcome (i.e., treatment failure) was the occurrence of any asthma exacerbation requiring prednisone, and co-secondary outcomes were the mean/median differences for both, (1) the pre-bronchodilator FEV_1 (% predicted) and (2) asthma control test (ACT/cACT) scores, from randomization to the last follow-up visit, and beclomethasone and albuterol consumption.

Results: Ninety-four subjects from each treatment arm were included. They were comparable regarding all baseline characteristics; prednisone was used by 10 (10.6%) and 7 (7.4%) patients, respectively (95% CI − 6.1 to 12.6%, for the difference; p = 0.47). Statistical analysis showed no statistically significant differences with respect to both FEV_1 (p = 0.39) and ACT/cACT scores (p = 0.38). As assessed through canister weighting, children used from 0.5 to 0.7 and from 1.6 to 1.8 puffs per day of beclomethasone in the intermittent and continuous regimens, respectively. Regarding albuterol, received 0.3–0.4 (intermittent) and 0.1–0.2 (continuous) inhalations per day. There were no relevant clinical or functional differences between the two treatment regimens.

Conclusion: Clinicians might consider intermittent inhaled steroid therapy as a therapeutic regimen for mild persistent asthma.

Keywords: Pediatric asthma, Asthma treatment, Asthma management

*Correspondence: pcamargs@medicina.ufmg.br
[1] Pediatric Pulmonology Unit, University Hospital, Federal University of Minas Gerais, Avenida Alfredo Balena 190, Room 267, Belo Horizonte 30130-100, Brazil
Full list of author information is available at the end of the article

Background

International guidelines consistently recommend daily use of inhaled corticosteroids (ICS) for mild persistent asthma, which accounts for the majority of persistent cases. However, three publications have evaluated the clinical benefits of an intermittent/as-needed strategy for the treatment of children with mild asthma, suggesting that although continuous treatment is associated with better disease control, the results for intermittent use were also clinically and functionally acceptable [1–3]. Studies have indicated that an on demand, intermittent regimen, combining inhaled [1, 2] or nebulized [3] corticosteroids with short acting beta 2-agonists is able to reduce the use of inhaled corticosteroids by almost 80% in these patients. In low and middle-income countries, where ICS is not widely available or affordable, reduced medication use can bring benefits for public health policies.

The present study aimed to study the efficacy of an intermittent regimen of beclomethasone dipropionate on exacerbations rate, as well as other clinical and lung function outcomes. Our hypothesis was that there would be a slight superiority in favor of the continuous regimen.

Methods

Study design

Two-arm, 16-week long, parallel, randomized open-label (i.e., with no placebo control) study, involving three centers. Participants were initially admitted to a 4-week run-in period, when they were prescribed two puffs (250 µg each) daily—even if they were given a lower dose of beclomethasone or equivalent previous to the run-in period—of HFA non-extrafine beclomethasone dipropionate (Clenil®, Chiesi, Brazil; hereafter beclomethasone), and albuterol as needed, every 4 h. Out of the two available options in Brazil, we decided to adopt the 250 µg formulation of beclomethasone instead of the 50 µg, in an attempt to reduce the number of daily puffs and achieve higher adherence rates.

In order to be included in the 16-week follow-up, patients with asthma had to be well controlled and without exacerbations during the run-in period, after which eligible patients were randomly allocated into two groups, i.e., intermittent or continuous treatment. From randomization until the end of the follow-up, patients were assessed clinically, with a complete physical examination and either the Asthma Control Test (ACT) [4] or the Childhood Asthma Control Test (cACT) [5] and pulmonary function tests. Due to the potential safety benefits regarding ICS' side effects in the case of reduction of total daily doses, height was also systematically evaluated at every follow-up visit.

Sampling site and randomization process

Children were recruited from the city's public health system facilities network, where they were initially evaluated by general pediatricians and then referred to and followed by a pediatric pulmonologist along with a multidisciplinary team allocated in three different secondary referral centers. Block randomization (30 patients per block) was used to assign participants into the two treatment regimens through a computer-generated random sequence of numbers.

Dosage and duration of the intervention

During the 16 weeks of the follow-up, subjects assigned to the continuous group were given 500 µg daily (250 µg bid) of beclomethasone, whereas those in the intermittent group received 1000 µg daily (1 puff of 250 µg every 6 h) of beclomethasone plus 4 puffs of albuterol every 4 h for 7 days, upon the worsening of asthma symptoms and/or the onset of any asthma exacerbation.

All inhaled medications were used through a pear-shaped, plastic, large volume (650 ml) valved spacer (Flumax®, Inside, Brazil). Subjects were instructed to assure proper use of the spacer and inhaler devices.

Inclusion criteria for admission into the run-in period

To ensure that only mild asthmatic patients would be recruited, we admitted participants that: had asthma symptoms but were naïve to controller treatment in the previous 2 years; had no asthma exacerbation in the previous 3 months; made regular use of inhaled corticosteroids in the previous 8 weeks (up to 500 µg daily of beclomethasone or equivalent); and their asthma was under control in the previous 8 weeks using 250–500 µg of beclomethasone (or equivalent) daily. Finally, in order to be included, children should have been able to perform spirometry and not have had smoked within the previous year.

Exclusion criteria

In order to preclude the recruitment of patients with other severity levels, we excluded patients that had had treatment with oral steroids in the 2 weeks prior to the run-in period or within 2 weeks of screening visits; forced expiratory volume in 1 s (FEV_1) less than 60% of predicted values [6] at the end of the run-in period; hospitalization for asthma in the previous year; presence of chronic or active disease other than asthma; asthma exacerbation in the previous 3 months or more than two in the last year; history of an exacerbation that required intensive care unit hospitalization; use of oral or injectable desensitizing immunotherapy for 3 months or more; inability to perform spirometry; and a nurse/physician impression that the family would not adhere to pre-scribed treatment.

Randomization process at the end of the run-in period

Participants were selected for randomization if after the run-in period their asthma symptoms (as assessed by ACT/cACT) were controlled and FEV_1 was equal or greater than 75% of predicted values [6].

Definition and management of exacerbations

Exacerbations were defined as (1) the use of more than 12 puffs of albuterol daily, (2) an acute attack that led to difficulty sleeping/nighttime asthma symptoms or doing daily activities for 2 or more consecutive days, and/or (3) an unscheduled visit to one of the three secondary referral center because of worsening of asthma symptoms.

To ensure a standardized approach in both arms of the study, a written action plan form was given to patients and their parents to collect and record relevant data during the study, with particular emphasis on how to: (1) recognize asthma worsening (including difficulty sleeping/nighttime symptoms or doing daily activities for 2 or more consecutive days) and (2) manage exacerbations at home including recording the number of administered doses of albuterol and beclomethasone.

The initial home management of exacerbations should be started with the use of albuterol (3 cycles of 4–6 inhalations every 20 min and then 4 puffs every 4 h); if no improvement had been observed within the next 2–4 h, then they were instructed to add beclomethasone provisionally (1 puff of 250 µg every 6 h, i.e., 1000 µg daily). If clinical improvement or control were not achieved within 2–4 h, patients were also instructed to seek assistance by the research team at the nearest study site. The final decision to prescribe beclomethasone for up to 7 days and prednisone (1–2 mg/kg/day for 5 days) was based solely on the assessment of the pediatric pulmonologist. He also was the solely responsible for withdrawing beclomethasone among patients that needed prednisone.

Primary and co-secondary endpoints

The primary endpoint was treatment failure, pre-defined as the occurrence of any asthma exacerbation requiring oral corticosteroid, in the two groups.

Co-secondary endpoints were also pre-defined as the mean/median difference for the pre-bronchodilator FEV_1 (% predicted) and for ACT/cACT scoring (20 or more points means asthma control) from randomization to the last follow-up visit, and beclomethasone and albuterol consumption (expressed as number of puffs per day). Adherence rate to inhaled medicines (firstly calculated in micrograms per day and then converted to number of puffs per day) was assessed by systematic

canister weighting (each actuation = 55.46 and 72.23 mg for beclomethasone and albuterol, respectively) through an analytical scale at every follow-up visit. A previous study from our group carried out in the same setting showed that the adherence assessment to beclomethasone through this method was comparable to electronic monitoring [7].

Spirometry

Forced expiratory spirometry with recording of FEV_1 values, was performed by an experienced technician who was blind to the treatment regimen, according to the American Thoracic Society recommendations [8]. To allow comparisons with the two previously published studies on the efficacy of on demand ICS treatment, FEV_1 values were expressed as a percentage of the predicted value according the equations reported by Polgar and Promadhat [6].

Height assessment

During the follow-up period, height was assessed every 2 months through a Harpenden stadiometer (ranging from 60.0 to 210.0 cm, length of 2 m, wall mounted, with a precision of 0.1 cm). Height was measured with the patient standing up, barefoot, positioned in such a way that the head, shoulders, buttocks and calves lightly touched the wall.

Allergic rhinitis assessment and treatment

Patients with allergic rhinitis (AR) enrolled in both groups were assessed through the score reported by Wilson et al. [9] and treated with continuous intranasal budesonide (32 µg/dose, bid). Each of the typical signs and symptoms of AR received a number of points, ranging from 0 (best) to 3 (worst). The total score could range from 0 to 18 points.

Statistics

Sample size

Assuming that the two regimens are in fact different, sample size calculation took into account the following parameters: (1) alpha and beta error equal to 0.05 and 0.20, respectively; (2) proportion of subjects with treatment failure of 5% (continuous arm) and 15% (intermittent arm), and a ratio of 1:1 between the two groups. A total of 282 participants were required, 141 in each group [10].

Analysis

Descriptive statistics was used to compare demographic, clinical and functional characteristics between the two groups. For longitudinal analysis of FEV_1, comparisons between the two groups were done by generalized estimating equations regression model for binary response, i.e., intermittent versus continuous treatment [11]. In that case, curve fitting was plotted to demonstrate its variations during the follow-up.

Because of the specificity of its longitudinal data characteristics, comparisons of the ACT/cACT between the two groups consisted of developing linear regression with random effects model for longitudinal data, to explain the variation throughout the follow-up of each of their items [12].

The underlying assumption for these models is that the outcome is a linear function of the regression coefficients obtained for the explanatory variables.

Results

Figure 1 displays the study design and Fig. 2 the flow of the participants throughout the trial. As shown, 279 children were initially assessed for eligibility. Due to operational and funding constraints, only 188 were enrolled into the trial, and out of those, 94 were assigned to each of the two treatment regimens.

The baseline characteristics of the studied subjects are displayed on Table 1.

The two groups were similar regarding demographic, socioeconomic, clinical, and functional characteristics.

Exacerbations were assessed at the end of follow-up and occurred in the 2nd and 3rd months of the follow-up when prednisone use was required in 10 (10.6%) and 7 (7.4%) patients of the intermittent and continuous regimen, respectively (p = 0.47). The 95% confidence interval for the difference (i.e., 3.2%) between the two (10.6 and 7.4%) proportions was − 6.1 to 12.6%.

Figures 3 and 4 show the curve fitting for FEV_1 and ACT/cACT scores for the entire population and for the two treatment regimen groups and Table 2 the monovariate analysis from randomization to the end of the follow-up.

Median FEV_1 ranged from 87 to 88% of predicted values from randomization to the end of the follow-up. In the multivariate regression analysis with time (in months) and treatment regimen as covariate, only the duration of the follow-up explained FEV_1 values, i.e., there were no statistically significant differences with respect to this functional parameter between groups (p value = 0.39). Also, they were not statistically different (p = 0.71) also for mean FEV_1 values of 87.1% (SD 15%; median of 87%) and 87.2% (SD 17.7%; median of 87%), for intermittent and continuous regimen, respectively.

As for ACT/cACT mean and median scores, they ranged from 21 to 23 points from randomization to the end of the follow-up. Again, after multivariate regression analysis, only the duration of the follow-up determined changes in ACT/cACT (p = 0.38).

Canister weighting revealed that children allocated to the intermittent regimen used from 0.5 to 0.7 puffs/day of beclomethasone, whereas those in the continuous group used from 1.6 to 1.8 puffs/day. The overall amount of beclomethasone administered throughout the study was approximately 210 for the continuous group and 80 for the intermittent group, 60% less. Regarding the intake of albuterol, intermittent arm patients received 0.3–0.4 inhalations per day, against 0.1–0.2 for the continuous one.

As for linear growth, there was no statistically significant difference (p = 0.35) between groups. The intermittent gained 1.6 cm (SD 1.4 cm) whereas the continuous, 1.4 cm (SD 1.6 cm).

Finally, Wilson's score of allergic rhinitis[9] at the end of the follow-up was 5.3 (SD 3.6) for the intermittent group, and 4.8 (SD 3.4) for the continuous one. There was no statistically significant difference (p = 0.34) in comparing changes, i.e., the treatment of allergic rhinitis led to a comparable degree of control of nasal symptoms in either treatment group.

Discussion

In the present study, we did not find any statistically significant difference in clinical and functional characteristics between the two groups. Our results suggest that the intermittent use of beclomethasone is an alternative to reduce future risk of asthma exacerbations, currently recognized as the main patient-related outcome to assess asthma control. Results also suggest that the intermittent regimen can reduce the frequency of exacerbations, even if to a lesser degree than the continuous one. Throughout the follow-up, asthma control, measured through ACT/

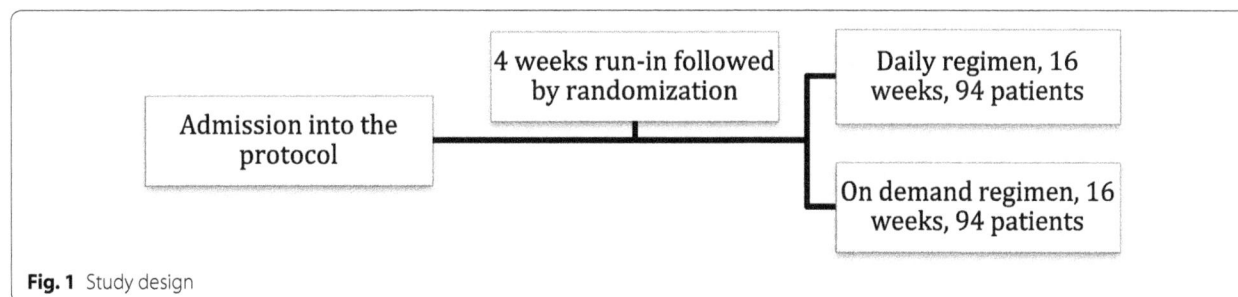

Fig. 1 Study design

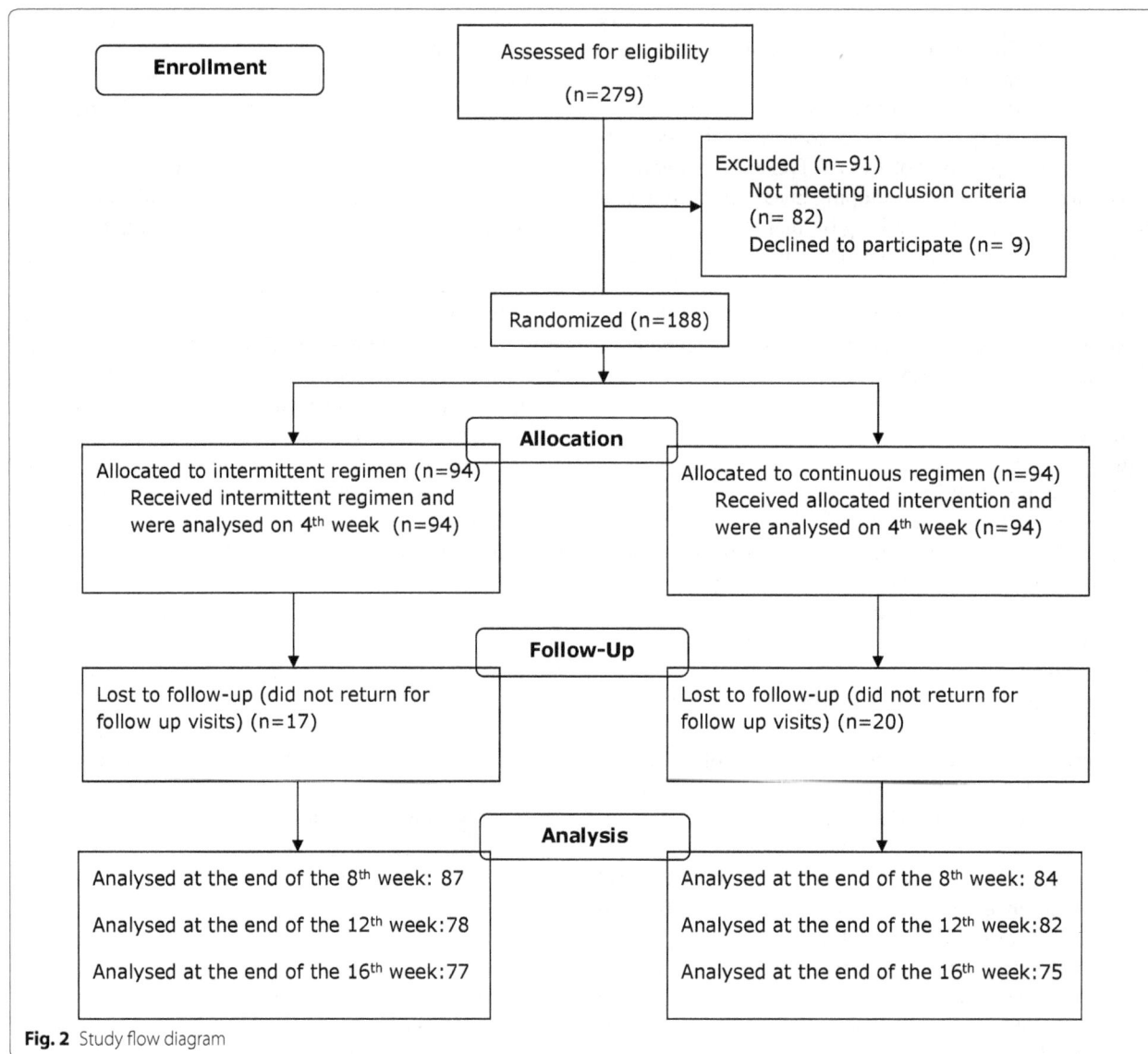

Fig. 2 Study flow diagram

cACT and FEV_1, was achieved at a satisfactory level in both groups.

Our results are comparable to those observed by Turpeinen et al. [1] and Martinez et al. [2], who carried out studies with similar methodologies, but among affluent populations, and with a longer follow-up. Their main endpoints were lung function, number of exacerbations and growth. They concluded that regular use of inhaled corticosteroids led to better asthma control than the intermittent regimen. In turn, Turpeinen et al. compared the effect of inhaled budesonide given daily (59 patients) or on-demand (58 patients) for mild persistent asthma patients, aged 5–10 years [1].

Martinez et al. [2] assessed the effectiveness of beclomethasone as rescue treatment, through a placebo-controlled study where two out of four groups also received (a) twice daily beclomethasone with beclomethasone plus albuterol as rescue (71 patients), or (b) twice daily beclomethasone with placebo plus albuterol as rescue (72 patients). They concluded that, daily beclomethasone was the most effective treatment to prevent exacerbations, and ICS as rescue medication with albuterol may be an effective step-down strategy for children with well-controlled, mild asthma.

Papi et al. [3] carried out a randomized controlled trial with a similar approach. Rather than inhaled, they used nebulized beclomethasone in 276 pre-school children assigned to three groups. At the end of the 3-month follow-up, the percentage of symptom-free days was higher with regular beclomethasone (69.6%) than with

Table 1 Baseline characteristics by treatment group at randomization

	Intermittent (n = 94)	Continuous (n = 94)	p value
Age in years, mean (SD)	10.6 (2.8)	9.9 (2.7)	0.09
Sex (boys)	55 (58.5)	50 (53.2)	0.55
Height (cm)	145.1 (15.3)	142.1(14.1)	0.12
Family monthly income (Brazilian minimum wage)	2.4 (1.6)	2.3 (1.5)	0.55
Mother's schooling (literate)	93 (99.0)	92 (97.9)	0.75
Ethnic group (white)	84 (89.3)	52 (55.3)	0.20
Number of siblings (up to three)	68 (72.3)	73 (77.6)	0.84
Parental history of allergic rhinitis (yes)	60 (63.8)	64 (68.0)	0.87
Parental history of asthma	54 (57.4)	52 (55.3)	0.81
Exposure to mould (yes)	38 (40.4)	38 (40.4)	0.88
Exposure to house dust mite (yes)	72 (76.6)	72 (76.6)	0.96
ACT/cACT score, mean (SD)	21.9 (3.0)	22.0 (2.7)	0.80
Previous ICS treatment (250–500 µg of beclomethasone or equivalent)	87 (92.5)	91 (96.8)	0.33
Allergic rhinitis/continuous intranasal budesonide (yes)	36 (38.2)	29 (30.8)	0.28
Allergic rhinitis scoring (points)[a]	6.6 (3.7)	6.1 (4.1)	0.44
Pre-bronchodilator FEV$_1$ (%), mean (SD)	88.2 (12.1)	89.8 (12.0)	0.39
Bronchodilator response (%), mean (SD)	7.7 (8.5)	7.2 (7.6)	0.95

Data are proportions (%) or means (SD) unless stated otherwise; one Brazilian minimum wage corresponded approximately to US$ 250.00 during the study period

ACT/cACT asthma control test/childhood-asthma control test, *FEV$_1$* forced expiratory volume in 1 s

[a] Described by Wilson et al. [9]

prn combination (64.9%, p = 0.03). As with the two previously mentioned studies, regular ICS was the most effective treatment for frequent wheezing in preschool children, with on-demand bronchodilator/ICS combination as an alternative.

It is worth noting that in our setting, similar to other low and middle-income countries, shortage and limited access to inhaled corticosteroids brings on the need to look for strategies to optimize the required dose to maintain asthma control and avoid exacerbations.

One of our main findings was that the amount of beclomethasone used by the intermittent group was 60% that of the continuous one. As most asthmatic children requiring continuous use of inhaled corticosteroids suffer from mild persistent asthma, we can estimate that this strategy could reduce by nearly 50% the consumption of beclomethasone used by mild asthmatic patients in a given setting. In other words, as many as double the amount of patients could benefit from the intermittent regimen in low-income settings.

Adherence rate to continuous treatment regimens is a major problem in real life, and it is invariably lower than the prescribed dose because families tend to use these medications intermittently, only to resume therapy when symptoms reappear [13]. Even in more affluent societies, where at least in a part of the population, mean rates can be lower than 60% [14, 15] a rate relatively similar to the consumption of beclomethasone in our intermittent

group, patients unwittingly make use of an informal intermittent therapeutic regimen. Therefore, the intermittent strategy is already part of the patients' or their parents' habits.

The negative impact of untreated AR on asthma control is well known, since they are pathophysiologically

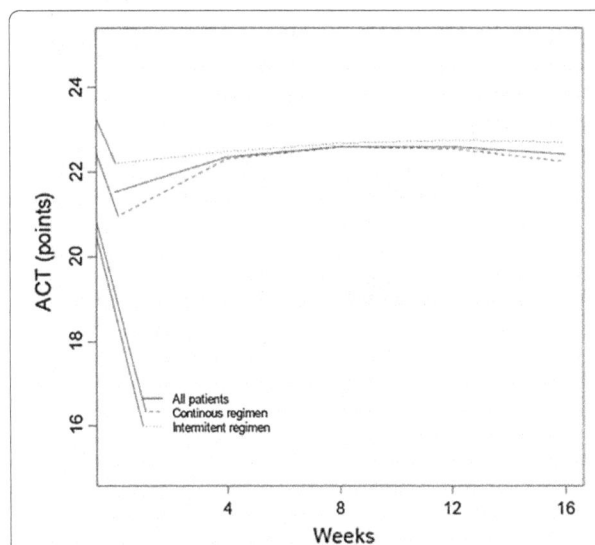

Fig. 3 Curve fitting for ACT/cACT scores from randomization to the end of the follow up of all (continuous line), intermittent (dotted line) and continuous (dashed line) participants.

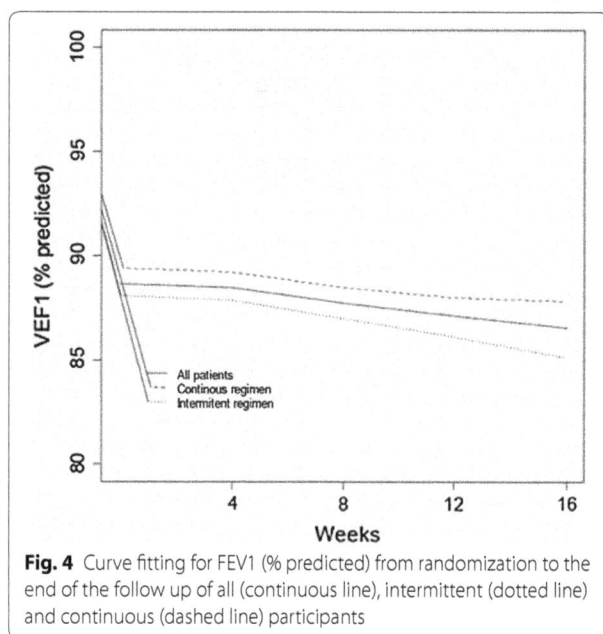

Fig. 4 Curve fitting for FEV1 (% predicted) from randomization to the end of the follow up of all (continuous line), intermittent (dotted line) and continuous (dashed line) participants

and clinically related. For this reason, intranasal corticosteroids do improve asthma outcomes in patients suffering from both AR and asthma. To avoid the confounder role of untreated AR among AR patients in the two arms, and differently from the previously mentioned studies [1–3], we included the diagnosis and treatment of all participants with this comorbidity to prevent the negative influence of untreated AR on the pre-defined endpoints in both arms. For instance, in a previous study carried out in the same setting, the presence of allergic rhinitis (OR 2.98, 95% CI 1.10–8.06) was an independent factor for unscheduled emergency departments visits [16]. As expected, the treatment of allergic rhinitis led to a comparable level of control of nasal symptoms in both groups and, at least theoretically, could have contributed to a better asthma control.

Our study have some limitations. The first one is related to the small population; due to financial and operational constraints, we recruited less individuals than the planned sample size. The fact that there was no difference in exacerbation rates could have been caused by lack of power. Secondly, a 16-week follow-up is suboptimal for a study assessing asthma exacerbations as primary outcome. Thus, a longer follow-up would be ideal, as seen in Martinez et al. [2] and Turpeinen et al. [1]. In the Turpeinen study [1], a difference in exacerbation rates was only noted during the second year of the treatment strategy. Likewise, the lack of growth effects and further increases in ACT/cACT and FEV_1 values might also be due to lack of power. All in all, the trial is underpowered, and no firm conclusions can be made.

However, as the 95% CI for the difference (3.2%) between the two groups, shows a range that might favor both regimens, we could speculate that adding more patients would not make that much of a difference. It is reasonable to presume that at least one exacerbation may occur within 16 weeks among patients suffering from undertreated/uncontrolled mild persistent asthma. The shape of the longitudinal curves for FEV_1 and ACT/cACT showed a homogenous pattern throughout the follow-up, demonstrating a comparable level of clinical and functional control in the two treatment groups.

Conclusion

Our results are in line and confirm those obtained in the three previously mentioned works and, therefore suggest that the intermittent strategy might be used as an alternative regimen for children suffering from mild persistent asthma.

Our study was conducted in a real life primary and secondary public health system facilities network with children from low-income families, which is more likely to increase the clinical applicability of our findings. As pointed out by Martinez et al. [2], this approach might also be an alternative for stepping down beclomethasone after asthma control is achieved among patients suffering from mild persistent asthma especially in poor resource settings.

Table 2 FEV$_1$ values and ACT/CACT score at randomization and at the end of the follow up by treatment group

	Intermittent			Continuous			p value
	Mean	SD	Median	Mean	SD	Median	
FEV$_1$ (% predicted)							
At randomization	87.1	15.0	87.0	87.2	17.7	87.0	0.71
At the end of follow up	91.2	23.0	88.0	82.9	22.5	87.0	0.42
ACT/cACT (points)							
At randomization	21.9	3.0	23.0	22.0	2.7	23.0	0.80
At the end of follow up	22.1	3.4	24.0	21.7	3.5	23.0	0.34

Finally, clinicians/pediatricians should carefully weigh the potential advantages and disadvantages of each of the two treatment strategies in individualized assessments and possibly in the context of a shared decision-making [17].

Abbreviations
ICS: inhaled corticosteroids; ACT: asthma control test; cACT: childhood asthma control test; FEV$_1$: forced expiratory volume in 1 s; AR: allergic rhinitis; SD: standard deviation.

Authors' contributions
PC and RS designed the study, interpreted the results and drafted the manuscript; AA, GC, LR, MR, NJ, SS, recruited, and followed the subjects, reviewed and approved the final version of the manuscript.

Author details
[1] Pediatric Pulmonology Unit, University Hospital, Federal University of Minas Gerais, Avenida Alfredo Balena 190, Room 267, Belo Horizonte 30130-100, Brazil. [2] Municipal Public Health Department, Belo Horizonte, Brazil. [3] Laboratory of Pediatric Respirology, Infant Center, Institute of Biomedical Research, Pontifícia Universidade Católica do Rio Grande do Sul, Porto Alegre, Brazil.

Acknowledgements
The authors are indebted with Prof. Fernando D Martinez, who discussed with us the original TREXA study protocol, which was duly adapted to the working conditions of our setting, the Belo Horizonte Municipal Health Department that provided the main infrastructural support for the study, and Prof. Álvaro Cruz for reviewing a previous version of the manuscript.

Competing interests
The authors declare that they have no competing interests.

Funding
This study was partially supported by a specific Grant (#558332/2009-9) from the Brazilian Council for Research and Technological Development (CNPq) to P. Camargos. P. Camargos is also supported by Minas Gerais State Foundation for Research Development (FAPEMIG, Grant #PPM0065-14). That Brazilian research agency had no influence in the design and conduct of the study; in the collection, management, analysis, and data interpretation; in the writing, review, or approval of the manuscript, and in the decision to submit the paper for publication.

References
1. Turpeinen M, Nikander K, Pelkonen AS, Syvanen P, Sorva R, Raitio H, Malmberg P, Juntunen-Backman K, Haahtela T. Daily versus as-needed inhaled corticosteroid for mild persistent asthma (The Helsinki early intervention childhood asthma study). Arch Dis Child. 2008;93:654–9.
2. Martinez FD, Chinchilli VM, Morgan WJ, Boehmer SJ, Lemanske RF Jr, Mauger DT, Strunk RC, Szeffler SJ, Zeiger RS, Bacharier LB, et al. Use of beclomethasone dipropionate as rescue treatment for children with mild persistent asthma (TREXA): a randomised, double-blind, placebo-controlled trial. Lancet. 2011;377:650–7.
3. Papi A, Nicolini G, Baraldi E, Boner AL, Cutrera R, Rossi GA, Fabbri LM, on behalf of the BEclomethasone and Salbutamol Treatment (BEST) for Children Study Group. Regular vs prn nebulized treatment in wheeze preschool children. Allergy. 2009;64:1463–71.
4. Nathan RA, Sorkness CA, Kosinski M, Schatz M, Li JT, Marcus P, Murray JJ, Pendergraft TB. Development of the asthma control test: a survey for assessing asthma control. J Allergy Clin Immunol. 2004;113:59–65.
5. Liu AH, Zeiger R, Sorkness C, Mahr T, Ostrom N, Burgess S, Rosenzweig JC, Manjunath R. Development and cross-sectional validation of the childhood asthma control test. J Allergy Clin Immunol. 2007;119:817–25.
6. Polgar G, Promadhat V. Standard values. Pulmonary function testing in children: techniques and standards. Philadelphia: W.B. Saunders; 1971. p. 87–212.
7. Jentzsch NS, Camargos P, Colosimo E, Bousquet J. Monitoring adherence to beclomethasone in asthmatic children and adolescents through four different methods. Allergy. 2009;64:1458–62.
8. American Thoracic Society. Standartization of spirometry, 1994 update. Am J Respir Crit Care Med. 1995;152:1107–36.
9. Wilson AM, Dempsey OJ, Sims EJ, Lipworth BJ. A comparison of topical budesonide and oral montelukast in seasonal allergic rhinitis and asthma. Clin Exp Allergy. 2001;31:616–24.
10. Dean AG, Sullivan KM, Soe MM. OpenEpi: open source epidemiologic statistics for public health, Version. www.OpenEpi.com. Updated 4 May 2015. Accessed 10 Dec 2016.
11. Liang KY, Zeger SL. Longitudinal data analysis for discrete and continuous outcomes. Biometrika. 1986;73:13–22.
12. Molenberghs G, Verbeke G. Models for discrete longitudinal data. New York: Springer; 2005.
13. Naspitz CK, Cropp GJ. Recommendations for treatment of intermittent mild persistent asthma in children and adolescents. Pediatr Pulmonol. 2009;44:205–8.
14. Engelkes M, Janssens HM, de Jongste JC, Sturkenboom MC, Verhamme KM. Prescription patterns, adherence and characteristics of non-adherence in children with asthma in primary care. Pediatr Allergy Immunol. 2016;27:201–8.
15. Bender BG, Cvietusa PJ, Goodrich GK, Lowe R, Nuanes HA, Rand C, Shetterly S, Tacinas C, Wagner N, Waboldt FS, et al. Pragmatic trial of health care technologies to improve adherence to pediatric asthma treatment: a randomized clinical trial. JAMA Pediatr. 2015;169:317–23.
16. Lasmar LMLB, Camargos PAM, Ordones AB, Gaspar GR, Campos EG, Ribeiro GA. Prevalence of allergic rhinitis and its impact on the use of emergency care services in a group of children and adolescents with moderate to severe persistent asthma. J Pediatr (Rio J). 2007;83:555–61.
17. Chauhan BF, Chartrand C, Ducharme FM. Intermittent versus daily inhaled corticosteroids for persistent asthma in children and adults. Cochrane Database Syst Rev. 2013;2:CD009611.

8

Is there a sex-shift in prevalence of allergic rhinitis and comorbid asthma from childhood to adulthood? A meta-analysis

M. Fröhlich[1,2] ⓘ, M. Pinart[1,3,4,5,6,7], T. Keller[1], A. Reich[8], B. Cabieses[9], C. Hohmann[1], D. S. Postma[10], J. Bousquet[11,12,13], J. M. Antó[4,5,6,7], T. Keil[1,14]* and S. Roll[1]

Abstract

Background: Allergic rhinitis and asthma as single entities affect more boys than girls in childhood but more females in adulthood. However, it is unclear if this prevalence sex-shift also occurs in allergic rhinitis and concurrent asthma. Thus, our aim was to compare sex-specific differences in the prevalence of coexisting allergic rhinitis and asthma in childhood, adolescence and adulthood.

Methods: Post-hoc analysis of systematic review with meta-analysis concerning sex-specific prevalence of allergic rhinitis. Using random-effects meta-analysis, we assessed male–female ratios for coexisting allergic rhinitis and asthma in children (0–10 years), adolescents (11–17) and adults (> 17). Electronic searches were performed using MEDLINE and EMBASE for the time period 2000–2014. We included population-based observational studies, reporting coexisting allergic rhinitis and asthma as outcome stratified by sex. We excluded non-original or non-population-based studies, studies with only male or female participants or selective patient collectives.

Results: From a total of 6539 citations, 10 studies with a total of 93,483 participants met the inclusion criteria. The male–female ratios (95% CI) for coexisting allergic rhinitis and asthma were 1.65 (1.52; 1.78) in children (N = 6 studies), 0.61 (0.51; 0.72) in adolescents (N = 2) and 1.03 (0.79; 1.35) in adults (N = 2). Male–female ratios for allergic rhinitis only were 1.25 (1.19; 1.32, N = 5) in children, 0.80 (0.71; 0.89, N = 2) in adolescents and 0.98 (0.74; 1.30, N = 2) in adults, respectively.

Conclusions: The prevalence of coexisting allergic rhinitis and asthma shows a clear male predominance in childhood and seems to switch to a female predominance in adolescents. This switch was less pronounced for allergic rhinitis only.

Keywords: Allergic rhinitis, Asthma, Multimorbidity, Prevalence, Systematic review

Background

Increasing prevalence in allergic diseases has been observed in many countries, especially in Western but also many developing countries [1]. Sex specific differences in prevalence of allergic rhinitis and asthma over the life span were recognized, showing a higher prevalence of allergic rhinitis and asthma as single entities in boys than in girls during childhood followed by an equal distribution in adolescence [2, 3]. In adulthood more women than men are affected by asthma [4, 5]. In a prospective cohort study, the prevalence of coexisting eczema, allergic rhinitis, and asthma in the same child was more common than expected by chance alone and was not only attributable to IgE sensitization, suggesting that these diseases share causal mechanisms [6]. In a systematic review of studies across the globe we showed a sex-switch in prevalence of allergic rhinitis in population-based studies [3]. Since research on multimorbidity, i.e. the coexistence of 2 or more allergic diseases in

*Correspondence: Thomas.Keil@charite.de
[1] Institute of Social Medicine, Epidemiology and Health Economics, Charité - Universitätsmedizin Berlin, Berlin, Germany
Full list of author information is available at the end of the article

the same individual, is sparse, the aim of this systematic review with meta-analyses was to examine sex specific differences in the prevalence of coexisting allergic rhinitis and asthma, from childhood through adolescence into adulthood.

Methods

Data sources, search strategy, and selection criteria

We conducted a systematic literature search using the online databases MEDLINE and EMBASE. MeSH terms were used in conjunction with keywords searched in the title and abstract. We restricted our search to studies published between January 2000 and April 2014. There was no restriction to the language of publication. The protocol for our systematic review was developed with guidance from the Preferred Reporting Items for Systematic Review and Meta-Analysis (PRISMA) statement [7]. It can be accessed at PROSPERO (http://www.crd.york.ac.uk/PROSPERO/, registration number CRD42016036105). To manage the identified publications, we used EndNote X7® (Thomson Reuters) bibliographic database.

Inclusion and exclusion criteria

The selection of studies was performed along with pre-set criteria for in- or exclusion. Since the present study is a post hoc analysis of a larger review considering the difference in prevalence for allergic rhinitis only [3], we chose broad inclusion criteria to reach most of the available information and to increase generalisability. The present analysis included studies of the previous comprehensive review that (1) recruited participants of both sexes from the general population, (2) reported the prevalence of coexisting allergic rhinitis and asthma, asthma only, and allergic rhinitis only stratified by sex and age if the population under study included both children and adults, and (3) were designed as longitudinal or cross-sectional studies.

We excluded (1) non-original studies (e.g. reviews or guidelines), (2) studies that selected participants by special occupation, (3) studies with only male or female participants, (4) studies analysing selective patient collectives (e.g. from special allergy clinics), or (5) non-population-based study designs e.g. ecological studies, case reports, case series, case–control studies, experimental studies, intervention studies, and clinical studies.

We evaluated prevalence estimates of allergic rhinitis, asthma and coexisting allergic rhinitis and asthma regarding the following endpoints: allergic rhinitis only was defined as having symptoms of allergic rhinitis (i.e. runny nose without having a cold) without having symptoms of asthma. In analogy, asthma only was defined as having symptoms of asthma (i.e. wheezing or whistling in the chest) but no symptoms of allergic rhinitis. An

individual who named both symptoms of allergic rhinitis and symptoms of asthma was included in the group of coexisting allergic rhinitis and asthma. If selected studies reported prevalence rates for having symptoms ever or current, we chose 'current', which was defined as reporting symptoms in the last 12 months.

Study selection, data extraction and quality assessment

A detailed protocol of the selection process for the initial review was published elsewhere [3]. In short a two-step review process was performed with scanning titles of identified studies first independently by two reviewers (MP and CH), followed by a second screening of all abstracts of articles rated as 'include' or 'unclear'. A disagreement between the two reviewers was resolved by discussion to meet a consensus. If consensus was not reached, a third independent reviewer (TKei or MF) was asked to assess the relevance.

Prior to data extraction, two reviewers (MP and MF) independently reviewed full texts of all selected publications rated as 'include' or 'unclear'. A pre-designed data extraction form was piloted with five studies selected from the pool of included studies. At least two reviewers (TKel, CH, BC, TKei, AR, MP and MF) extracted data from the selected full texts independently with disagreements through referral to a third reviewer (TKei).

For data extraction we used a self-designed (MP) SoSci-Survey questionnaire (https://www.soscisurvey.de/) retrieving information on country, study design, description of the process of recruitment of participants, age of participants, sample size, residency, response rate, observation period, definition of disease and measurement, method of data collection, prevalence of allergic rhinitis only (i.e. subjects without asthma) and asthma only (i.e. subjects without allergic rhinitis) as well as coexisting allergic rhinitis and asthma stratified by sex. Prevalences for each study were calculated using the number of participants with the respective disease as numerator and the total number of participants as denominator.

To evaluate the quality of identified literature and the heterogeneity between different studies we used an evaluation score based on previously published studies [8]. For this score every included article was reviewed on sampling method, response rate, sample size, and data collection method. A maximum of five points would account for 'high quality', three to four points would be 'moderate' and zero to two would be 'low quality'.

Quantitative data synthesis

Study populations were divided into age ranges of childhood (0–10 years of age), adolescence (11–17 years), or adulthood (18–79 years). For each study, we extracted the prevalence rates of coexisting allergic rhinitis and asthma, as well as of allergic rhinitis only, and asthma only separately for male and female participants. We then calculated male–female ratios for each study, as well as pooled male–female-ratio estimates with 95% confidence intervals (95% CI) using random-effects meta-analyses with the inverse variance method (SR). Heterogeneity between the studies was measured by I^2. Statistical analyses were done using Review Manager (RevMan), Version 5.3. Copenhagen (The Nordic Cochrane Centre, The Cochrane Collaboration, 2014) and R (R Foundation for Statistical Computing, Vienna, Austria).

Results

Characteristics of included studies

1222 out of 6539 publications were selected by title screening. Of those, 247 studies were eligible for data extraction since they reported prevalence of allergic rhinitis stratified by sex. Finally, 10 studies reporting the prevalence of asthma alone and allergic rhinitis with coexisting asthma were included into the systematic review (Fig. 1, Table 1) [8–16]. Six studies provided sex-specific prevalence of coexisting allergic rhinitis and asthma, allergic rhinitis only, and asthma only in children (0–10 years), two studies in adolescents (11–17 years), and two studies in adults (18–79 years). Studies with a broad age range were categorised as closely as possible to the targeted age groups, using the mean age of the participants for one study [16]. The assessment of allergic symptoms was questionnaire-based, mainly using the International Study of Asthma and Allergies in Childhood (ISAAC) [17] questionnaire for 8 studies in children and adolescents [8, 10–15, 18], or the European Community Respiratory Health Survey (ECRHS) [19] for 2 studies in adults [9, 20]. See Additional file 1: Tables E1–E3 for further description of study characteristics and Additional file 1: Table E5 for study results.

Male–female ratios of coexisting allergic rhinitis and asthma

We included 6 studies with a total of 34,365 males and 31,611 females for children (0–10 years), 2 studies with 1803 males and 2152 females for adolescents (11–17 years) and 2 studies with 11,573 males and 11,979 females for adults (18–79 years). The pooled estimates for the male–female ratio (males vs. females) of the prevalence of coexisting allergic rhinitis and asthma were 1.65 (95% CI 1.52–1.78) in children, 0.61 (0.51–0.72) in adolescents, and 1.03 (0.79–1.35) in adults (Fig. 2).

The studies reported a male predominance of coexisting allergic rhinitis and asthma in children and a female predominance in adolescents. Desalu et al. [9] and Konno et al. [20] showed heterogeneous results for adulthood.

Male–female ratios of allergic rhinitis without asthma

We included 5 studies with 29,775 males and 27,071 females for children (0–10 years), 2 studies with 1803 males and 2152 females for adolescents (11–17 years) and 2 studies that included 11,573 males and 11,979 females for adults (18–79 years). The pooled estimates for the male–female ratio of the prevalence of allergic rhinitis only were 1.25 (1.19–1.32) in children, 0.80 (0.71–0.89) in adolescents and 0.98 (0.74–1.30) in adults.

None of the studies reported a female predominance in the prevalence of allergic rhinitis only among children. In contrast both studies providing information on adolescents showed a female predominance. Concerning the prevalence among adults the two analysed studies again showed heterogeneous results.

Male–female ratios of asthma without allergic rhinitis

We included 5 studies with 29,775 males and 27,071 females for children (0–10 years), 2 studies with 1803 males and 2152 females for adolescents (11–17 years). We found only one study providing information on asthma only in adults. The pooled estimates for the male–female-ratio of the prevalence of asthma only were 1.20 (0.99–1.45) in children and 1.03 (0.62–1.71) in adolescents. Konno et al. [20] reported in a study with 11,132 males and 11,687 females a male–female ratio for the prevalence of asthma only of 1.61 (1.44–1.81) in adults (Fig. 3).

Four of five included studies for asthma only in children reported a male predominance, whereas Nahhas et al. [15] showed a female predominance. Two studies analysed the prevalence of asthma only in adolescents and found heterogeneous results. De Brito et al. [8] reported a female predominance, whereas Luna et al. [14] showed a male predominance.

Heterogeneity and quality of studies

While no statistical heterogeneity was detected among the lower age groups, moderate heterogeneity existed among the studies in the adult group ($I^2_{18-79} = 41\%$) for coexisting allergic rhinitis and asthma. In the meta-analysis for the prevalence of asthma only, considerable heterogeneity was found ($I^2_{0-10} = 75\%$; $I^2_{11-17} = 81\%$) resulting in an overall of $I^2 = 85\%$. Little or no heterogeneity was seen in studies reporting results for allergic rhinitis only in children and adolescents ($I^2_{0-10} = 27\%$; $I^2_{11-17} = 0\%$) compared to studies including adults ($I^2_{18-79} = 73\%$). All studies were of moderate quality (4 points) except from Desalu et al., which was rated as high quality (5 points), see Additional file 1: Table E4.

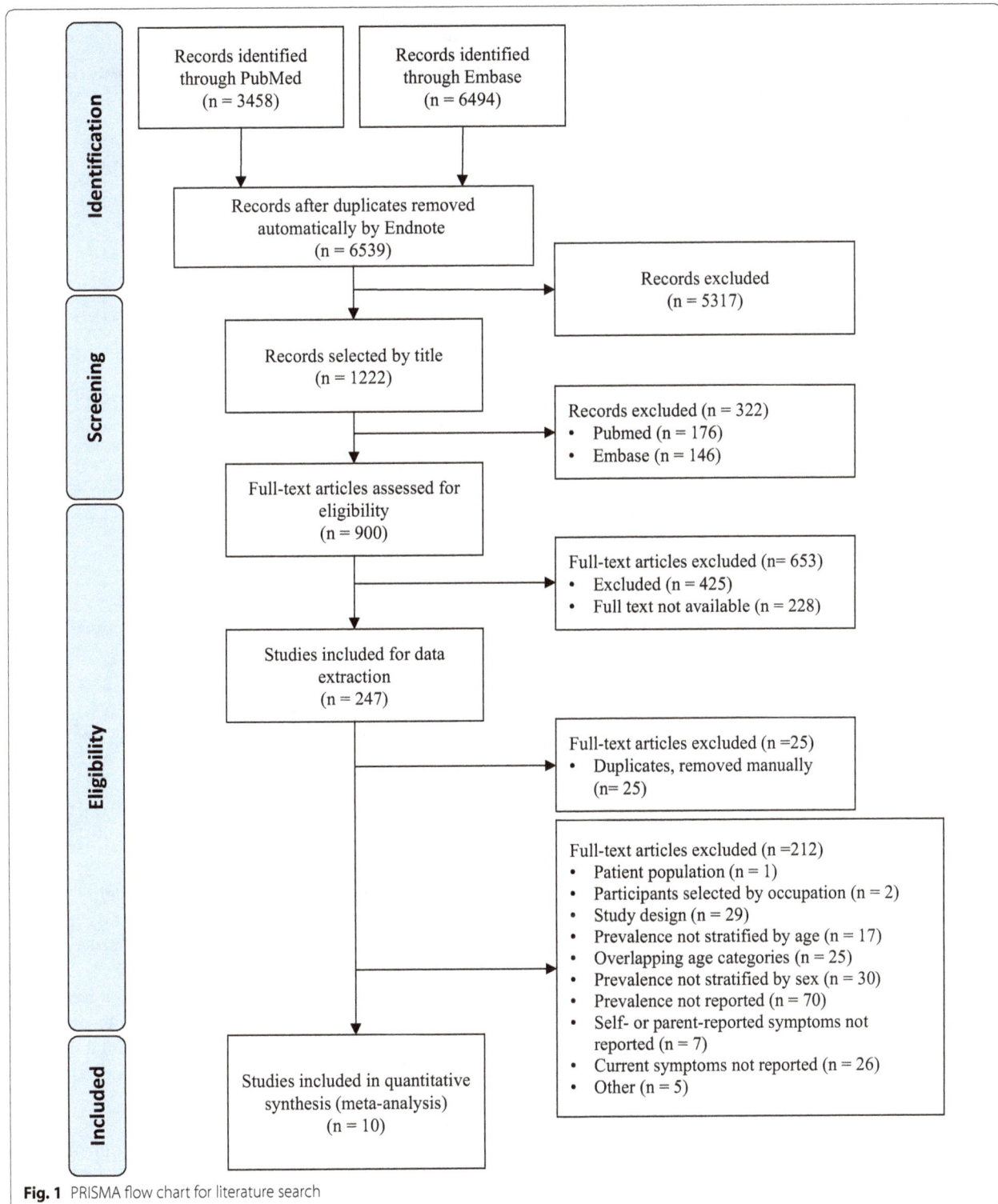

Fig. 1 PRISMA flow chart for literature search

Discussion

Main findings

We found a clear 'sex-switch' in the prevalence of coexisting allergic rhinitis and asthma from a male predominance in childhood to a female predominance in adolescence. Similar trends of these sex-specific prevalence patterns were observed in participants with asthma only and those with allergic rhinitis only. Two studies in adults showed similar prevalence rates in both sexes.

Comparison with other studies

In a global systematic review with meta-analysis we showed sex-related differences in rhinitis prevalence with a prevalence shift from a male predominance at around puberty to a female predominance thereafter [3]. Similarly, a retrospective analysis of the ECRHS data from 16 European countries showed a transition for asthma from a male predominance in childhood (0–10 years) followed by an equal gender distribution in adolescence (10–15 years) leading to a female predominance in adults (> 15 years) [21]. Sex-specific rhinitis and comorbid asthma prevalence data for older men and women are very scarce. Interestingly, according to a large observational all-female cohort, the Nurses' Health Study in USA, the age-adjusted risk of asthma seems to be increased in postmenopausal women who ever or currently used hormone replacement therapy (i.e. conjugated estrogens with or without progesterone) compared to those who never used such hormones. However, allergic rhinitis with and without comorbid asthma has not been examinated [22]. In a cohort study of 509 children with allergic rhinitis from Turkey (mean age 7.2 ± 3.5 years, age range 1.5–18 years) Dogru showed that asthma was prevalent in the majority (53.2%) of these children [23]. In a French observational study of patients with asthma more than 50% of participants had concomitant allergic rhinitis [24]. Several narrative reviews showed this change in sex predominance favoring females during the transition from childhood to adulthood for diverse allergy-related diseases [4, 5, 25, 26]. Therefore, and since asthma and rhinitis coexist more often than expected [6], we hypothesized that also concomitant allergic rhinitis and asthma may undergo a similar sex-shift in prevalence during puberty.

Our results support this hypothesis to some extent. However, the limited number of studies found in adults did not allow us to clearly establish a clear tendency towards a male or female predominance but rather a balance between the sexes. Our pooled estimates relied only upon data from studies conducted in Asia (N = 7), South America (N = 2) and Africa (N = 1). In Pinart et al. a sex switch for allergic rhinitis prevalence around puberty was not found in studies conducted in Asia [3]. Five of six studies in the youngest age group (0–10 years) were from Asia, whereas no Asian studies were found for adolescents (11–17 years), suggesting a considerable bias.

Concerning possible mechanisms underlying a higher prevalence of allergic diseases in women during and after adolescence, higher levels of sex hormones such as estrogen and progesterone were suggested to be of central importance [27]. Sex hormones play a role in the

Table 1 Main characteristics of studies included in the systematic review

Study characteristics	Number of studies
Total	10
Study period	
2000–2007	7
2008–2014	3
Region	
Africa	1
Asia	7
South America	2
Sample size analysed	
< 1000	2
1001–5000	1
5001–10,000	3
10,001–100,000	4
Age category (in years)	
0–10	6
11–17	2
18–79	2
Urbanicity	
Urban	7
Rural/urban	1
Unclear/not reported	2
Method for assessing prevalence	
ISAAC questionnaire	8
ECHRS questionnaire	2

ISAAC International Study of Asthma and Allergies in Childhood, *ECRHS* European Community Respiratory Health Survey

homeostasis of immunity [28]. Estrogen and progesterone enhance type 2 and suppress type 1 responses in females, whereas testosterone suppresses type 2 responses in males [29]. Experiments in rodents showed an effect of estrogens on mast cell activation and the development of allergic sensitization, while progesterone can suppress histamine release but potentiate IgE induction [28]. Similarly for asthma sex differences have been reported for different phenotypes and symptom profiles in epidemiological, clinical and experimental studies, however, the aetiology remains largely unclear [30–33].

Risk of bias

We tried to identify all population based studies reporting prevalence of coexisting allergic rhinitis and asthma. Given that such observational studies require large samples, it seems unlikely that a study of this dimension will have been published and not identified by our search. Furthermore, in population-based prevalence studies publication bias seems to be less of a concern than e.g. in interventional studies. Thus, we believe that a bias due to unpublished data is unlikely.

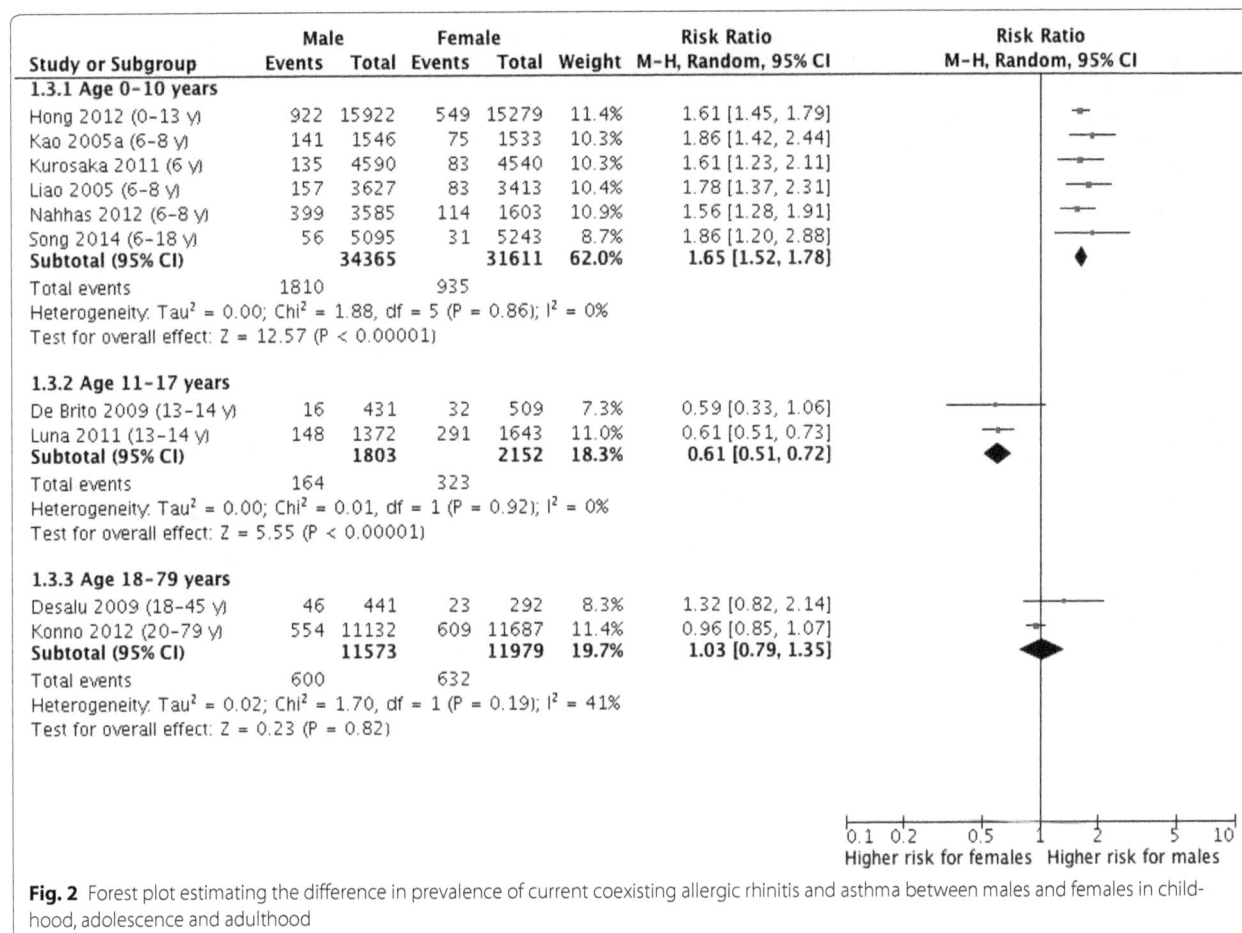

Fig. 2 Forest plot estimating the difference in prevalence of current coexisting allergic rhinitis and asthma between males and females in childhood, adolescence and adulthood

Our systematic review was embedded in a larger review considering the difference in prevalence for rhinitis only [3]. Although we used broad inclusion criteria, we may have missed studies that provided information on prevalence of having allergic rhinitis and asthma but did not provide information of having allergic rhinitis only or were published in journals that are not listed in the 2 major databases of medical literature, MEDLINE and EMBASE. Primary care-based studies including e.g. only out-patients were excluded because of a possible gender-related bias considering that women seek medical treatment, screening programs and other health care offers more often than men [34]. Restricting our search to studies published between 2000 and 2014 does not allow us to conclude on possibly different findings from earlier studies. The prevalence of allergies has dramatically increased in the second half of the twentieth century but reasons for these temporal trends are not clear [35]. We therefore wanted to avoid the rather speculative comparisons of prevalence studies across 5 and more decades and focused our evaluation on the 2 recent decades where the prevalence of allergies may

have reached a plateau in many regions around the world [36].

Most of the included studies, especially in children, were conducted in Asia, which may limit the generalisability of the results, because of specific genetic differences between ethnic groups as well as different environmental factors for allergic diseases such as air pollution.

Our results showed that a sex switch from a male to a female predominance in the coexistence of allergic rhinitis and asthma is reported in population-based studies; however, further research is needed to study the underlying mechanisms. The definition of allergic rhinitis and asthma in our study is based on answers to validated questions from the ISAAC and ECRHS projects. Though these instruments are widely used globally and well validated in many languages especially for asthma, a possible overestimation of asthma or allergic rhinitis prevalence cannot be excluded. However, we do not think that this affects the male–female-ratios of the prevalence estimates used in our analysis since there is no indication for different overestimation between male and female responders of the included questions.

Study or Subgroup	Male Events	Total	Female Events	Total	Weight	Risk Ratio M-H, Random, 95% CI	Risk Ratio M-H, Random, 95% CI
1.1.1 Age 0-10 years							
Hong 2012 (0-13 y)	5545	15922	4359	15279	12.9%	1.22 [1.18, 1.26]	
Kao 2005a (6-8 y)	333	1546	267	1533	11.6%	1.24 [1.07, 1.43]	
Liao 2005 (6-8 y)	568	3627	386	3413	12.0%	1.38 [1.23, 1.56]	
Nahhas 2012 (6-8 y)	558	3585	186	1603	11.4%	1.34 [1.15, 1.57]	
Song 2014 (6-18 y)	494	5095	430	5243	11.9%	1.18 [1.04, 1.34]	
Subtotal (95% CI)		**29775**		**27071**	**59.8%**	**1.25 [1.19, 1.32]**	
Total events	7498		5628				
Heterogeneity: Tau² = 0.00; Chi² = 5.52, df = 4 (P = 0.24); I² = 27%							
Test for overall effect: Z = 8.58 (P < 0.00001)							
1.1.2 Age 11-17 years							
De Brito 2009 (13-14 y)	36	431	55	509	6.8%	0.77 [0.52, 1.15]	
Luna 2011 (13-14 y)	346	1372	518	1643	12.1%	0.80 [0.71, 0.90]	
Subtotal (95% CI)		**1803**		**2152**	**18.8%**	**0.80 [0.71, 0.89]**	
Total events	382		573				
Heterogeneity: Tau² = 0.00; Chi² = 0.03, df = 1 (P = 0.87); I² = 0%							
Test for overall effect: Z = 3.98 (P < 0.0001)							
1.1.3 Age 18-79 years							
Desalu 2009 (18-45 y)	95	441	53	292	8.5%	1.19 [0.88, 1.60]	
Konno 2012 (20-79 y)	3312	11132	3951	11687	12.9%	0.88 [0.85, 0.91]	
Subtotal (95% CI)		**11573**		**11979**	**21.4%**	**0.98 [0.74, 1.30]**	
Total events	3407		4004				
Heterogeneity: Tau² = 0.03; Chi² = 3.72, df = 1 (P = 0.05); I² = 73%							
Test for overall effect: Z = 0.12 (P = 0.91)							

```
        0.1 0.2      0.5    1     2      5   10
        Higher risk for females  Higher risk for males
```

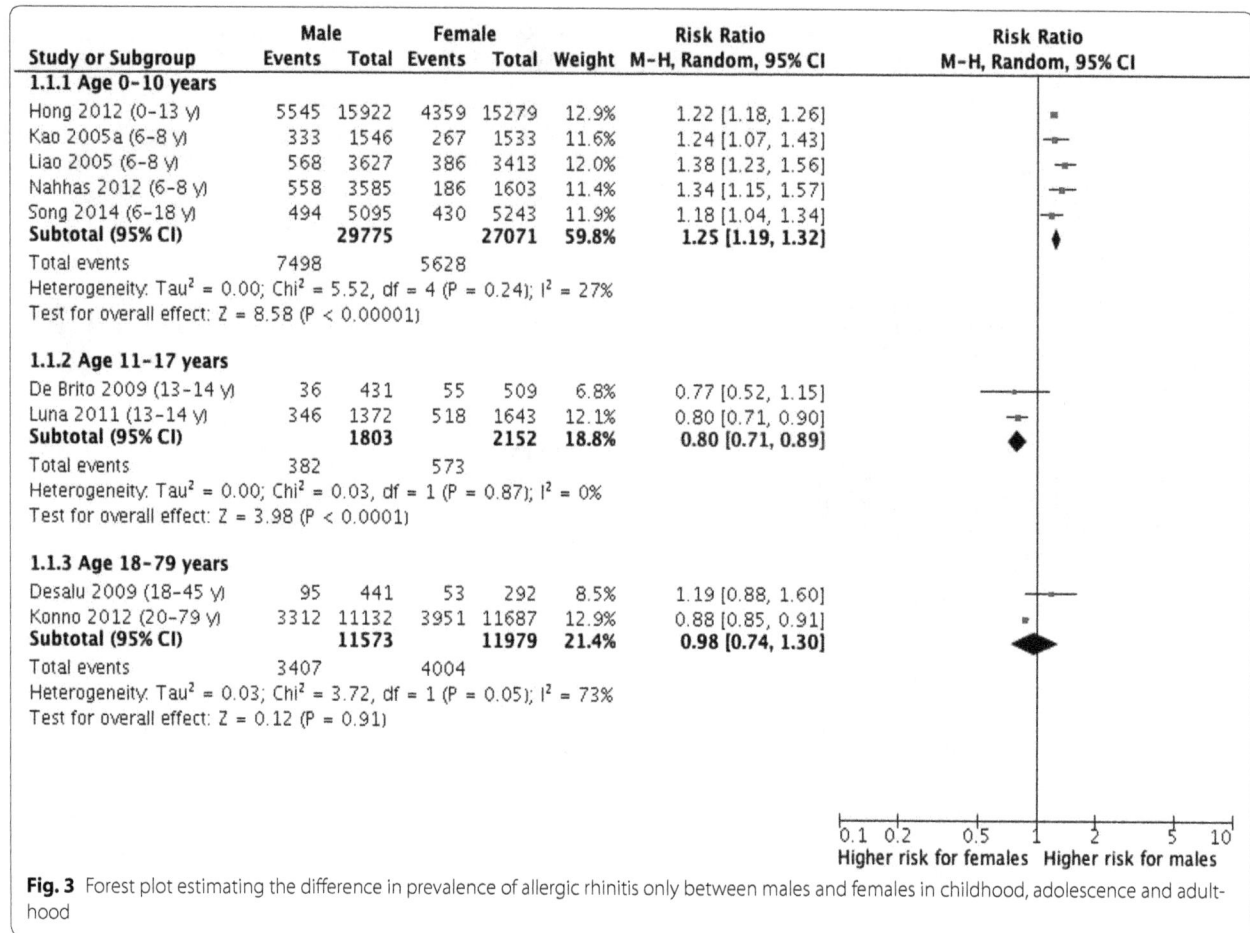

Fig. 3 Forest plot estimating the difference in prevalence of allergic rhinitis only between males and females in childhood, adolescence and adulthood

Using *current symptoms* of asthma and allergic rhinitis as outcome definition may cause misclassification if classifying individuals without symptoms because of successful symptom control for example as negative. However, we consider it unlikely that a person using e.g. anti-obstructive medication on a daily basis would answer negative to the question for having wheeze during the last 12 months. While, on the contrary, we judge the usage of doctor's diagnosis to result in an underestimation of the number of subjects with allergic diseases.

Though there were many studies using the ISAAC study-design only few studies fulfilled our stringent inclusion criteria. This shows that there is a need for a more multimorbid perspective in population-based studies. For this work, we identified only cross-sectional studies. Although this study design is adequate for estimating population-based prevalences, longitudinal studies would be of interest to examine possible mechanisms underlying these differences in prevalence. Therefore, birth cohort studies in particular, are currently being evaluated regarding sex-specific allergy prevalence differences in childhood and early adolescence within the MeDALL project [37, 38].

Considerable inconsistency was found solely in our meta-analyses for asthma only and for the 2 adult studies as indicated by the Higgins' I²-tests. These summary measures of the meta-analyses should be interpreted with extra caution. Potential sources of heterogeneity include study design, study area or analysed age groups, but the specific influence cannot be examined due to the limited number of studies.

Conclusions

Based on a systematic review with meta-analysis of cross-sectional population-studies from across the globe we found a clear male predominance for the prevalence of coexisting allergic rhinitis and asthma in childhood. This seems to shift towards a female predominance in adolescents. Such a shift was less pronounced for allergic rhinitis as a single entity. Our results suggest that the effect of puberty seems to be particularly present in the most severely affected patients who have both allergic rhinitis and concurrent asthma. However, sex- and gender-specific evaluations beyond 14 years of age are scarce and further allergic multimorbidity studies in different population settings, particularly in adults, are required. In clinical, epidemiological and basic research more sex- and gender-specific analyses are needed to develop better prevention and treatment strategies.

Abbreviations
ECRHS: European Community Respiratory Health Survey; ISAAC: International Study of Asthma and Allergies in Childhood; PRISMA: Preferred Reporting Items for Systematic Reviews and Meta-Analyses.

Authors' contributions
Conceived and designed the experiments: MF, MP, TKei and SR. Performed the experiments: MF, MP, CH, AR, TKel, BC. Data analysis and/or interpretation of the systematic review: MF, TKel, AR, Tkei and SR. Wrote the paper: all authors. All authors read and approved the final manuscript.

Author details
[1] Institute of Social Medicine, Epidemiology and Health Economics, Charité - Universitätsmedizin Berlin, Berlin, Germany. [2] Clinic for Neonatology, Charité - Universitätsmedizin Berlin, Berlin, Germany. [3] Max-Delbrück-Centrum für Molekulare Medizin, Research Team Molecular Epidemiology, Berlin, Germany. [4] ISGlobal, Centre for Research in Environmental Epidemiology (CREAL), Barcelona, Spain. [5] IMIM (Hospital del Mar Research Institute), Barcelona, Spain. [6] Universitat Popmpeu Fabra (UPF), Barcelona, Spain. [7] CIBFR Epidemiología y Salud Pública (CIBERESP), Barcelona, Spain. [8] Epidemiology, German Rheumatism Research Centre, Berlin, Germany. [9] Facultad de Medicina Clínica Alemana, Universidad del Desarrollo, Santiago, Chile. [10] Department of Pulmonology, University Medical Center Groningen, University of Groningen, Groningen, The Netherlands. [11] University Hospital, Montpellier, France. [12] MACVIA-LR, Contre les Maladies Chroniques pour un Vieillissement Actifen Languedoc Roussillon, European Innovation Partnership on Active and Healthy Ageing Reference Site, and INSERM, VIMA: Ageing and Chronic Diseases, Epidemiological and Public Health Approaches, U1168, Paris, France. [13] UVSQ, UMR-S 1168, Université Versailles, St-Quentin-en-Yvelines, France. [14] Institute of Clinical Epidemiology and Biometry, University of Wuerzburg, Würzburg, Germany.

Acknowledgements
This work was initiated and supported by MeDALL, a collaborative project conducted within the European Union under the Health Cooperation Work Programme of the 7th Framework Programme (Grant Agreement No. 261357).

Competing interests
The authors declare that they have no competing interests.

Funding
Mariona Pinart is a recipient of a 'Sara Borrell' postdoctoral contract (CD11/00090) from the Fondo de Investigaciones Sanitarias (FIS), Ministry of Economy and Competitiveness, Spain.

References
1. Eder W, Ege MJ, von Mutius E. The asthma epidemic. N Engl J Med. 2006;355:2226–35.
2. Kurukulaaratchy RJ, Karmaus W, Arshad SH. Sex and atopy influences on the natural history of rhinitis. Curr Opin Allergy Clin Immunol. 2012;12:7–12.
3. Pinart M, Keller T, Reich A, Fröhlich M, Cabieses B, Hohmann C, Postma D, Bousquet J, Antó J, Keil T. Sex-related allergic rhinitis prevalence switch from childhood to adulthood: a systematic review and meta-analysis. Int Arch Allergy Immunol. 2017;172:224–35.
4. Becklake MR, Kauffmann F. Gender differences in airway behaviour over the human life span. Thorax. 1999;54:1119–38.
5. Postma DS. Gender differences in asthma development and progression. Gend Med. 2007;4 Suppl B:S133–46.
6. Pinart M, Benet M, Annesi-Maesano I, von Berg A, Berdel D, Carlsen KCL, Carlsen KH, Bindslev-Jensen C, Eller E, Fantini MP, et al. Comorbidity of eczema, rhinitis, and asthma in IgE-sensitised and non-IgE-sensitised children in MeDALL: A population-based cohort study. Lancet Respir Med. 2014;2:131–40.
7. Moher D, Liberati A, Tetzlaff J, Altman DG. Preferred reporting items for systematic reviews and meta-analyses: the PRISMA statement. Int J Surg. 2010;8:336–41.
8. Brito Rde C, da Silva GA, Motta ME, Brito MC. The association of rhino-conjunctivitis and asthma symptoms in adolescents. Rev Port Pneumol. 2009;15:613–28.
9. Desalu OO, Salami AK, Iseh KR, Oluboyo PO. Prevalence of self reported allergic rhinitis and its relationship with asthma among adult Nigerians. J Investig Allergol Clin Immunol. 2009;19:474–80.
10. Hong S, Son DK, Lim WR, Kim SH, Kim H, Yum HY, Kwon H. The prevalence of atopic dermatitis, asthma, and allergic rhinitis and the comorbidity of allergic diseases in children. Environ Health Toxicol. 2012;27:e2012006.
11. Kao CC, Huang JL, Ou LS, See LC. The prevalence, severity and seasonal variations of asthma, rhinitis and eczema in Taiwanese schoolchildren. Pediatr Allergy Immunol. 2005;16:408–15.
12. Kurosaka F, Terada T, Tanaka A, Nakatani Y, Yamada K, Nishikawa J, Oka K, Takahashi H, Mogami A, Yamada T, et al. Risk factors for wheezing, eczema and rhinoconjunctivitis in the previous 12 months among six-year-old children in Himeji City, Japan: food allergy, older siblings, day-care attendance and parental allergy history. Allergol Int. 2011;60:317–30.
13. Liao MF, Huang JL, Chiang LC, Wang FY, Chen CY. Prevalence of asthma, rhinitis, and eczema from ISAAC survey of schoolchildren in Central Taiwan. J Asthma. 2005;42:833–7.
14. Luna Mde F, Almeida PC, Silva MG. Asthma and rhinitis prevalence and co-morbidity in 13-14-year-old schoolchildren in the city of Fortaleza, Ceara State, Brazil. Cad Saude Publica. 2011;27:103–12.
15. Nahhas M, Bhopal R, Anandan C, Elton R, Sheikh A. Prevalence of allergic disorders among primary school-aged children in Madinah, Saudi Arabia: two-stage cross-sectional survey. PLoS ONE. 2012;7:e36848.
16. Song N, Shamssain M, Zhang J, Wu J, Fu C, Hao S, Guan J, Yan X. Prevalence, severity and risk factors of asthma, rhinitis and eczema in a large group of Chinese schoolchildren. J Asthma. 2014;51:232–42.
17. Asher MI, Keil U, Anderson HR, Beasley R, Crane J, Martinez F, Mitchell EA, Pearce N, Sibbald B, Stewart AW, et al. International Study of Asthma and Allergies in Childhood (ISAAC): rationale and methods. Eur Respir J. 1995;8:483–91.
18. Song WJ, Kim MY, Jo EJ, Kim MH, Kim TH, Kim SH, Kim KW, Cho SH, Min KU, Chang YS. Rhinitis in a community elderly population: relationships with age, atopy, and asthma. Ann Allergy Asthma Immunol. 2013;111:347–51.
19. Burney PG, Luczynska C, Chinn S, Jarvis D. The European community respiratory health survey. Eur Respir J. 1994;7:954–60.
20. Konno S, Hizawa N, Fukutomi Y, Taniguchi M, Kawagishi Y, Okada C, Tanimoto Y, Takahashi K, Akasawa A, Akiyama K, Nishimura M. The prevalence of rhinitis and its association with smoking and obesity in a nationwide survey of Japanese adults. Allergy. 2012;67:653–60.
21. de Marco R, Locatelli F, Sunyer J, Burney P. Differences in incidence of reported asthma related to age in men and women. A retrospective analysis of the data of the European Respiratory Health Survey. Am J Respir Crit Care Med. 2000;162:68–74.
22. Troisi RJ, Speizer FE, Willett WC, Trichopoulos D, Rosner B. Menopause,

postmenopausal estrogen preparations, and the risk of adult-onset asthma. A prospective cohort study. Am J Respir Crit Care Med. 1995;152:1183–8.

23. Dogru M. Investigation of asthma comorbidity in children with different severities of allergic rhinitis. Am J Rhinol Allergy. 2016;30:186–9.

24. Magnan A, Meunier JP, Saugnac C, Gasteau J, Neukirch F. Frequency and impact of allergic rhinitis in asthma patients in everyday general medical practice: a French observational cross-sectional study. Allergy. 2008;63:292–8.

25. Almqvist C, Worm M, Leynaert B. Impact of gender on asthma in childhood and adolescence: a GA2LEN review. Allergy. 2008;63:47–57.

26. Chen W, Mempel M, Schober W, Behrendt H, Ring J. Gender difference, sex hormones, and immediate type hypersensitivity reactions. Allergy Eur J Allergy Clin Immunol. 2008;63:1418–27.

27. Bonds RS, Midoro-Horiuti T. Estrogen effects in allergy and asthma. Curr Opin Allergy Clin Immunol. 2013;13:92–9.

28. Chen W, Mempel M, Schober W, Behrendt H, Ring J. Gender difference, sex hormones, and immediate type hypersensitivity reactions. Allergy. 2008;63:1418–27.

29. Roved J, Westerdahl H, Hasselquist D. Sex differences in immune responses: Hormonal effects, antagonistic selection, and evolutionary consequences. Horm Behav. 2017;88:95–105.

30. Fuseini H, Newcomb DC. Mechanisms driving gender differences in asthma. Curr Allergy Asthma Rep. 2017;17:19.

31. Keller T, Hohmann C, Standl M, Wijga AH, Gehring U, Melen E, Almqvist C, Lau S, Eller E, Wahn U, et al.: The sex-shift in single disease and multimorbid asthma and rhinitis during puberty—a study by MeDALL. Allergy. 2017. https://doi.org/10.1111/all.13312.

32. Kynyk JA, Mastronarde JG, McCallister JW. Asthma, the sex difference. Curr Opin Pulm Med. 2011;17:6–11.

33. McCallister JW, Mastronarde JG. Sex differences in asthma. J Asthma. 2008;45:853–61.

34. Vaidya V, Partha G, Karmakar M. Gender differences in utilization of preventive care services in the United States. J Womens Health (Larchmt). 2012;21:140–5.

35. Worldwide variation in prevalence of symptoms of asthma, allergic rhinoconjunctivitis, and atopic eczema: ISAAC. The International Study of Asthma and Allergies in Childhood (ISAAC) Steering Committee. Lancet 1998; 351:1225–32.

36. Asher MI, Montefort S, Bjorksten B, Lai CK, Strachan DP, Weiland SK, Williams H. Worldwide time trends in the prevalence of symptoms of asthma, allergic rhinoconjunctivitis, and eczema in childhood: ISAAC Phases One and Three repeat multicountry cross-sectional surveys. Lancet. 2006;368:733–43.

37. Anto JM, Bousquet J, Akdis M, Auffray C, Keil T, Momas I, Postma DS, Valenta R, Wickman M, Cambon-Thomsen A, et al. Mechanisms of the Development of Allergy (MeDALL): introducing novel concepts in allergy phenotypes. J Allergy Clin Immunol. 2017;139:388–99.

38. Bousquet J, Anto JM, Akdis M, Auffray C, Keil T, Momas I, Postma DS, Valenta R, Wickman M, Cambon-Thomsen A, et al. Paving the way of systems biology and precision medicine in allergic diseases: the MeDALL success story: Mechanisms of the Development of ALLergy; EU FP7-CP-IP; Project No: 261357; 2010-2015. Allergy 2016.

9

Having concomitant asthma phenotypes is common and independently relates to poor lung function in NHANES 2007–2012

Rita Amaral[1,2]*[iD], João A. Fonseca[1,3,4], Tiago Jacinto[1,2,4], Ana M. Pereira[1,4], Andrei Malinovschi[5], Christer Janson[6] and Kjell Alving[7]

Abstract

Background: Evidence for distinct asthma phenotypes and their overlap is becoming increasingly relevant to identify personalized and targeted therapeutic strategies. In this study, we aimed to describe the overlap of five commonly reported asthma phenotypes in US adults with current asthma and assess its association with asthma outcomes.

Methods: Data from the National Health and Nutrition Examination Surveys (NHANES) 2007–2012 were used (n = 30,442). Adults with current asthma were selected. Asthma phenotypes were: B-Eos-high [if blood eosinophils (B-Eos) ≥ 300/mm³]; FeNO-high (FeNO ≥ 35 ppb); B-Eos&FeNO-low (B-Eos < 150/mm³ and FeNO < 20 ppb); asthma with obesity (AwObesity) (BMI ≥ 30 kg/m²); and asthma with concurrent COPD. Data were weighted for the US population and analyses were stratified by age (< 40 and ≥ 40 years old).

Results: Of the 18,619 adults included, 1059 (5.6% [95% CI 5.1–5.9]) had current asthma. A substantial overlap was observed both in subjects aged < 40 years (44%) and ≥ 40 years (54%). The more prevalent specific overlaps in both age groups were AwObesity associated with either B-Eos-high (15 and 12%, respectively) or B-Eos&FeNO-low asthma (13 and 11%, respectively). About 14% of the current asthma patients were "non-classified". Regardless of phenotype classification, having concomitant phenotypes was significantly associated with (adjusted OR, 95% CI) ≥ 2 controller medications (2.03, 1.16–3.57), and FEV_1 < LLN (3.21, 1.74–5.94), adjusted for confounding variables.

Conclusions: A prevalent overlap of commonly reported asthma phenotypes was observed among asthma patients from the general population, with implications for objective asthma outcomes. A broader approach may be required to better characterize asthma patients and prevent poor asthma outcomes.

Keywords: Asthma, Asthma-related outcomes, Epidemiological study, Overlap, Phenotypes

Background

Profiling asthma phenotypes is becoming increasingly relevant to choose the most appropriate therapeutic strategy for individual patients, and to provide optimal improvement of disease control and quality of life [1, 2].

The predominant pathophysiological mechanism of asthma is type 2-mediated, associated with atopy and eosinophilic inflammation [3, 4]. However, it has been shown that asthma is a heterogeneous disease that involves other mechanisms that are not so well understood and respond poorly to corticosteroid therapy (e.g. non-type 2-mediated) [3, 5, 6].

There has been a recent rise in the number of studies that try to identify asthma phenotypes based on non-invasive type 2-markers, such as blood eosinophils (B-Eos) count, fraction of exhaled nitric oxide (FeNO), serum IgE, and/or serum periostin [7–10]. Moreover, there appears to be an additive role of biomarkers, such as B-Eos and FeNO, in relation to recent asthma morbidity [7, 11, 12].

*Correspondence: rita.s.amaral@gmail.com
[1] CINTESIS- Center for Health Technology and Services Research, Faculty of Medicine, University of Porto, Edifício Nascente, Piso 2, Rua Dr. Plácido da Costa, s/n, 4200-450 Porto, Portugal
Full list of author information is available at the end of the article

However, there is little information regarding the appropriate use of these biomarkers in asthma phenotype classification, particularly when a significant overlap occurs. Also, the importance of having concomitant asthma phenotypes for disease outcomes has scarcely been studied in the general population. This information may be useful to identify personalized and targeted therapeutic strategies [13, 14].

Recently, an extensive overlap of asthma phenotypes was described [15]. However, only type 2-high, atopic, and eosinophilic asthma were examined. The extent of overlap with other phenotypes commonly reported in the literature, among adults with asthma from the general population remains unknown. Asthma phenotypes are frequently reported in the literature according to the high levels of systemic and local type 2-markers (B-Eos high and FeNO-high, respectively) [1–4, 16–18]. However, other distinct subgroups of asthma phenotypes are increasingly being reported due to its characteristics of steroid therapy resistance and lack of inflammatory markers: e.g. subjects with asthma without evidence of type 2 inflammation (Th2-low phenotype); obese asthmatic subjects (obesity-related asthma phenotype); and patients with asthma-COPD overlap syndrome [19–22]. Therefore, we hypothesized that if, in general population, occurs a high proportion of overlap of commonly reported asthma phenotypes, there may be a need for improving the definition of asthma phenotypes. Additionally, asthma subjects with multiple phenotypes may have poorer asthma-related outcomes.

The aims of this study were to describe the proportion of overlap of five commonly reported asthma phenotypes: asthma with obesity (AwObesity), asthma with concurrent COPD (AwCOPD), B-Eos-high, FeNO-high and B-Eos&FeNO-low asthma, and to examine the association of their overlap with asthma-related outcomes, using population-based data from the National Health and Nutrition Examination Surveys (NHANES), 2007–2012.

Methods
Study design
The NHANES is a nationally representative survey of the civilian, non-institutionalized U.S. population that uses a complex stratified, multistage probability sampling. Further details on NHANES survey design databases can be found in Additional file 1: Supplementary methods. The National Center for Health Statistics, Ethics Review Board approved NHANES protocol, and all participants gave written informed consent.

Subjects selection
Six survey years (NHANES 2007–2012) were analyzed, resulting in 30,442 individuals of all ages (Fig. 1). We included adults (≥ 18 years-old) with current asthma (n = 1059), defined by a positive answer to the questions: "Has a doctor ever told you that you have asthma?" together with "Do you still have asthma?", and either "wheezing/whistling in the chest in the past 12 months" or "asthma attack in the past 12 months."

Variables
Demographic characteristics, such as age, gender, body mass index (BMI), race/ethnicity, and educational status were analyzed. B-Eos count, FeNO and spirometric measurements, collected at the NHANES Mobile Examination Center were also examined. A detailed description of the procedures can be found elsewhere [23–25]. FeNO and spirometric measurements not fulfilling ATS/ERS recommendations [26, 27] were excluded (n = 653). After predicted values of basal FEV_1 and FEV_1/FVC were calculated [28], with a correction factor for ethnicity [29], abnormal lung function was defined if either one of them were less than the lower limit of normal (LLN), defined as lower fifth percentile of the reference population [30].

Prescription medications used last month were also analyzed [31]. More details regarding the inclusion of reliever and controller medications for asthma and the definitions of each asthma-related variable included in the analysis (asthma attack, asthma-related emergency department (ED) visit, work/school absenteeism, asthma symptoms, smoking status and rhinitis) are provided in the supplementary material (see Additional file 1: Supplementary methods).

Asthma phenotypes definition
A B-Eos count $\geq 300/mm^3$ was used to define an B-Eos-high asthma phenotype [32, 33], while FeNO-high was defined as FeNO ≥ 35 ppb [34]. Asthma patients with both B-Eos $< 150/mm^3$ and FeNO < 20 ppb were categorized as B-Eos&FeNO-low asthma [35]. Additionally, we considered subjects with either B-Eos-high or FeNO-high as having "Type 2-high" asthma.

The AwObesity phenotype was defined by a BMI ≥ 30 kg/m^2 in individuals with current asthma [36]. Finally, the AwCOPD phenotype was considered if participants ≥ 40 years-old had concurrent asthma and COPD, defined by a positive answer to "Has a doctor ever told you that you have chronic bronchitis/emphysema", with age of diagnosis ≥ 40 years and having self-reported smoking history (being either a current or ex-smoker) [37, 38].

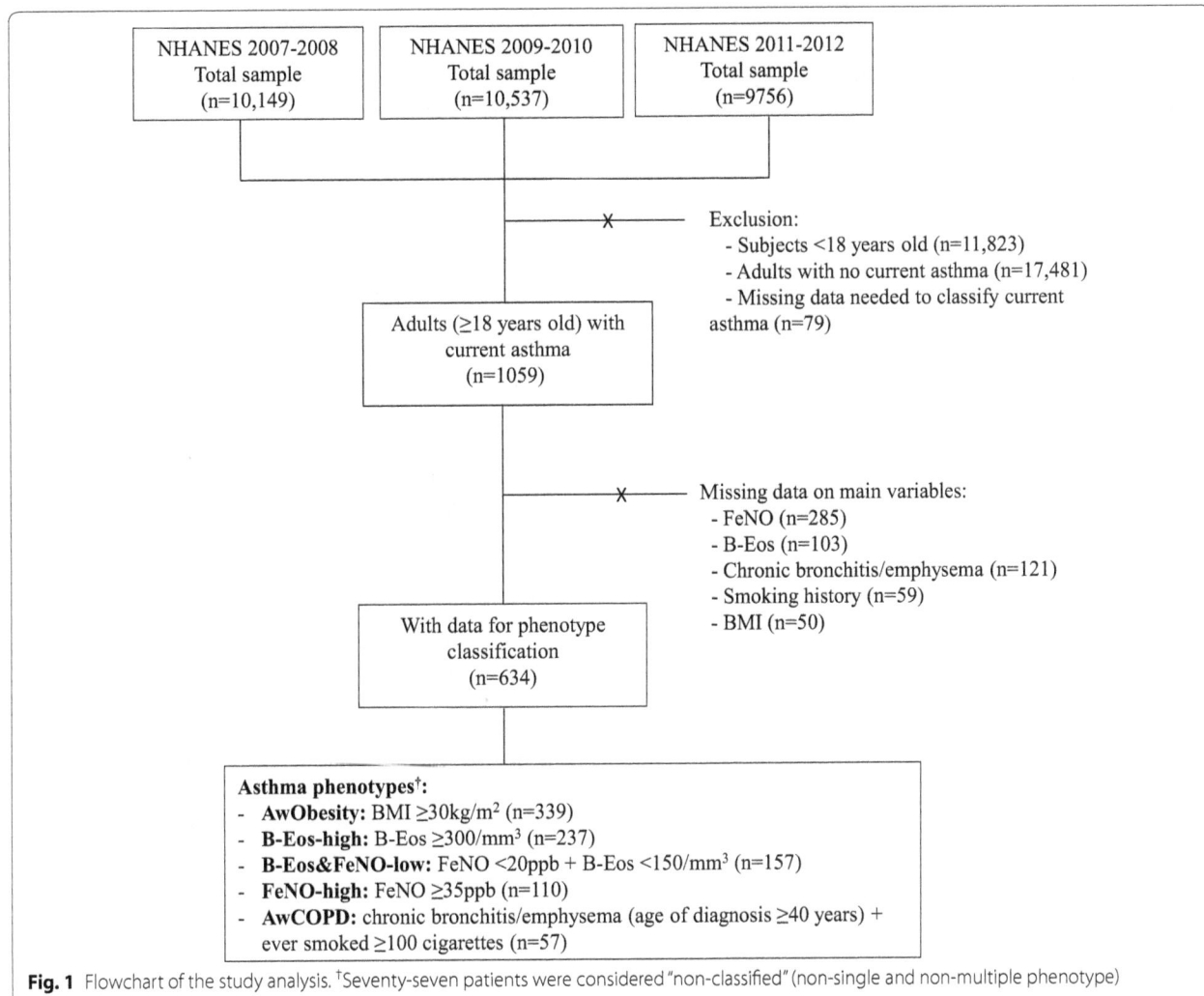

Fig. 1 Flowchart of the study analysis. †Seventy-seven patients were considered "non-classified" (non-single and non-multiple phenotype)

Statistical analysis

In accordance with the NHANES sampling design, the weights for each full sample 2-year mobile examination center were used to obtain weighted percentages adjusted to the US adult population.

Categorical variables were described as frequencies and weighted proportions, and continuous variables were described as median and first and third quartiles (Q1–Q3). Chi square test and Mann–Whitney U-test were used to compare groups. To explore the association of concomitant (having at least 2 concurrent) phenotypes with each asthma-related outcome we performed multivariate logistic regression modelling. Separate models were run using each asthma-related outcome and abnormal lung function as dependent variable and having multiple phenotypes as independent variables. Adjustments were also made for potential confounders: sex, age, race, current smoking and rhinitis. Adjusted odds ratios (aOR)

with 95% confidence intervals (95% CI) were presented, and model fit was assessed using the *svylogitgof* function [39].

According to age (< 40 or ≥ 40 years-old), a four- or five-set Venn-Euler diagram was used to quantify the proportion of individuals with different asthma phenotypes and to illustrate the overlap.

The diagrams were created using R software version 3.2.0 ("VennDiagram", "venneuler" and "reshape2" packages) and all statistical analyses were performed in Stata version 13.1 (StataCorp, TX, USA), using the *survey* command to account for the complex sampling design and weights in the NHANES. The *MI* command was used to perform sensitivity analysis by multiple-imputation of missing values; however, to create the Venn-Euler diagrams, a listwise deletion for missing data was applied. A p value < 0.05 was considered statistically significant.

Results

Of the 18,619 adults included in NHANES 2007–2012 datasets, 1059 (5.6% [95% CI 5.1–5.9]) had current asthma (Fig. 1). Of these, 63% were female, and the median (Q1–Q3) age was 48.0 (32.0–62.0) years. After excluding subjects with missing data on the main variables, 634 individuals were included for phenotype classification (Fig. 1). Despite having all information available, 77 patients did not meet the criteria for any of the defined asthma phenotypes and were considered "non-classified". These were non-obese subjects with asthma who did not meet the criteria for COPD, had B-Eos values ranging between 150 and 300/mm^3, and FeNO ranging 20–34 ppb.

Demographic characteristics of adults with current asthma included and excluded from the analysis and patients with single (n = 271) and multiple phenotypes (n = 286) are described in Table 1.

There is a female predominance in both groups (64 and 66%, respectively). Subjects with multiple phenotypes were older ($p = 0.003$), had higher BMI ($p < 0.001$), were more often obese ($p < 0.001$) and ex-smokers ($p = 0.003$), and a higher proportion of patients were treated with inhaled corticosteroids (ICS) ($p = 0.01$), than those with only one phenotype. Females were more obese, regardless the number of concomitant asthma phenotypes (data not shown).

Phenotypes and overlap description

The weighted proportions of asthma phenotypes were (in descending order): 49% for AwObesity, 36% for B-Eos-high asthma, 26% for B-Eos&FeNO-low asthma, 18% for FeNO-high asthma, and 8% for AwCOPD (Table 1).

Demographic and clinical characteristics among all 5 asthma phenotypes and the "non-classified" group are described in Table 2.

There is a female predominance among all phenotypes, particularly in the B-Eos&FeNO-low (78%). Subjects with AwCOPD phenotype were the oldest group (median [Q1–Q3]: 61.0 [52.0–69.0] years-old), with the lowest proportion of individuals that had ≥ high school and lowest FEV$_1$/FVC (0.63 [0.50–0.75]), comparing to the other phenotypes.

When categorized by age, < 40 (n = 227) and ≥ 40 years-old (n = 330), the most prevalent phenotypes were AwObesity (42 and 53%, respectively) and B-Eos-high asthma (34 and 37%). The less ones were FeNO-high asthma (18 and 19%) and AwCOPD (19% in the older group) (Fig. 2).

The areas of intersection in the four- and five-set Venn-Euler diagrams revealed 5 and 12 overlapping categories, and proportions of 17 and 12% of non-classified asthma subjects, respectively.

In both diagrams, a substantial total overlap was observed: 44% in subjects < 40 years-old and 54% in subjects ≥ 40 years-old. About 40% of the individuals in both age groups had two concomitant asthma phenotypes, 4% of the younger group had 3 concomitant phenotypes and 13% of the older group had ≥ 3 (Table 3 and Fig. 2). Furthermore, 1% of the older subjects had four concomitant asthma phenotypes: AwObesity, AwCOPD, FeNO-high, and B-Eos-high asthma.

The most prevalent overlaps in both groups (< 40 and ≥ 40 years-old) were AwObesity together with either B-Eos-high (15 and 12%, respectively) or B-Eos&FeNO-low asthma (13 and 11%) (Fig. 2).

Moreover, the proportions of subjects having AwObesity together with other phenotypes were high: 53% for the B-Eos-high phenotype, 48% for AwCOPD, 45% for the B-Eos&FeNO-low, and 44% for the FeNO-high phenotype. Also, the proportion of individuals having AwCOPD together with the B-Eos-high phenotype was high (36%), whereas the proportions were lower for the B-Eos&FeNO-low and the FeNO-high asthma phenotypes (15 and 10%, respectively) (data not shown).

In this population, only 12 and 15% of asthma subjects (< 40 and ≥ 40 years-old, respectively) with high B-Eos count had a concomitant high FeNO values (Fig. 2). Moreover, the two biomarkers were non-congruent across cut-offs. For example, when comparing groups with B-Eos count < 150/mm^3 and 150–300/mm^3, the proportion of asthma subjects having low FeNO (< 20 ppb), was not significantly different (Additional file 2: Table S1).

Associations between asthma-related outcomes and phenotype overlap

A comparison of the clinical characteristics of participants with one, two or three or more asthma phenotypes, stratified by age, is presented in Table 3 and no significant differences were observed in any age groups with regard to asthma attacks, asthma-related ED, ≥ 2 asthma symptoms, and use of ≥ 1 reliever. In the older group, the proportion of individuals with work/school absenteeism, ≥ 2 controller medications and with FEV$_1$/FVC < LLN was significantly higher in participants with concomitant phenotypes than in those with a single phenotype (Table 3). In both age groups, the proportion of patients with FEV$_1$ < LLN was significantly higher when participants presented multiple phenotypes, as well as they presented lower median FEV$_1$% predicted values.

When analyzing the asthma-related outcomes in subjects with a single phenotype with those having specific combination of asthma phenotypes, the overall findings were that subjects having multiple phenotypes had significantly higher proportion of using ≥ 1 reliever and ≥ 2

Table 1 Characteristics of adults with current asthma: included and excluded from phenotype classification, and stratified by single or multiple phenotypes

Demographic characteristics n (wt%)	Included subjects n = 634	Excluded subjects n = 425	p value*	Single phenotype[†] n = 271	Multiple phenotypes[†] n = 286	p value*
Female gender	410 (63)	261 (64)	0.93	174 (64)	192 (66)	0.68
Age (yrs), median (Q1–Q3)	44.0 (31.0–57.0)	48.9 (33.7–68.0)	*<0.001*	42.0 (30.0–55.0)	47.5 (34.0–60.0)	*0.003*
BMI (kg/m^2), median (Q1–Q3)	30.8 (25.4–35.9)	31.4 (24.4-35.7)	0.99	28.7 (24.2–35.0)	33.7 (30.7–39.0)	*<0.001*
Obesity status						
Underweight (≤ 18.4 kg/m^2)	2 (0.3)	13 (4)	*<0.001*	1 (0.2)	1 (0.5)	0.41
Normal (18.5–24.9 kg/m^2)	142 (25)	98 (27)	0.44	78 (30)	20 (8)	*<0.001*
Overweigh (25–29.9 kg/m^2)	151 (26)	77 (19)	0.07	80 (32)	38 (15)	*<0.001*
Obese (≥ 30 kg/m^2)	339 (49)	187 (49)	0.94	112 (38)	227 (77)	*<0.001*
Race and/or ethnicity						
Hispanic	105 (8)	85 (10)	0.30	38 (8)	56 (9)	0.24
Non-Hispanic white	323 (74)	184 (63)	*0.005*	135 (72)	138 (72)	0.93
Non-Hispanic black	167 (14)	117 (18)	*0.03*	76 (14)	81 (16)	0.71
Other Race	39 (4)	39 (7)	0.06	22 (6)	11 (3)	0.11
Smoking status						
Current smoker	199 (29)	114 (32)	0.40	89 (31)	87 (27)	0.46
Ex-smoker	163 (29)	98 (23)	0.13	56 (20)	89 (36)	*0.003*
Non-smoker	272 (43)	154 (45)	0.53	126 (49)	110 (37)	*0.02*
Education						
≥ High school	478 (84)	225 (69)	*<0.001*	205 (86)	209 (81)	0.13
Asthma-related medication[‡]						
Reliever medication**	276 (41)	202 (48)	0.16	113 (37)	132 (47)	0.10
Oral corticosteroids	33 (8)	29 (3)	*0.001*	12 (3)	15 (4)	0.75
Inhaled corticosteroids[§]	153 (25)	122 (30)	0.14	55 (19)	81 (32)	*0.01*
Other control medications[‖]	53 (9)	63 (14)	0.19	15 (8)	33 (10)	0.50
Asthma phenotype						
AwObesity	339 (49)	–		112 (38)	227 (76)	*<0.001*
B-Eos-high	237 (36)	–		61 (22)	176 (62)	*<0.001*
B-Eos&FeNO-low	157 (26)	–		74 (30)	83 (30)	0.95
FeNO-high	110 (18)	–		18 (8)	92 (34)	*<0.001*
AwCOPD	57 (8)	–		6 (2)	51 (17)	*<0.001*
Non-classified[††]	77 (14)	–		–	–	

Data presented as absolute numbers and proportions weighted for the U.S. population. *p* values <0.05 are presented in italic

Yrs years, *BMI* body mass index, *Q1* first quartile, *Q3* third quartile, *BMI* body mass index, *AwObesity* Asthma with obesity, *AwCOPD* Asthma with concurrent COPD

* Chi square test or Mann–Whitney U-test was used

[†] Seventy seven subjects included in the "non-classified" group were considered as missing

[‡] Prescribed medication taken in the past 30 days

[§] Alone or in combination with long-acting inhaled β$_2$-agonist

[‖] Included long-acting inhaled β$_2$-agonist (without corticosteroids), leukotriene inhibitors, and mast cell stabilizers

**Short-acting β$_2$-agonist and/or anticholinergic

[††] Subjects with non-single and non-multiple asthma phenotype

controller medications and had decreased lung function, with the exception of those with the B-Eos&FeNO-low phenotype combined with any of the other phenotypes (Additional file 3: Table S2, and Additional file 4: Table S3).

Moreover, a lower proportion of subjects reporting asthma attacks was observed in subjects with AwObesity and either FeNO-high (26%) or AwCOPD (20%), compared to those with a single phenotype (67%) (Additional file 3: Table S2). Subjects with concomitant AwCOPD and B-Eos&FeNO-low phenotypes had the lowest

Table 2 Demographic and clinical characteristics among all 5 phenotypes and in the "Non-classified" group

Characteristics n (wt%)	AwObesity n=339	B-Eos-high n=237	B-Eos&FeNO-low n=157	FeNO-high n=110	AwCOPD n=57	Non-classified[††] n=77
Female gender	366 (67)	196 (55)	138 (78)	78 (52)	71 (58)	44 (56)
Age (yrs), median (Q1–Q3)	48.0 (34.0–59.0)	47.0 (31.0–59.0)	41.0 (27.0–57.0)	45.0 (30.0–54.0)	61.0 (52.0–69.0)	39.0 (28.0–53.0)
BMI (kg/m²), median (Q1–Q3)	35.4 (32.5–40.4)	30.3 (25.9–36.8)	28.9 (24.2–33.0)	27.6 (24.9–33.4)	30.3 (25.1–35.1)	24.3 (22.8–27.5)
Race and/or ethnicity						
Hispanic	94 (9)	78 (11)	30 (8)	29 (10)	18 (4)	11 (6)
Non-Hispanic white	230 (65)	175 (73)	79 (69)	65 (75)	80 (81)	50 (86)
Non-Hispanic black	177 (21)	74 (12)	62 (17)	38 (13)	27 (11)	10 (6)
Other race	25 (5)	21 (4)	13 (6)	6 (2)	10 (4)	6 (2)
Smoking status						
Current smoker	150 (27)	104 (32)	48 (23)	18 (13)	65 (52)	23 (28)
Ex-smoker	134 (27)	100 (32)	35 (25)	42 (39)	70 (48)	18 (30)
Non-smoker	229 (45)	124 (35)	88 (51)	66 (49)	0 (0)	36 (42)
Education						
≥ High school	358 (79)	227 (80)	125 (81)	102 (87)	73 (59)	64 (91)
Asthma-related medication[‡]						
Reliever medication**	234 (42)	172 (51)	82 (44)	65 (46)	69 (57)	31 (36)
Oral corticosteroids	36 (5)	17 (5)	4 (2)	10 (7)	15 (7)	2 (2)
Inhaled corticosteroids[§]	144 (27)	103 (32)	36 (20)	36 (33)	60 (47)	17 (19)
Asthma-related outcomes						
Asthma attack	363 (68)	252 (74)	125 (68)	98 (71)	85 (63)	54 (75)
Asthma-related ED	130 (27)	80 (23)	41 (23)	26 (13)	37 (32)	9 (8)
> 2 asthma symptoms	311 (66)	199 (65)	92 (55)	80 (57)	90 (74)	42 (59)
Work/school absenteeism	66 (18)	43 (16)	25 (18)	23 (14)	12 (20)	10 (14)
Lung function						
FEV₁% predicted, median (Q1–Q3)	89.0 (75.6–99.2)	84.1 (75.2–95.4)	93.2 (83.8–100.8)	82.7 (75.9–95.4)	74.0 (62.9–90.1)	89.9 (80.5–103.5)
FEV₁/FVC, median (Q1–Q3)	0.77 (0.62–0.82)	0.74 (0.65–0.80)	0.79 (0.72–0.83)	0.72 (0.66–0.79)	0.63 (0.50–0.75)	0.76 (0.69–0.82)

Data presented as absolute numbers and proportions weighted for the U.S. population

Yrs years, *BMI* body mass index, *Q1* first quartile, *Q3* third quartile, *BMI* body mass index, *AwObesity* Asthma with obesity, *AwCOPD* Asthma with concurrent (COPD), *ED* emergency-department, *FEV1* Forced expiratory volume in 1 s, *FEV1/FVC* forced expiratory volume in 1 s and functional vital capacity ratio, *LLN* lower limit of normality

[††] Subjects with non-single and non-multiple asthma phenotype

[‡] Prescribed medication taken in the past 30 days

** Short-acting β₂-agonist and/or anticholinergic

[§] Alone or in combination with long-acting inhaled β₂-agonist

proportion of ≥2 asthma symptoms (20%), but had the highest proportion of using ≥1 reliever medication (84%) as well as having $FEV_1 < LLN$ (71%).

In multivariate regression analysis, adjusting for co-variables, having multiple phenotypes was significantly associated with using ≥2 controller medications (aOR, 95% CI 2.03, 1.16–3.57), and having reduced FEV_1 (3.21, 1.73–5.94) (Table 4). However, no associations were seen with asthma attacks, asthma-related ED, ≥2 asthma symptoms, work/school absenteeism, use of reliever medication or $FEV_1/FVC < LLN$ (Additional file 5: Table S4).

Furthermore, subjects aged ≥40 years-old, had significantly higher odds of using ≥2 controller medications and having $FEV_1 < LLN$ predicted, compared to those <40 years-old, adjusted for covariates (Table 4). Being a current smoker was significantly associated with using ≥1 reliever medication (1.95, 1.35–2.83) and with reduced lung function: $FEV_1 < LLN$ predicted (2.01, 1.21–3.33) and $FEV_1/FVC < LLN$ (2.02, 1.16–3.51) and not associated with any other asthma-related outcomes (Table 4 and Additional file 5: Table S4).

The association between having concomitant phenotypes and using multiple controller medications was consistent when considering oral corticosteroids (OCS) separated from other controller medications (1.87, 1.09–3.21) (data not shown).

Having concomitant asthma phenotypes is common and independently relates to poor lung...

85

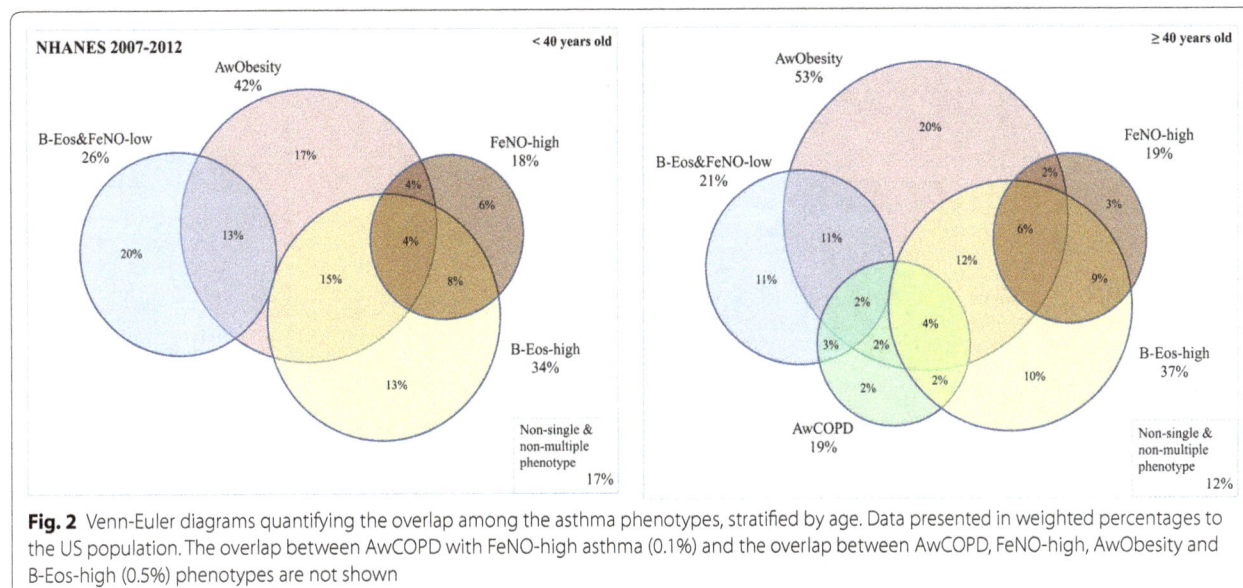

Fig. 2 Venn-Euler diagrams quantifying the overlap among the asthma phenotypes, stratified by age. Data presented in weighted percentages to the US population. The overlap between AwCOPD with FeNO-high asthma (0.1%) and the overlap between AwCOPD, FeNO-high, AwObesity and B-Eos-high (0.5%) phenotypes are not shown

We also analyzed the potential bias of controller medications in the phenotype classification, particularly in the B-Eos-high and FeNO-high phenotypes (Additional file 6: Fig. S1). No significant differences in asthma-related treatment were found between the phenotypes, with exception for a higher proportion of patients treated with ICS within the FeNO-high and B-Eos-high phenotypes compared to those with B-Eos&FeNO-low phenotype ($p = 0.03$). When restricting to subjects with a single asthma phenotype no significant differences were found.

Moreover, sensitivity analyses showed that the proportion of total overlap (weighted 53%), and the associations between having multiple phenotypes and asthma outcomes were similar when imputing all missing values (data not shown). The goodness-of-fit test revealed adequate fitting for all regression models, except when using $FEV_1/FVC < LLN$ as dependent variable (Additional file 5: Table S4) and no statistically significant interactions between co-variables were observed.

Discussion

We report a substantial overlap of commonly reported asthma phenotypes among adults with current asthma in a large population sample, with almost half of them having two or more concomitant phenotypes. Furthermore, having multiple asthma phenotypes, regardless of their classification, was associated with poorer asthma outcomes, particularly the use of more controller medication and reduced lung function.

These findings illustrate the complexity and unique features of the concomitant asthma phenotypes when categorizing asthma in adults, using only the "classical"

(hypothesis-driven) approach, based on measures readily available in the clinic (such as non-invasive biomarkers and medical records).

Hypothesis-driven asthma phenotypes are usually based on single dimensions of the disease, such as clinical symptoms, triggers, pathology or patterns of airway obstruction [16–18, 40–42]. However, evidence has shown that this approach is highly heterogenous, as it depends on the a priori assumptions and target population [43–45]. Also, it is of note that the 77 subjects with asthma that could not be classified as having any of the studied phenotypes, supports the fact that there is a considerable number of asthma patients whose clinical phenotype is not easily classified (e.g. asthmatics with irreversible airflow obstruction, patients with similar airways symptoms but with different pattern of airway inflammation), suggesting the presence of sub-phenotypes [1, 22, 44, 45].

In an attempt to explore the pathophysiology of specific asthma subgroups, and help stratify patients for targeted therapies, data-driven or unsupervised approaches (such as k-means, hierarchical clustering, partition-around-medoids methods or latent class analysis) are being applied in airways disease to identify "novel" accurate and distinct phenotypes, taking into account the heterogeneity and multidimensional characteristics of the disease [8, 46–52].

Our study results seem to be in line with the view of those that argue for a combination of both hypothesis- and data-driven approaches as a way forward to progress our knowledge on asthma endotypes and clinical phenotypes in an iterative way [52–54]. The data-driven

Table 3 Distribution and comparisons of the asthma-related outcomes among asthma phenotypes, stratified by age

	Total n (wt%)	Asthma attack	Asthma-related ED	≥2 asthma symptoms	Work/school absenteeism	Asthma medication		Lung function		
						≥1 reliever medication[†]	≥2 controller medication	FEV$_1$<LLN	FEV$_1$% predicted[§]	FEV$_1$/FVC<LLN
<40 yrs										
1 phenotype	118 (56)	85 (70)	27 (20)	59 (56)	15 (21)	55 (43)	17 (11)	10 (7)	95.6 (90.2–102.1)	26 (20)
2 phenotypes	97 (40)	69 (75)	26 (32)	57 (73)	12 (9)	41 (40)	8 (9)	19 (23)	91.8 (81.3–99.2)	25 (29)
3 phenotypes	12 (4)	10 (73)	5 (40)	8 (72)	4 (25)	9 (68)	1 (4)	3 (36)	81.9 (75.3–84.6)	4 (29)
*p value**										
1 versus 2		0.43	0.10	0.052	0.04	0.72	0.64	0.006	0.07	0.25
2 versus 3		0.92	0.55	0.96	0.07	0.15	0.46	0.43	0.009	0.98
1 versus 3		0.86	0.11	0.39	0.73	0.20	0.34	0.01	<0.001	0.48
≥40 yrs										
1 phenotype	153 (46)	104 (65)	35 (23)	76 (62)	20 (15)	58 (33)	26 (17)	29 (20)	91.2 (81.6–99.2)	34 (26)
2 phenotypes	136 (41)	92 (69)	28 (21)	70 (55)	12 (9)	60 (46)	43 (36)	31 (37)	80.4 (70.0–91.7)	27 (32)
≥3 phenotypes	41 (13)	26 (72)	4 (9)	30 (70)	8 (40)	22 (60)	16 (40)	12 (46)	74.0 (63.0–85.8)	16 (53)
*p value**										
1 versus 2		0.56	0.82	0.38	0.41	0.12	0.02	0.01	0.007	0.46
2 versus ≥3		0.80	0.27	0.30	0.002	0.24	0.67	0.47	0.22	0.09
1 versus ≥3		0.50	0.21	0.54	0.03	0.053	0.02	0.01	0.006	0.02

Data presented as absolute numbers and proportions weighted for the U.S. population. *p* values <0.05 are considered as missing. The 77 subjects included in the "non-classified" group were presented in italic. The 77 subjects included in the "non-classified" group were considered as missing

ED emergency-department, *FEV$_1$* forced expiratory volume in 1 s, *FEV$_1$/FVC* forced expiratory volume in 1 s and functional vital capacity ratio, *LLN* lower limit of normality, *Q1* first quartile; *Q3*: third quartile

* Chi square test or Mann–Whitney U-test was used

† Short-acting β$_2$-agonist or/and anticholinergic

§ Presented as median (Q1–Q3)

Table 4 Regression models with significant associations between having multiple asthma phenotypes and asthma-related outcomes, adjusted for co-variates

	≥ 2 controller medications		$FEV_1 < LLN$	
	aOR	95% CI	aOR	95% CI
Multiple versus single phenotype	*2.03*	*1.16–3.57*	*3.21*	*1.74–5.94*
Female gender	1.39	0.77–2.50	1.51	0.81–2.81
Age ≥ 40 yrs	*3.01*	*1.52–5.95*	2.55	*1.29–5.03*
Caucasian versus others	1.38	0.86–2.23	1.37	0.78–2.42
Current smoker versus non-/ex-smokers	1.02	0.52–2.02	*2.01*	*1.21–3.33*
Rhinitis	1.08	0.57–2.16	0.94	0.54–1.63
Goodness-of-fit test				
χ^2 (p value)	0.86 (0.56)		0.80 (0.61)	

Multivariate logistic regression models adjusted for gender, age, race, current smoking and rhinitis. The aOR values with $p < 0.05$ are presented in italic

FEV_1 forced expiratory volume in 1 s, *LLN* lower limit of normal, *CI* confidence interval, *aOR* adjusted odds ratio, χ^2 Chi square goodness-of-fit

phenotypes studies obtained some of the phenotypes already defined by hypothesis-driven approaches (e.g. obese, non-eosinophilic asthmatics [8]; persistent airway inflammation [46]; low type-2 inflammation [49]; fixed obstructive, non-eosinophilic and neutrophilic [50]), but, importantly, they identified other phenotypes that differ by certain characteristics: clinical parameters [8, 47–49], clinical response to treatment [46, 52], and airway inflammation [49, 51]. Therefore, further studies are required to compare and validate the asthma phenotypes obtained using different unsupervised methods.

The high overlap of asthma phenotypes seen in this study was similar to the findings of Tran et al. [15], who used datasets from previous NHANES surveys to evaluate the overlap of asthma phenotypes. However, Tran et al. study focused on allergic asthma phenotypes, based on IgE levels, and was therefore limited to the 2005–2006 survey that lacks data on FeNO. We provided a broader analysis of phenotypes that included not only the eosinophil-based phenotype (associated more closely with IL-5-driven) and the one based on FeNO values (mostly dependent on IL-4/IL-13-driven) [12], but also other phenotypes not defined by biomarkers and in a much larger dataset.

In this study, we extended previous observations [7, 11] suggesting that FeNO and B-Eos count partially reflect different inflammatory pathways, representing a local and a systemic type 2-marker, respectively. We observed that only 12–15% of asthma subjects with high B-Eos count had concomitant high FeNO levels, in this population. Also, a similar proportion of subjects with multiple

phenotypes was obtained when considering the "Type 2-high" phenotype, supporting the view that these two biomarkers are not interchangeable and that the use of both biomarkers in combination may allow for better targeted and personalized treatment for at least certain subsets of asthma patients [7, 10, 11].

The more prevalent combinations of phenotypes observed in this study were AwObesity together with either B-Eos-high or B-Eos&FeNO-low phenotypes. This supports the view that obesity-related asthma, despite often suggested to be a separate asthma phenotype associated with non-eosinophilic airway inflammation [9, 55, 56], may also be associated to eosinophilic inflammation.

Given the high prevalence in the US population, in this sample, obesity is likely to be a comorbidity, rather than the primary reason for asthma [57]; however, we defined the AwObesity phenotype as a separate group, since the interdependence on inflammatory markers to targeting different asthma therapies makes essential the accurate characterization of inflammation in obese asthmatic subjects [19, 58]. In addition, the relevance of defining the AwObesity phenotype is supported by the data as the weighted proportion of overlap is similar when excluding AwObesity or B-Eos-high phenotype from the analysis (data not shown). Moreover, the weighted proportion of subjects with "non-classified" asthma doubled when excluding the AwObesity phenotype (increasing to 32% in the < 40 years-old and 29% in ≥ 40 years old).

Having multiple asthma phenotypes was more common in older subjects and in non- and former- smokers; whether this is due to a general increase of comorbidities with age [58–60] and/or an interaction with environmental factors [61] cannot be specifically addressed by this study design. Nevertheless, when interpreting these results one should bear in mind that AwCOPD is associated to older age and prior/current smoking while FeNO increases with age and decreases with smoking [62, 63].

Interestingly, subjects with a higher number of concomitant asthma phenotypes presented reduced lung function and this association remained when controlling for potential confounders by multiple regression analysis. This shows that having multiple phenotypes is independently associated with reduced lung function, suggesting a cumulative effect of different disease processes.

Moreover, patients having several commonly reported asthma phenotypes had higher odds of using more controller medications, supporting the view that these patients are those with more complex disease and higher asthma morbidity [9, 15]. This also suggests that these asthma patients have an inadequate response to prescribed therapies, since lung function was reduced, and that they may represent a group of patients with the need for add-on treatment. However, the choice of specific treatments, such as biological therapies, will be more difficult considering the complexity introduced by having multiple phenotypes.

The lack of significant associations between multiple phenotypes and the other asthma-related outcomes may be difficult to understand. A possible explanation could be that the prescribed medication is effective against asthma symptoms and attacks but less effective against (subclinical) processes that cause long-term reduction in lung function. However, the results could also be related to data collection methods, as lung function measurement and the way medication use was ascertained, were less dependent on patient recall than the self-reported variables that were used for the outcomes with null results in the present study. Further studies should be done, adding the quantitative assessment of asthma attacks/asthma-related ED visits, and also including the age of asthma onset, that could have an influence on asthma-related outcomes.

This study has several limitations. First, because of its cross-sectional design, it was not possible to evaluate interactions between phenotypes over time in patients with concomitant phenotypes, nor was it possible to determine which phenotype occurred first. Second, although there were differences between the included and excluded groups in the variables age, BMI, non-Hispanic white/black subjects, having finished high school and OCS use, the majority were not used for phenotypic classification and did not affect the outcomes, as shown in sensitivity analysis. Third, as our asthma and COPD definitions were based on self-reported diagnosis, rather than relying on lung function tests, the acquired information is subject to recall bias and misclassification. However, these definitions have been commonly used in NHANES reports [7, 11, 15] and have proven to be reasonably reliable [64, 65]. Moreover, we have used the most frequent combination of questions seen in epidemiological studies [65, 66], and we also included questions on recent wheeze and/or asthma attacks, which should reduce the risk of including individuals without true disease. Also, we stratified the analysis by age (at 40 years), as used in other COPD studies [37, 67], in order to improve the clinical value into the interpretation of phenotyping data, as the overlap among asthma phenotypes will be different among those less than age 40 and those older than 40 (with higher possibility of having COPD) [37]. Fourth, the lack of other biomarkers in the present NHANES years, prevented the analysis of other asthma phenotypes and the use of alternative definitions. However, we analyzed biomarkers of type 2-inflammation in both blood and exhaled air that previously have been shown to independently relate to asthma morbidity [7, 11]. Fifth, as there is no consensual definition of

biomarker-defined asthma phenotypes, we based our definitions on cut-offs used in previous studies to discriminate patients in single asthma phenotypes [32–35], rather than on any reported specificity or sensitivity for predicting asthma morbidity or response to therapeutics [68, 69]. For high probability of eosinophilic inflammation, the cut-off value for FeNO has been suggested to be >50 ppb for adults [70]. However, we chose a FeNO cut-off of 35 ppb, based on the mean baseline FeNO levels of patients included in randomized controlled trials of anti-IL-13 treatment [33, 69]. In spite of using this lower cut-off, 77 subjects with current asthma could not be classified as having any of the predefined phenotypes, indicating the need for better, and probably personalized, cut-offs for biomarkers in asthma.

Furthermore, we could not demonstrate a clear effect of ongoing controller medication in the phenotypic classification in our data. No significant associations were observed, probably at least partially explained with the exclusion of the participants with ICS/OCS use <48 h prior to the exhaled NO measurements. Also, contrary to the expected, we observed a higher proportion of patients treated with ICS/OCS within both B-Eos-high and FeNO-high phenotypes than the B-Eos&FeNO-low phenotype. A plausible explanation is that subjects with ongoing inflammation have more clear asthma, with more symptoms, and, thus, a higher need of treatment. B-Eos&FeNO-low asthma is a heterogeneous group with less need of controller treatment, and because the treatment is ineffective, it may be that medication use and even prescription has been stopped.

Finally, even though we did not specifically analyze the overlap of asthma phenotypes in patients with severe asthma, the significant association between presenting more than one phenotype and being treated with multiple asthma controller medications suggests higher asthma severity in this subset [71]. Also, we did not consider individual environmental factors, such as air pollution and/or indoor allergens, that could influence asthma phenotypes. Further studies describing the overlap in patients with severe asthma and studies examining asthma patients exposed to different environmental factors, such as subjects who live in cities versus in rural areas are needed.

This study indicates that the overlap of commonly reported asthma phenotypes is observed also in non-selected asthma patients from the general population. Our findings highlight the importance of classifying asthma patients with regard to applicable phenotypes, rather than using a single asthma phenotype, to enable the development of adequate targeted strategies to avoid lung function impairment. However, further data is required, such as that from higher order analysis, using data-mining methods possibly combined with those that rely on predefined hypotheses. This synergy is expected to improve the knowledge on asthma phenotypes and, ultimately, to lead to more personalized treatment strategies [53, 54].

Conclusions

In conclusion, a prevalent overlap of commonly reported phenotypes was observed in asthma patients identified from the general population. Subjects classified as having multiple phenotypes used more controller medications and had reduced lung function. Thus, the complexity and unique features of concomitant asthma phenotypes may require a broader data analysis approach, based on a combination of clinical information and biomarkers resulting in better characterization of patients. This could lead to better asthma outcomes, particularly preserved lung function.

Additional files

Additional file 1. Supplementary Methods.

Additional file 2: Table S1. Distribution and comparisons between the FeNO and B-Eos cut-offs used in this study, among individuals with current asthma.

Additional file 3: Table S2. Weighted percentages and comparisons of asthma-related outcomes among subjects with a single asthma phenotype versus: non-classified, and specific combinations of asthma phenotypes.

Additional file 4: Table S3. Weighted percentages and comparisons of asthma-related outcomes among subjects with a single asthma phenotype versus: non-classified, and specific combinations of asthma phenotypes.

Additional file 5: Table S4. Multivariable logistic regression models between each asthma-related outcome and having multiple asthma phenotypes, adjusted for co-variables.

Additional file 6: Fig. S1. Proportions (weighted to the US population) of subjects taking asthma controller medications stratified into the different phenotypes, among all participants included for asthma phenotype classification (left) and only in those with a single phenotype (right). P-values <0.05 were indicated. NA: Non-applicable (not possible to determine because some participants had both B-Eos-high and FeNO-high asthma phenotypes).

Abbreviations

aOR: adjusted odds ratios; ATS/ERS: American Thoracic Society/European Respiratory Society; AwCOPD: asthma with concurrent COPD; AwObesity: asthma with obesity; B-Eos: blood eosinophils; BMI: body mass index; COPD: chronic obstructive pulmonary disease; CI: confidence intervals; ED: emergency department; FeNO: fraction of exhaled nitric oxide; FEV_1: forced expiratory volume in 1 s; FEV_1/FVC: ratio of forced expiratory volume in 1 s to forced vital capacity; ICS: inhaled corticosteroids; IgE: immunoglobulin E; IL: interleukin; LLN: lower limit of normal; NHANES: National Health and Nutrition Examination Survey (USA); OCS: oral corticosteroids; Q1: first quartile; Q3: third quartile; Th2: T helper cell type 2.

Authors' contributions

RA, JAF, AM and KA contributed to study conception and design, analysis and interpretation of data, writing and revising the article. TJ, AMP and CJ

contributed to data interpretation, writing and revising the article. All authors read and approved the final version of the manuscript.

Author details

[1] CINTESIS- Center for Health Technology and Services Research, Faculty of Medicine, University of Porto, Edifício Nascente, Piso 2, Rua Dr. Plácido da Costa, s/n, 4200-450 Porto, Portugal. [2] Department of Cardiovascular and Respiratory Sciences, Porto Health School, Porto, Portugal. [3] MEDCIDS- Department of Community Medicine, Information, and Health Sciences, Faculty of Medicine, University of Porto, Porto, Portugal. [4] Department of Allergy, Instituto & Hospital CUF, Porto, Portugal. [5] Department of Medical Sciences: Clinical Physiology, Uppsala University, Uppsala, Sweden. [6] Department of Medical Sciences: Respiratory Medicine and Allergology, Uppsala University, Uppsala, Sweden. [7] Department of Women's and Children's Health: Paediatric Research, Uppsala University, Uppsala, Sweden.

Acknowledgements

RA is supported by Fundação para a Ciência e Tecnologia (PhD grant – Ref. PD/BD/113659/2015), Portugal.

Competing interests

The authors declare that they have no competing interests.

Funding

Project "NORTE-01-0145-FEDER-000016" is financed by the North Portugal Regional Operational Programme (NORTE 2020), under the PORTUGAL 2020 Partnership Agreement, and through the European Regional Development Fund (ERDF).

References

1. Froidure A, Mouthuy J, Durham SR, Chanez P, Sibille Y, Pilette C. Asthma phenotypes and IgE responses. Eur Respir J. 2016;47:304–19.
2. Corren J. Asthma phenotypes and endotypes: an evolving paradigm for classification. Discov Med. 2013;15(83):243–9.
3. Woodruff PG, Modrek B, Choy DF, Jia G, Abbas AR, Ellwanger A, Koth LL, Arron JR, Fahy JV. T-helper type 2-driven inflammation defines major subphenotypes of asthma. Am J Respir Crit Care Med. 2009;180(5):388–95.
4. Robinson D, Humbert M, Buhl R, Cruz AC, Inoue H, Korom S, Hanania NA, Nair P. Revisiting Type 2-high and Type 2-low airway inflammation in asthma: current knowledge and therapeutic implications. Clin Exp Allergy. 2017;47(2):161–75.
5. Hastie AT, Moore WC, Li H, Rector BM, Ortega VE, Pascual RM, Peters SP, Meyers DA, Bleecker ER, National Heart, Lung, and Blood Institute's Severe Asthma Research Program. Biomarker surrogates do not accurately

predict sputum eosinophil and neutrophil percentages in asthmatic subjects. J Allergy Clin Immunol. 2013;132(1):72.e12–80.e12.

6. Green RH, Brightling CE, Woltmann G, Parker D, Wardlaw AJ, Pavord ID. Analysis of induced sputum in adults with asthma: identification of subgroup with isolated sputum neutrophilia and poor response to inhaled corticosteroids. Thorax. 2002;57(10):875–9.

7. Malinovschi A, Fonseca JA, Jacinto T, Alving K, Janson C. Exhaled nitric oxide levels and blood eosinophil counts independently associate with wheeze and asthma events in National Health and Nutrition Examination Survey subjects. J Allergy Clin Immunol. 2013;132(4):821.e5–27.e5.

8. Jia G, Erickson RW, Choy DF, Mosesova S, Wu LC, Solberg OD, et al. Periostin is a systemic biomarker of eosinophilic airway inflammation in asthmatic patients. J Allergy Clin Immunol. 2012;130(3):647.e10–54.e10.

9. Haldar P, Pavord ID, Shaw DE, Berry MA, Thomas M, Brightling CE, et al. Cluster analysis and clinical asthma phenotypes. Am J Respir Crit Care Med. 2008;178(3):218–24.

10. Jia G, Erickson RW, Choy DF, Mosesova S, Wu LC, Solberg OD, Shikotra A, Carter R, Audusseau S, Hamid Q, et al. Identification of airway mucosal type 2 inflammation by using clinical biomarkers in asthmatic patients. J Allergy Clin Immunol. 2017;140(3):710–9.

11. Malinovschi A, Janson C, Borres M, Alving K. Simultaneously increased fraction of exhaled nitric oxide levels and blood eosinophil counts relate to increased asthma morbidity. J Allergy Clin Immunol. 2016;138(5):1301. e2–308.e2.

12. Katial RK, Bensch GW, Busse WW, Chipps BE, Denson JL, Gerber AN, Jacobs JS, Kraft M, Martin RJ, Nair P, et al. Changing paradigms in the treatment of severe asthma: the role of biologic therapies. J Allergy Clin Immunol Pract. 2017;5(2):S1–14.

13. Chung KF, Adcock IM. How variability in clinical phenotypes should guide research into disease mechanisms in asthma. Ann Am Thorac Soc. 2013;10(Suppl):S109–17.

14. Merritt F. Blood eosinophils: the Holy Grail for asthma phenotyping? Ann Allergy Asthma Immunol. 2016;116(2):90–1.

15. Tran TN, Zeiger RS, Peters SP, Colice G, Newbold P, Goldman M, Chipps BE. Overlap of atopic, eosinophilic, and TH2-high asthma phenotypes in a general population with current asthma. Ann Allergy Asthma Immunol. 2016;116(1):37–42.

16. Borish L. The immunology of asthma: asthma phenotypes and their implications for personalized treatment. Ann Allergy Asthma Immunol. 2016;117(2):108–14.

17. Hekking PPW, Bel EH. Developing and emerging clinical asthma phenotypes. J Allergy Clin Immunol Pract. 2014;2(6):671–80.

18. Wenzel SE. Asthma phenotypes: the evolution from clinical to molecular approaches. Nat Med. 2012;18(5):716–25.

19. Gibeon D, Batuwita K, Osmond M, Heaney LG, Brightling CE, Niven R, et al. Obesity-associated severe asthma represents a distinct clinical phenotype: analysis of the British Thoracic Society Difficult Asthma Registry Patient cohort according to BMI. Chest. 2013;143(2):406–14.

20. Kobayashi S, Hanagama M, Yamanda S, Ishida M, Yanai M. Inflammatory biomarkers in asthma-COPD overlap syndrome. Int J Chronic Obstr Pulm Dis. 2016;11:2117–23.

21. Carr TF, Zeki AA, Kraft M. Eosinophilic and noneosinophilic asthma. Am J Respir Crit Care Med. 2018;197(1):22–37.

22. Christenson SA, Steiling K, van den Berge M, Hijazi K, Hiemstra PS, Postma DS, Lenburg ME, Spira A, Woodruff PG, et al. Asthma-COPD overlap. Clinical relevance of genomic signatures of type 2 inflammation in chronic obstructive pulmonary disease. Am J Respir Crit Care Med. 2015;191(7):758–66.

23. Complete Blood Count. http://www.cdc.gov/nchs/data/nhanes/nhanes_11_12/cbc_g_met_he.pdf. Accessed 17 June 2017.

24. Respiratory Health ENO Procedures Manual. www.cdc.gov/nchs/data/nhanes/nhanes_11_12/Respiratory_Health_ENO_Procedures_Manual.pdf. Accessed 26 May 2017.

25. Respiratory Health Spirometry Procedures Manual. https://www.cdc.gov/nchs/data/nhanes/nhanes_11_12/spirometry_procedures_manual.pdf. Accessed 6 June 2017.

26. ATS/ERS. ATS/ERS Recommendations for Standardized Procedures for the Online and Offline Measurement of Exhaled Lower Respiratory Nitric Oxide and Nasal Nitric Oxide, 2005. Am J Respir Crit Care Med. 2005;171(8):912–30.

27. Miller MR. Standardisation of spirometry. Eur Respir J. 2005;26(2):319–38.

28. Hankinson JL, Odencrantz JR, Fedan KB. Spirometric reference values from a sample of the general U.S. population. Am J Respir Crit Care Med. 1999;159(1):179–87.

29. Hankinson JL, Kawut SM, Shahar E, Smith LJ, Stukovsky KH, Barr RG. Performance of American Thoracic Society-recommended spirometry reference values in a multiethnic sample of adults. Chest. 2010;137(1):138–45.

30. Pellegrino R, Viegi G, Brusasco V, Crapo RO, Burgos F, Casaburi R, Coates A, van der Grinten CP, Gustafsson P, Hankinson J, et al. Interpretative strategies for lung function tests. Eur Respir J. 2005;26(5):948–68.

31. Prescription Medications - Drug Information. http://wwwn.cdc.gov/Nchs/Nhanes/1999-2000/RXQ_DRUG.htm. Accessed 6 June 2017.

32. Castro M, Zangrilli J, Wechsler ME, Bateman ED, Brusselle GG, Bardin P, Murphy K, Maspero JF, O'Brien C, Korn S. Reslizumab for inadequately controlled asthma with elevated blood eosinophil counts: results from two multicentre, parallel, double-blind, randomised, placebo-controlled, phase 3 trials. Lancet Respir Med. 2015;3:355–66.

33. Wenzel S, Ford L, Pearlman D, Spector S, Sher L, Skobieranda F, Wang L, Kirkesseli S, Rocklin R, Bock B, et al. Dupilumab in persistent asthma with elevated eosinophil levels. N Engl J Med. 2013;368(26):2455–66.

34. Dweik RA, Sorkness RL, Wenzel S, Hammel J, Curran-Everett D, Comhair SA, Bleecker E, Busse W, Calhoun WJ, Castro M, et al. Use of exhaled nitric oxide measurement to identify a reactive, at-risk phenotype among patients with asthma. Am J Respir Crit Care Med. 2010;181(10):1033–41.

35. McGrath KW, Icitovic N, Boushey HA, Lazarus SC, Sutherland ER, Chinchilli VM, Fahy JV, Asthma Clinical Research Network of the National Heart, Lung, and Blood Institute. A large subgroup of mild-to-moderate asthma is persistently noneosinophilic. Am J Respir Crit Care Med. 2012;185(6):612–9.

36. Flegal KM, Carroll MD, Kuczmarski RJ, Johnson CL. Overweight and obesity in the United States: prevalence and trends, 1960–1994. Int J Obes Relat Metab Disord. 1998;22(1):39–47.

37. Buist AS, McBurnie MA, Vollmer WM, Gillespie S, Burney P, Mannino DM, et al. International variation in the prevalence of COPD (The BOLD Study): a population-based prevalence study. Lancet. 2007;370(9589):741–50.

38. Diagnosis of Diseases of Chronic Airflow Limitation: Asthma, COPD and Asthma-COPD Overlap Syndrome (ACOS). http://goldcopd.org/asthma-copd-asthma-copd-overlap-syndrome/. Accessed 3 Jan 2017.

39. Archer KJ, Lemeshow S. Goodness-of-fit test for a logistic regression model fitted using survey sample data. Stata J. 2006;6(1):97–105.

40. Hirano T, Matsunaga K. Late-onset asthma: current perspectives. J Asthma and Allergy. 2018;11:19–27.

41. Wenzel SE. Asthma: defining of the persistent adult phenotypes. Lancet. 2006;368:804–13.

42. Vonk JM, Jongepier H, Panhuysen CIM, Schouten JP, Bleecker ER, Postma DS. Risk factors associated with the presence of irreversible airflow limitation and reduced transfer coefficient in patients with asthma after 26 years of follow up. Thorax. 2003;58(4):322–7.

43. Bousquet J, Anto JM, Sterk PJ, Adcock IM, Chung KF, Roca J, et al. Systems medicine and integrated care to combat chronic noncommunicable diseases. Genome Med. 2011;3:43.

44. Agusti A, Bel E, Thomas M, Vogelmeier C, Brusselle G, Holgate S, Humbert M, Jones P, Gibson PG, Vestbo J, et al. Treatable traits: toward precision medicine of chronic airway diseases. Eur Respir J. 2016;47(2):410–9.

45. Zedan MM, Laimon WN, Osman AM, Zedan MM. Clinical asthma phenotyping: a trial for bridging gaps in asthma management. World J Clin Pediatr. 2015;4(2):13–8.

46. Wu W, Bleecker E, Moore W, Busse WW, Castro M, Chung KF, Calhoun WJ, Erzurum S, Gaston B, Israel E, et al. Unsupervised phenotyping of Severe Asthma Research Program participants using expanded lung data. J Allergy Clin Immunol. 2014;133(5):1280–8.

47. Moore WC, Meyers DA, Wenzel SE, Teague WG, Li H, Li X, D'Agostino R Jr, Castro M, Curran-Everett D, Fitzpatrick AM, et al. Identification of asthma phenotypes using cluster analysis in the Severe Asthma Research Program. Am J Respir Crit Care Med. 2010;181(4):315–23.

48. Siroux V, Basagaña X, Boudier A, Pin I, Garcia-Aymerich J, Vesin A, Slama R, Jarvis D, Anto JM, Kauffmann F, Sunyer J. Identifying adult asthma phenotypes using a clustering approach. Eur Respir J. 2011;38(2):310–7.

49. Lefaudeux D, de Meulder B, Loza MJ, Peffer N, Rowe A, Baribaud F, Bansal AT, Lutter R, Sousa AR, Corfield J, et al. U-BIOPRED clinical adult asthma clusters linked to a subset of sputum omics. J Allergy Clin Immunol. 2017;139:1797–807.

50. Loza MJ, Adcock I, Auffray C, Chung KF, Djukanovic R, Sterk PJ, Susulic VS, Barnathan ES, Baribaud F, Silkoff PE, et al. Longitudinally stable, clinically defined clusters of patients with asthma independently identified in the ADEPT and U-BIOPRED asthma studies. Ann Am Thorac Soc. 2016;13(Suppl 1):S102–3.

51. Loza MJ, Djukanovic R, Chung KF, Horowitz D, Ma K, Branigan P, Barnathan ES, Susulic VS, Silkoff PE, Sterk PJ, et al. Validated and longitudinally stable asthma phenotypes based on cluster analysis of the ADEPT study. Respir Res. 2016;17(1):165.

52. Clemmer GL, Wu AC, Rosner B, McGeachie MJ, Litonjua AA, Tantisira KG, Weiss ST. Measuring the corticosteroid responsiveness endophenotype in asthmatic patients. J Allergy Clin Immunol. 2015;136(2):274.e8–81.e8.

53. Belgrave D, Henderson J, Simpson A, Buchan I, Bishop C, Custovic A. Disaggregating asthma: big investigation vs. big data. J Allergy Clin Immunol. 2016;139(2):400–7.

54. Bousquet J, Anto JM, Akdis M, Auffray C, Keil T, Momas I, Postma DS, Valenta R, Wickman M, Cambon-Thomsen A, et al. Paving the way of systems biology and precision medicine in allergic diseases: the MeDALL success story. Allergy. 2016;71(11):1513–25.

55. Leiria LOS, Martins MA, Saad MJA. Obesity and asthma: beyond TH2 inflammation. Metabolism. 2015;64(2):172–81.

56. Bates JHT, Poynter ME, Frodella CM, Peters U, Dixon AE, Suratt BT. Pathophysiology to phenotype in the asthma of obesity. Ann Am Thorac Soc. 2017;14(Supplement 5):S395–8.

57. Gonzalez-Barcala FJ, Pertega S, Perez-Castro T, Sampedro M, Sanchez-Lastres J, San-Jose-Gonzalez MA, Bamonde L, Garnelo L, Valdés-Cuadrado L, Moure JD, et al. Obesity and asthma: an association modified by age. Allergol Immunopathol (Madr). 2013;41(3):176–80.

58. Amelink M, De Nijs SB, De Groot JC, Van Tilburg PMB, Van Spiegel PI, Krouwels FH, et al. Three phenotypes of adult-onset asthma. Allergy. 2013;68(5):674–80.

59. Ledford DK, Lockey RF. Asthma and comorbidities. Curr Opin Allergy Clin Immunol. 2013;13(1):78–86.

60. Yanez A, Cho S-H, Soriano JB, Rosenwasser LJ, Rodrigo GJ, Rabe KF, Peters S, Niimi A, Ledford DK, Katial R, et al. Asthma in the elderly: what we know and what we have yet to know. World Allergy Organ J. 2014;7(1):8.

61. Miller RL, Ho SM. Environmental epigenetics and asthma: current concepts and call for studies. Am J Respir Crit Care Med. 2008;177(6):567–73.

62. Jacinto T, Malinovschi A, Janson C, Fonseca J, Alving K. Evolution of exhaled nitric oxide levels throughout development and aging of healthy humans. J Breath Res. 2015;9(3):36005.

63. Jacinto T, Malinovschi A, Janson C, Fonseca J, Alving K. Differential effect of cigarette smoke exposure on exhaled nitric oxide and blood eosinophils in healthy and asthmatic individuals. J Breath Res. 2017;11(3):036006.

64. Halldin CN, Doney BC, Hnizdo E. Changes in prevalence of chronic obstructive pulmonary disease and asthma in the US population and associated risk factors. Chron Respir Dis. 2015;12(1):47–60.

65. Sá-Sousa A, Jacinto T, Azevedo LF, Morais-Almeida M, Robalo-Cordeiro C, Bugalho-Almeida A, Bousquet J, Fonseca JA. Operational definitions of asthma in recent epidemiological studies are inconsistent. Clin Transl Allergy. 2014;4:24.

66. de Marco R, Cerveri I, Bugiani M, Ferrari M, Verlato G. An undetected burden of asthma in Italy: the relationship between clinical and epidemiological diagnosis of asthma. Eur Respir J. 1998;11(3):599–605.

67. Menezes AMB, Perez-Padilla R, Jardim JRB, Muiño A, Lopez MV, Valdivia G, et al. Chronic obstructive pulmonary disease in five Latin American cities (the PLATINO study): a prevalence study. Lancet. 2005;366(9500):1875–81.

68. Hanania NA, Noonan M, Corren J, Korenblat P, Zheng Y, Fischer SK, Cheu M, Putnam WS, Murray E, Scheerens H, et al. Lebrikizumab in moderate-to-severe asthma: pooled data from two randomised placebo-controlled studies. Thorax. 2015;70(8):748–56.

69. Corren J, Lemanske RF, Hanania NA, Korenblat PE, Parsey MV, Arron JR, Harris JM, Scheerens H, Wu LC, Su Z, et al. Lebrikizumab treatment in adults with asthma. N Engl J Med. 2011;365(12):1088–98.

70. Dweik RA, Boggs PB, Erzurum SC, Irvin CG, Leigh MW, Lundberg JO, Olin AC, Plummer AL. Taylor DR; American Thoracic Society Committee on Interpretation of Exhaled Nitric Oxide Levels (FENO) for Clinical Applications. An official ATS clinical practice guideline: interpretation of exhaled nitric oxide levels (FENO) for clinical applications. Am J Respir Crit Care Med. 2011;184(5):602–15.

71. Global Strategy for Asthma Management and Prevention 2016. http://ginasthma.org/2016-gina-report-global-strategy-for-asthma-management-and-prevention/. Accessed 12 May 2017.

10

The state of asthma epidemiology: an overview of systematic reviews and their quality

Jon Genuneit[1]*[iD], Annina M. Seibold[1], Christian J. Apfelbacher[2], George N. Konstantinou[3], Jennifer J. Koplin[4], Stefania La Grutta[5], Kirsty Logan[6], Carsten Flohr[7], Michael R. Perkin[8] and for the Task Force "Overview of Systematic Reviews in Allergy Epidemiology (OSRAE)" of the EAACI Interest Group on Epidemiology

Abstract

Background: Recently, we have published an overview of systematic reviews in allergy epidemiology and identified asthma as the most commonly reviewed allergic disease. Building on this work, we aimed to investigate the quality of systematic reviews in asthma using the AMSTAR checklist and to provide a reference for future, more in-depth assessment of the extent of previous knowledge.

Methods: We included all 307 systematic reviews indexed with asthma, including occupational asthma, and/or wheeze from our previous search in PubMed and EMBASE up to December 2014 for systematic reviews on epidemiological research on allergic diseases. Topics of the included systematic reviews were indexed and we applied the AMSTAR checklist for methodological quality to all. Statistical analyses include description of lower and upper bounds of AMSTAR scores and variation across publication time and topics.

Results: Of 43 topics catalogued, family history, birth weight, and feeding of formula were only covered once in systematic reviews published from 2011 onwards. Overall, at least one meta-analysis was conducted for all topics except for "social determinants", "perinatal", "birth weight", and "climate". AMSTAR quality scores were significantly higher in more recently published systematic reviews, in those with meta-analysis, and in Cochrane reviews. There was evidence of variation of quality across topics even, after accounting for these characteristics. Genetic factors in asthma development were often covered by systematic reviews with some evidence of unsubstantiated updates or repetition.

Conclusions: We present a comprehensive overview with an indexed database of published systematic reviews in asthma epidemiology including quality scores. We highlight some topics including active smoking and pets, which should be considered for future systematic reviews. We propose that our search strategy and database could be a basis for topic-specific overviews of systematic reviews in asthma epidemiology.

Background

The state of current knowledge of asthma epidemiology has been summarised in numerous narrative expert reviews including the Global Atlas of Asthma of the European Academy of Allergy and Clinical Immunology and the European Lung White Book of the European Respiratory Society [1, 2]. With an ever increasing number of systematic reviews on asthma epidemiology, systematic overviews of these systematic reviews become more and more important to keep track of the evidence, to prevent redundancy, and to provide comprehensive summaries informing decision makers. However, to date there are only two overviews of systematic reviews in asthma epidemiology and both only cover specific aspects of asthma epidemiology [3, 4].

One overview of systematic reviews, providing a meta-analysis of risk and protective factors on childhood asthma, included 42 systematic reviews published up to January 2016 [3]. Of note, this was focused on childhood, on non-genetic factors, and on systematic reviews with

---

*Correspondence: jon.genuneit@uni-ulm.de
[1] Institute of Epidemiology and Medical Biometry, Ulm University, Helmholtzstr. 22, 89081 Ulm, Germany
Full list of author information is available at the end of the article

meta-analysis. Another overview of systematic reviews was restricted to the association of diet with asthma [4]. We are also aware of three systematic reviews which have examined the original literature rather than systematic reviews on some areas of asthma epidemiology: The first searched for articles describing risk factors for asthma incidence and the second aimed at comprehensively reviewing the original literature on selected risk and protective factors for asthma [5, 6]. The third conducted a more specific search to identify original articles on the genetic predisposition to asthma and atopy over a period of 6 years [7].

Recently, we have published a comprehensive overview on systematic reviews in allergy epidemiology which has identified a total of 307 systematic reviews covering asthma and wheeze [8]. Building on our previous work, we aimed here to investigate the systematic reviews' quality using the AMSTAR checklist [9] and to provide a reference for future, more in-depth assessments of individual topic areas.

Methods

The complete search strategy has been published previously [8]. In brief, we searched PubMed and EMBASE (via OVID, including conference abstracts) for systematic reviews on epidemiological research on allergic diseases. The databases were searched from their inception without restrictions, in particular with regard to language, publication period, or data on humans; the last update of the search was carried out on December 17, 2014.

Following removal of duplicates, titles and abstracts were screened for potential relevance and in that case full-text was obtained. Exclusion criteria were: (1) clear indication of lack of a systematic search (e.g. narrative reviews or meta-analyses of data from multiple study centres), (2) no human data presented (e.g. animal data, in vitro studies, simulation studies), (3) outcome definition that did not include asthma or wheeze, and (4) the investigated topic was the management of existing disease (e.g. therapeutic intervention, patient education, secondary and tertiary prevention). References of overviews of systematic reviews were scrutinised for systematic reviews and these were included if not already identified through the search strategy. All evaluation of entries and full texts was conducted by two members of the review team independently and the senior author settled cases of disagreement. The studied diseases and topics covered by the systematic reviews were indexed as previously described; here we analyse all 307 systematic reviews covering asthma, including occupational asthma, and/or wheeze [8].

Complete citations of the included reviews were extracted; we categorized the year of (print) publication into three periods: before 2006, 2006–2010, after 2010 (bands chosen with consideration of the number of articles in each period at the time of analysis). The type of systematic review, i.e. systematic review, systematic review with meta-analysis, or overview of systematic reviews, and the studied topics covered were taken from the previously published index [8]. For the outcomes and the topics, we extracted the definitions presented in the systematic reviews and any age restrictions that were applied. Data extraction was conducted independently by two members of the review team. The lead author settled any cases of disagreement.

In addition, two members of the review team independently applied the AMSTAR checklist to all relevant full-text entries [9, 10]. This is the most frequently used validated checklist to evaluate the methodological quality of systematic reviews. It has been previously noted that the wording of the AMSTAR items and instructions is a trade-off between feasibility and reliability [11]. Because of the subjective interpretation, inter-rater agreement on some AMSTAR items may be lower than on others. Rather than solving disagreement between raters and producing one averaged AMSTAR score, we deliberately instructed one rater to be more liberal and the other rater to be more conservative in applying the AMSTAR checklist. Thus, we documented an upper bound (liberal) and a lower bound (conservative) of the total AMSTAR score that may be achieved by each systematic review. Details of the liberal and conservative criteria for each AMSTAR item are shown in Additional file 1: Table S1.

For two of the systematic reviews, the extracted data were based on the abstract and those parts of the full text that could be translated [12, 13]. Full application of the AMSTAR checklist was not possible due to the limited information included in the abstracts. Therefore, these two articles were excluded from the analyses of the AMSTAR scores.

All evaluation, data extraction, and indexing was performed using a relational database (Microsoft Access 2010©, Microsoft Corporation, Redmond, Washington, United States). Counts, percentages, and distributions as well as correlations and p values were analysed using SAS® 9.3 (The SAS Institute, Cary, NC, USA). To assess differences in the systematic reviews' quality across topics, we modelled linear regression with AMSTAR scores as the dependent variable and separate independent dummy variables per topic (each yes/no) since some systematic review were indexed with multiple topics. We report p values for the likelihood ratio test of the global association of topics with AMSTAR scores from these models and after further adjustment for other variables influencing the AMSTAR score. Also, we visualized the predicted mean AMSTAR scores per topic after centring all topic dummy variables and all co-variables at their respective arithmetic mean. Data visualisation in Fig. 1 was produced using Gephi© (https://gephi.org/), a non-profit open-source software for network visualization and analysis created by the Gephi Consortium.

Results

Additional file 2: Appendix S2 contains the full list of the included 307 systematic reviews, including the indexed diseases and topics as well as the AMSTAR checklist in a single spreadsheet, which can be searched and sorted. Overall, 57.0% of the systematic reviews included a meta-analysis. There were two overviews of systematic reviews, both not confined to asthma: one on second-hand smoke exposure and child health and the other on occupational safety and health interventions [14, 15].

Figure 1 depicts the aggregated topics (see Additional file 1: Table S2) indexed along with asthma or wheeze. If the line thickness matches the bubble diameter, this

means that all articles indexed with that topic were indexed with asthma; if the line is thinner than the bubble diameter, the topic is also indexed solely with other allergic diseases as previously published [8]. E.g. for "obesity", almost all systematic reviews displayed data on asthma, whereas for "pre-/probiotics", most systematic reviews covered only other allergic diseases. Of the full list of 43 topics catalogued (see Additional file 1: Table S2), "family history", "birth weight", and feeding of "formula" were only covered once in systematic reviews published from 2011 onwards. The other topics were covered at least twice. Overall, at least one meta-analysis was conducted for all topics except for "social determinants", "perinatal", "birth weight", and "climate".

Overall, following the liberal and the conservative instructions, 63.0 and 13.1% respectively, had an AMSTAR score ≥8 which suggests good methodological quality. The AMSTAR score increased over the time period studied (Fig. 2; liberal AMSTAR:

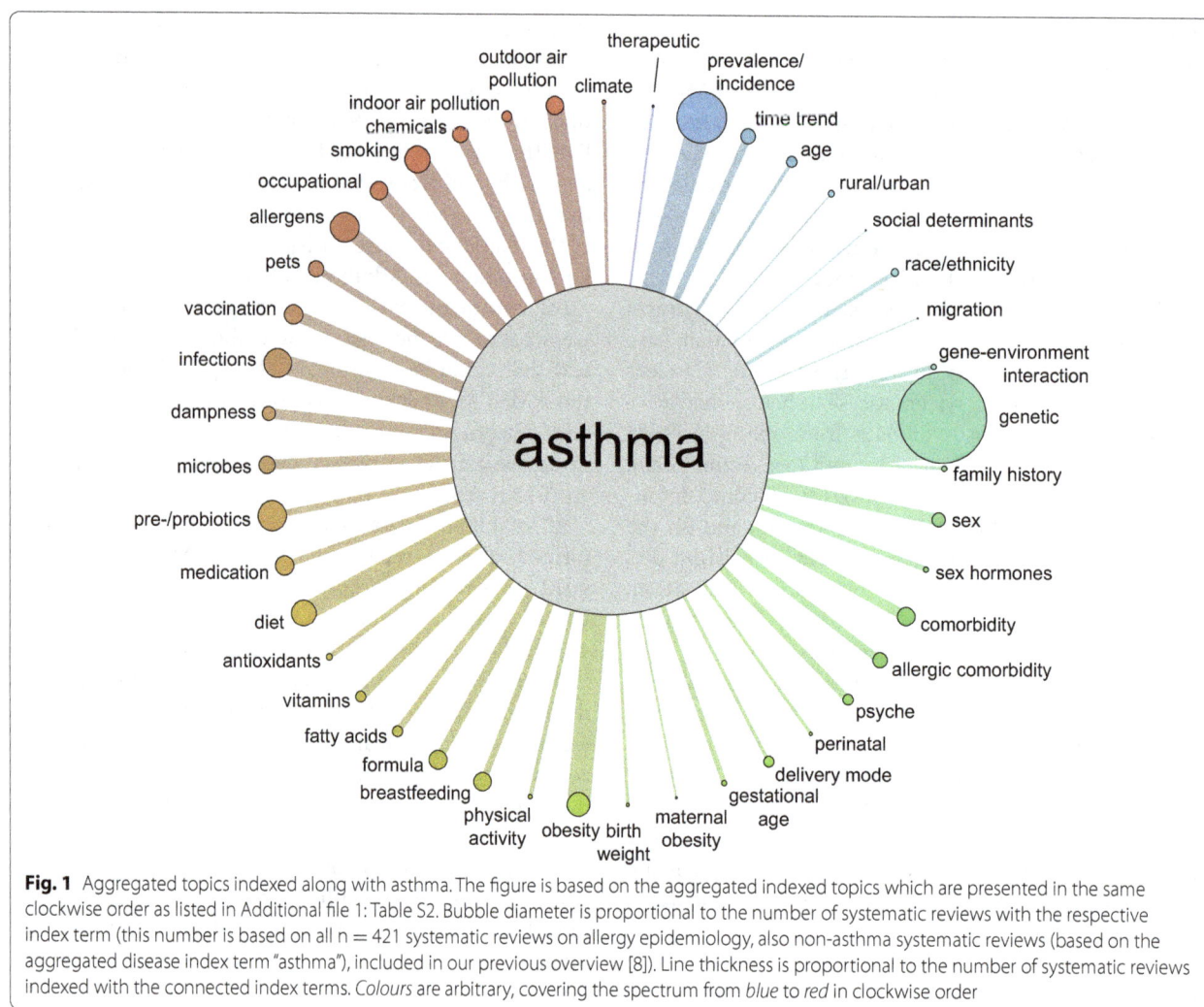

Fig. 1 Aggregated topics indexed along with asthma. The figure is based on the aggregated indexed topics which are presented in the same clockwise order as listed in Additional file 1: Table S2. Bubble diameter is proportional to the number of systematic reviews with the respective index term (this number is based on all n = 421 systematic reviews on allergy epidemiology, also non-asthma systematic reviews (based on the aggregated disease index term "asthma"), included in our previous overview [8]). Line thickness is proportional to the number of systematic reviews indexed with the connected index terms. *Colours* are arbitrary, covering the spectrum from *blue* to *red* in clockwise order

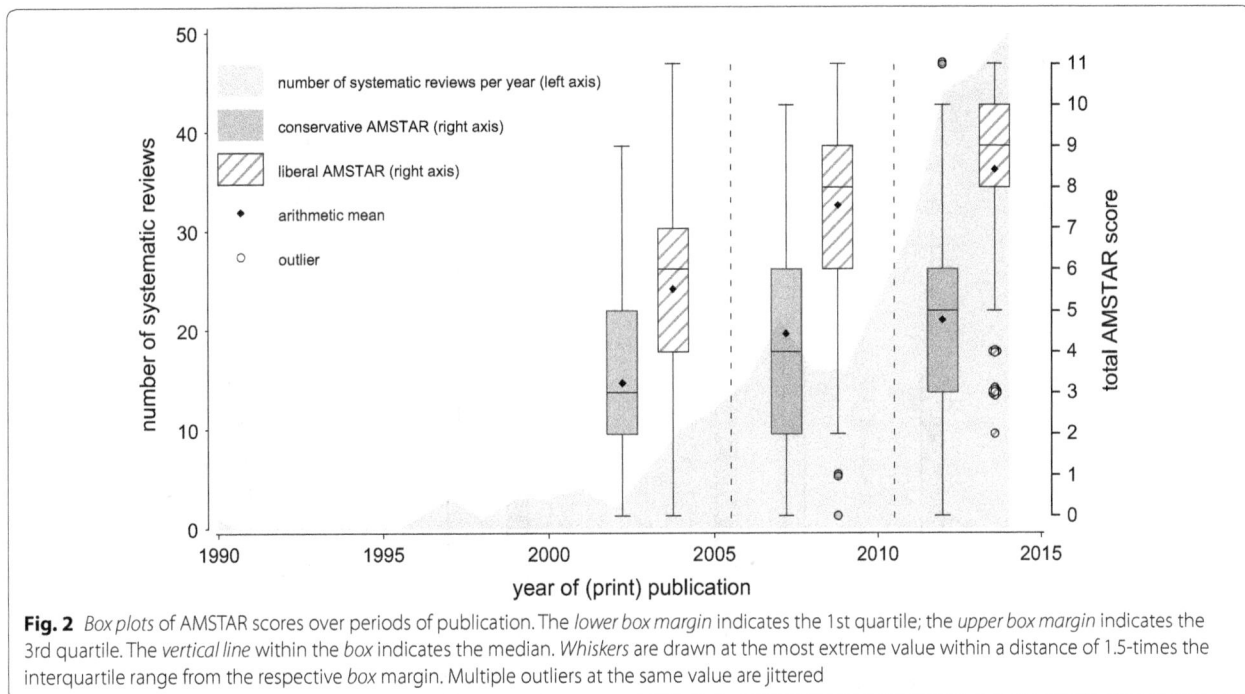

Fig. 2 *Box plots* of AMSTAR scores over periods of publication. The *lower box margin* indicates the 1st quartile; the *upper box margin* indicates the 3rd quartile. The *vertical line* within the *box* indicates the median. *Whiskers* are drawn at the most extreme value within a distance of 1.5-times the interquartile range from the respective *box* margin. Multiple outliers at the same value are jittered

$p_{\text{Kruskal–Wallis,2DF}} < 0.001$, Spearman $\rho = 0.34$; conservative AMSTAR: $p_{\text{Kruskal–Wallis,2DF}} < 0.001$, Spearman $\rho = 0.21$). This trend happened against the background of an increasing number of systematic reviews per year over time (Fig. 2). Also, the proportion of systematic reviews with meta-analysis increased over time up to 65.5% in the most recent period from 2011 to 2014 ($p_{\chi^2} < 0.001$). In the same years, 76.3 and 11.8% had high (AMSTAR ≥ 8) and 5.3 and 27.2% had low (AMSTAR <4) methodological quality following the liberal and the conservative instructions, respectively. Systematic reviews with meta-analysis had a 3.0- and 2.0-points higher liberal and conservative AMSTAR score, respectively, compared to systematic reviews without meta-analysis (data not shown).

The AMSTAR score also differed across aggregated topics (Fig. 3; Additional file 1: Figure S1; for information on aggregation of topics see Additional file 1: Table S2). This difference was not explained by effects of publication period or methodology (Additional file 1: Figure S1). Further adjustment for Cochrane versus non-Cochrane reviews resulted in decreasing average AMSTAR scores for topics with Cochrane reviews (2 for "allergens", 7 for "diet", 4 for "microbes"; data not shown). The global test for association of topics with AMSTAR scores in these fully adjusted models was $p_{\text{LR-test}} = 0.063$ and $p_{\text{LR-test}} = 0.040$ for the liberal and conservative AMSTAR score, respectively. The proportion of variance in AMSTAR scores explained by topics, measured as r^2 in the linear regression models, reduced from

15.3 and 10.4% in the crude models to 3.9 and 5.1% in the fully adjusted models for the liberal and conservative AMSTAR score, respectively. Overall, 48.4 and 36.4% of the variance were explained in the fully adjusted models for the liberal and the conservative AMSTAR, respectively.

Of the full list of 43 topics (see Additional file 1: Table S2), only "birth weight" did not include a systematic review reaching a liberal AMSTAR of at least 8 which indicates good methodological quality. Restricting to more recent systematic reviews published after 2010, "pets" was another topic in which the systematic review published in this period achieved a liberal AMSTAR below 8 as well. Using the conservative AMSTAR, the list of topics with all systematic reviews achieving scores below 8 is much longer: "therapeutic", "prevalence/incidence", "time trend", "age", "rural/urban", "race/ethnicity", "genetic", "family history", "sex", "sex hormones", "allergic comorbidity", "perinatal", "delivery mode", "birth weight", "obesity", "physical activity", "breastfeeding", "dampness", "pets", "chemical", "indoor air pollution", "outdoor air pollution", and "climate".

The topic covered most often was "genetic" (n = 76) although this would have been outnumbered if all "environmental" topics were aggregated. Table 1 shows the number of systematic reviews pertaining to the respective genes that were investigated. Of note, most of these systematic reviews only included case–control studies and family studies were typically excluded or not discussed.

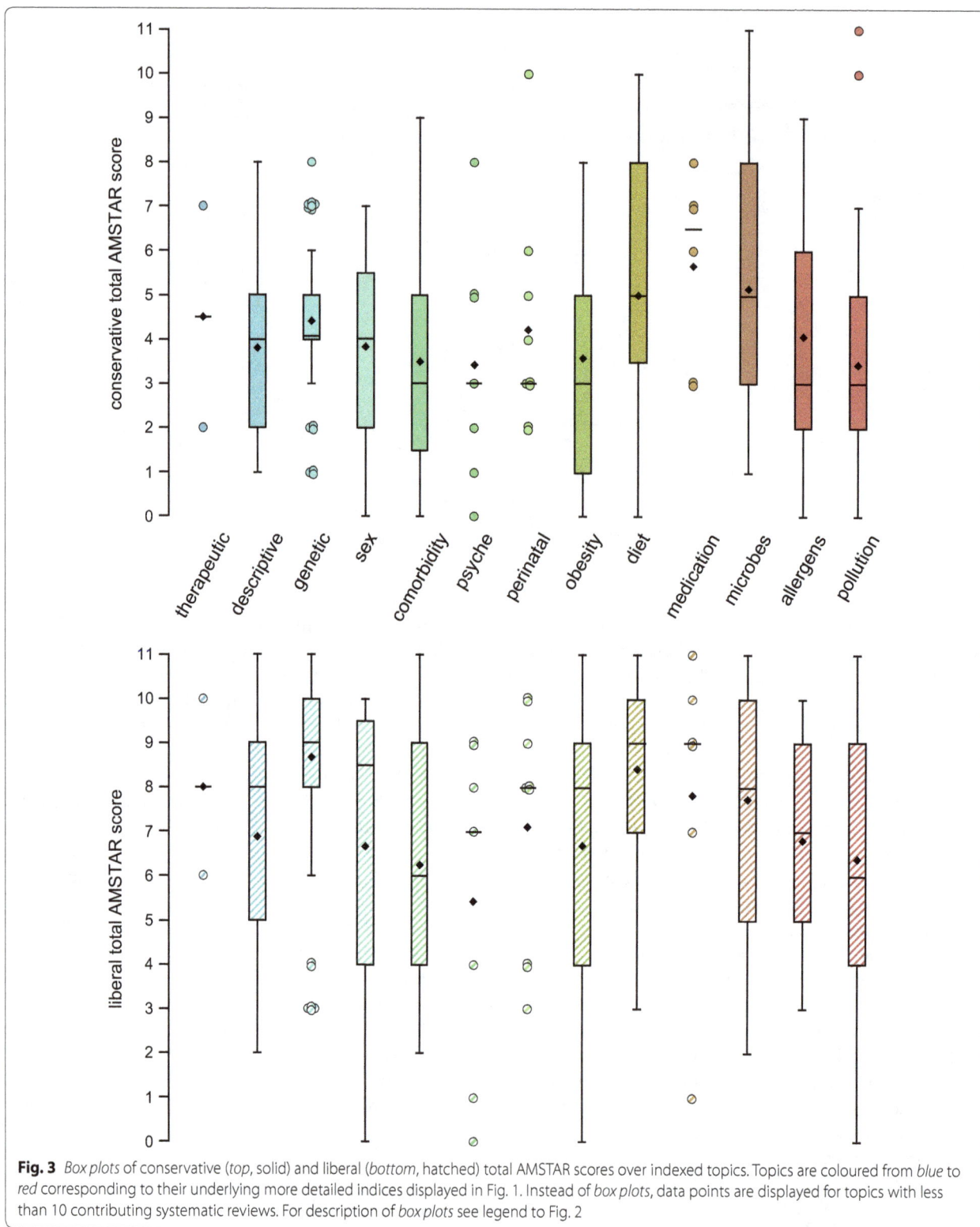

Fig. 3 *Box plots* of conservative (*top*, solid) and liberal (*bottom*, hatched) total AMSTAR scores over indexed topics. Topics are coloured from *blue* to *red* corresponding to their underlying more detailed indices displayed in Fig. 1. Instead of *box plots*, data points are displayed for topics with less than 10 contributing systematic reviews. For description of *box plots* see legend to Fig. 2

Following mutual adjustment for the other topics, 87.8% of the systematic reviews on genetics had performed meta-analyses, a significantly higher proportion than for other topics. Several systematic reviews concentrated on single polymorphisms rather than all polymorphisms in a given gene or location.

Table 1 Genes along with the frequency they were covered by systematic reviews

Gene(s)	Number of systematic reviews
IL4	12
IL13	8
ADAM33, CCL5, TNF	7
ADRB2, CD14, IL4R	6
GST[a], IL10, TGFB1	4
ACE, CXCL8, IFNG, IL18, MS4A2, TLR4	3
CTLA4, FLG, LTA, LTC4S, STAT6	2
CFTR, HLA, IL1B, IL9, MBL2, NAT2, PTGDR, SCGB1A1, SERPINE1, SFTPD, TLR2	1

[a] Including GSTT1 (n = 4), GSTM1 (n = 3), and GSTP1 (n = 2)

Four systematic reviews investigated gene-environment interactions: one on multiple genes and respiratory syncytial virus (RSV) infection [16], one on glutathione S-transferase genes and smoking [17], one on multiple genes and exposure to outdoor air pollution [18], and one on CD14 and exposure to microbes [19]. In addition, there were two systematic reviews with meta-analysis of genome-wide linkage studies [20, 21] and one systematic review with meta-analysis of studies on the effects of maternal and paternal asthma [22]. A further systematic review investigated the association between migration status and asthma with the aim of providing information on genetic and environmental components of the disease risk [23].

Discussion

We present a comprehensive overview of systematic reviews in asthma epidemiology including their methodological quality which demonstrates that there are systematic reviews for most of the topics identified as relevant in recent expert opinion pieces [1, 2]. Most topics have been covered by more than one systematic review and have also been covered since 2010. However, a substantial number of published systematic reviews fall short in methodological quality.

Compared to the only previous overview of systematic reviews across several topics in asthma epidemiology [3], we miss 9 systematic reviews identified by the other overview due to its 13 month longer search period up to January 2016. However, we also include 15 systematic reviews this overview failed to identify despite matching its inclusion criteria. Because this other overview was restricted to systematic reviews with meta-analysis, on childhood, and on non-genetic factors [3], our more comprehensive search identified 256 additional articles. Inevitably, such a comprehensive effort is outdated upon publication. Our previously published overview [8] suggests that

about 70 systematic reviews on allergy epidemiology are published per year from 2014 on, of which about 75% are on asthma. Nonetheless and while most of the topics we identified were discussed in the previous two overviews [3, 4], our to date most extensive overview of systematic reviews on asthma epidemiology enables us to make some additions:

First, we identified 19 systematic reviews on the effects of smoking on asthma, principally covering environmental tobacco smoke exposure which is discussed in the previous overview [3]. In addition, we identified 6 systematic reviews on active smoking: one on asthma in women [24], one on gene-environment interaction with Glutathione-S-Transferase genes [17], one on marijuana smoking [25], one on the effects of smoke-free legislation [26], one evidence-based guideline on occupational asthma [27], and one on risk and protective factors [5]. The latter was published in 2004 and is the only one with a focus on the main effects of active smoking in a general population, suggesting an update is warranted.

Second, we identified several systematic reviews on the effects of specific infections other than RSV infection which is the only infection discussed in the previous overview [3]. A total of four systematic reviews on Helicobacter pylori infection were included, one of poor quality [28]. The other three all conducted their search up to April to July 2012 [29–31]. However, one included only five studies and found no association [29]. The other two had 12 studies in common, including the aforementioned five studies and found weaker evidence for an inverse association between H. pylori infection and asthma [30, 31]. This example documents how differing search and inclusion criteria may affect the overall interpretation of the assembled body of evidence. Our previous overview of systematic reviews in allergy epidemiology includes a discussion towards this issue [8].

Third, topics not covered by the previous overview include genetics (by methodology, n = 76 systematic reviews), effects of physical activity or sedentary behaviour (n = 4), pet exposure (n = 6), and formula rather than breastfeeding (n = 8, including updates). Our primary purpose was not to discuss these systematic reviews in depth but to index them and provide quality scores for future reference. Still, our results indicate that specifically birth weight was covered by systematic reviews with low methodological quality. Here, the authors of the other overview [3] identified a further systematic review [32] published after our search period which achieved an AMSTAR score of 9 in their evaluation which potentially closes this gap. Moreover, the second topic with only low quality systematic reviews published after 2010 was "pets" which was not covered by the other overview and for which a high-quality update may be warranted.

In particular our conservative AMSTAR scores and our more comprehensive list may help to guide selection of further topics which may require new or updated systematic reviews. Whether an overview of systematic reviews for a specific topic or an update of an existing systematic review is warranted will also depend on scientific interest and closer investigation of the body of evidence covered by each individual systematic review.

Fourth, in our overview of systematic reviews on genetic factors implicated in asthma development, we were able to demonstrate that evidence from family-based designs has largely been ignored, even though methodology to statistically combine this evidence with that from other study designs has been suggested and applied elsewhere [33]. Moreover, as we previously discussed [8], the nature of the search for articles covering genetics may make these more amenable to quick and efficient systematic review. Furthermore, the underlying original articles have very homogenous definitions of the exposure variable (i.e. the genetic trait) and often report odds ratios which facilitates meta-analysis. For example, the effects of *IL4* polymorphisms have been investigated in 12 systematic reviews published from 2008 on with four of them in 2013 and three of them in 2014. Four of these 12 reviews included only a single polymorphism within the gene. While there may be scientific rationale to concentrate on specific polymorphisms (e.g. due to considerations of biology or those of linkage disequilibrium), it may be more appropriate to summarize evidence at the gene level. Of note, our list of genes is not a comprehensive list of genetic factors implicated in asthma development but a reflection of which of these have been investigated by systematic reviews. There are many examples of large-scale meta-analyses on genetic factors (and also other factors as we discuss in our previous publication [8]) which we did not include and which may provide high-quality evidence.

Operational definitions of asthma have previously been shown to be heterogeneous [34, 35]. In systematic reviews on asthma, its definition in the underlying original articles needs to be extracted, displayed, and discussed. This was done in a substantial number of the systematic reviews included in our overview (data not shown). Additionally, atopic and non-atopic asthma were separated in some systematic reviews. Here, specific focus should be devoted to the definition of the comparison or reference groups in the original articles, as these definitions may dramatically influence resulting associations [36]. We advocate that future systematic reviews continue to take a holistic approach with regard to specifying asthma definitions as an inclusion criterion and that they evaluate and discuss potential heterogeneity of the asthma definitions used.

While the methodological quality of the systematic reviews has been generally increasing over the past decades, there were still up to 27% with low quality scores among those published after 2010. This may of course be a high estimate due to conservative application of the AMSTAR checklist and due to inclusion of a few articles in which the authors described a systematic search but did not aim at writing a systematic review. We have deliberately applied the AMSTAR checklist twice with more liberal and with more conservative instructions rather than averaging two replicate sets to produce a range of AMSTAR scores for each systematic review. The quality score from a consensus procedure would be likely to lie within this range. Indeed, for the 33 systematic reviews included in both our list and the only previous overview supplying AMSTAR scores [3], our conservative AMSTAR was consistently lower and our liberal AMSTAR was mostly equal or higher.

The AMSTAR checklist has been previously shown to yield higher scores for Cochrane reviews, if a meta-analysis was conducted, and for more recently published systematic reviews [10, 37], all of which is reflected in our analyses. While these characteristics explained a larger portion of the overall variance in AMSTAR scores than our indexed aggregated topics, we could still detect some consistent differences across topics for both our AMSTAR definitions. The AMSTAR has also been shown to be associated with the number of pages of a systematic review [10] and the journal's impact factor [37], but we refrained from evaluating these as we deemed them of lower importance to our aims. The AMSTAR interval we provide may guide future updates of existing systematic reviews in particular for those topics for which high quality systematic reviews are lacking as discussed above.

In conclusion, we present a comprehensive overview and an indexed database of published systematic reviews in asthma epidemiology including quality scores. We highlight some topics and issues which we believe should be considered in future systematic reviews. We propose that our results could be a basis for topic-specific overviews of systematic reviews in asthma epidemiology.

Abbreviations

AMSTAR: a measurement tool to assess systematic reviews; *H. pylori: Helicobacter pylori*; IL: interleukin; RSV: respiratory syncytial virus.

Authors' contributions
All authors have designed the project, the search strategy, and the criteria used during evaluation. JG and AS have contributed to the evaluation of the search results. JG, MRP, and CF have written the first draft of the manuscript. All authors read and approved the final manuscript.

Author details
[1] Institute of Epidemiology and Medical Biometry, Ulm University, Helmholtzstr. 22, 89081 Ulm, Germany. [2] Institute of Epidemiology and Preventive Medicine, University of Regensburg, Regensburg, Germany. [3] Department of Allergy and Clinical Immunology, 424 General Military Training Hospital, Thessaloniki, Greece. [4] Murdoch Children's Research Institute, University of Melbourne, Melbourne, Australia. [5] Institute of Biomedicine and Molecular Immunology, National Research Council of Italy, Palermo, Italy. [6] Division of Asthma, Allergy and Lung Biology, Children's Allergies Department, King's College London, London, UK. [7] Unit for Population-Based Dermatology Research, St John's Institute of Dermatology, King's College London and Guy's and St Thomas' NHS Foundation, London, UK. [8] Population Health Research Institute, St George's, University of London, London, UK.

Acknowledgements
We thank Elizabeth Stovold, Information Specialist from the Cochrane Airways Group (Population Health Research Institute, St George's, University of London, United Kingdom), for assistance in designing the search terms and for retrieving the search results from the databases. We also thank David Rothenbacher for his help in evaluating the search results and Raphael Peter, MSc, for his assistance in the creation of images with Gephi (both Institute of Epidemiology and Medical Biometry, Ulm University, Germany).

Competing interests
CA reports personal fees and non-financial support from Cogitando Healthcare Communication, outside the submitted work. None of the other authors declare that they have no competing interests.

Funding
This work has partly been funded by the European Academy of Allergy and Clinical Immunology (EAACI) through support of the Task Force "Overview of Systematic Reviews in Allergy Epidemiology (OSRAE)" of the EAACI Interest Group on Epidemiology (Chair: Jon Genuneit, Secretary: Carsten Flohr).

References
1. Akdis CA, Agache I, editors. Global atlas of asthma. Zürich: EAACI; 2013.
2. Gibson G, Loddenkemper R, Sibille Y, editors. The European lung white book. 2nd ed. Sheffield: European Respiratory Society; 2013.
3. Castro-Rodriguez JA, Forno E, Rodriguez-Martinez CE, Celedón JC. Risk and protective factors for childhood asthma: what is the evidence? J Allergy Clin Immunol Pract. 2016;4:1111–22.
4. Garcia-Larsen V, Del Giacco SR, Moreira A, Bonini M, Charles D, Reeves T, et al. Asthma and dietary intake: an overview of systematic reviews. Allergy. 2016;71:433–42.
5. King ME, Mannino DM, Holguin F. Risk factors for asthma incidence. A review of recent prospective evidence. Panminerva Med. 2004;46:97–110.
6. Dick S, Friend A, Dynes K, AlKandari F, Doust E, Cowie H, et al. A systematic review of associations between environmental exposures and development of asthma in children aged up to 9 years. BMJ Open. 2014;4:e006554.
7. Contopoulos-Ioannidis DG, Kouri IN, Ioannidis JPA. Genetic predisposition to asthma and atopy. Respir Int Rev Thorac Dis. 2007;74:8–12.
8. Genuneit J, Seibold AM, Apfelbacher CJ, Konstantinou GN, Koplin JJ, La Grutta S, Logan K, Perkin MR, Flohr C, Task Force 'Overview of Systematic Reviews in Allergy Epidemiology (OSRAE)' of the EAACI Interest Group on Epidemiology. Overview of systematic reviews in allergy epidemiology. Allergy. 2017. doi:10.1111/all.13123.
9. Shea BJ, Grimshaw JM, Wells GA, Boers M, Andersson N, Hamel C, et al. Development of AMSTAR: a measurement tool to assess the methodological quality of systematic reviews. BMC Med Res Methodol. 2007;7:10.
10. Shea BJ, Bouter LM, Peterson J, Boers M, Andersson N, Ortiz Z, et al. External validation of a measurement tool to assess systematic reviews (AMSTAR). PLoS ONE. 2007;2:e1350.
11. Shea BJ, Hamel C, Wells GA, Bouter LM, Kristjansson E, Grimshaw J, et al. AMSTAR is a reliable and valid measurement tool to assess the methodological quality of systematic reviews. J Clin Epidemiol. 2009;62:1013–20.
12. Jarahi L, Shojaie SRH. Long-term effects of sulfur mustard poisoning in iranian chemical warfare victims: a systematic review (English). J Isfahan Med Sch. 2013;30:2353–66.
13. Tang L, Chen J, Shen Y. [Meta-analysis of probiotics preventing allergic diseases in infants]. Zhonghua Er Ke Za Zhi Chin J Pediatr. 2012;50:504–9.
14. Himathongkam T, Nicogossian A, Kloiber O, Ebadirad N. Updates of secondhand smoke exposure on infants' and children's health. World Med Health Policy. 2013;5:124–40.
15. Verbeek J, Ivanov I. Essential occupational safety and health interventions for low- and middle-income countries: an overview of the evidence. Saf Health Work. 2013;4:77–83.
16. Drysdale SB, Milner AD, Greenough A. Respiratory syncytial virus infection and chronic respiratory morbidity: is there a functional or genetic predisposition? Acta Paediatr Oslo Nor. 1992;2012(101):1114–20.
17. Saadat M, Ansari-Lari M. Genetic polymorphism of glutathione S-transferase T1, M1 and asthma, a meta-analysis of the literature. Pak J Biol Sci. 2007;10:4183–9.
18. Vawda S, Mansour R, Takeda A, Funnell P, Kerry S, Mudway I, et al. Associations between inflammatory and immune response genes and adverse respiratory outcomes following exposure to outdoor air pollution: a HuGE systematic review. Am J Epidemiol. 2014;179:432–42.
19. Lau MY, Dharmage SC, Burgess JA, Lowe AJ, Lodge CJ, Campbell B, et al. CD14 polymorphisms, microbial exposure and allergic diseases: a systematic review of gene–environment interactions. Allergy. 2014;69:1440–53.
20. Denham S, Koppelman GH, Blakey J, Wjst M, Ferreira MA, Hall IP, et al. Meta-analysis of genome-wide linkage studies of asthma and related traits. Respir Res. 2008;9:38.
21. Bouzigon E, Forabosco P, Koppelman GH, Cookson WOCM, Dizier M-H, Duffy DL, et al. Meta-analysis of 20 genome-wide linkage studies evidenced new regions linked to asthma and atopy. Eur J Hum Genet. 2010;18:700–6.
22. Lim RH, Kobzik L, Dahl M. Risk for asthma in offspring of asthmatic mothers versus fathers: a meta-analysis. PLoS ONE. 2010;5:e10134.
23. Cabieses B, Uphoff E, Pinart M, Antó JM, Wright J. A systematic review on the development of asthma and allergic diseases in relation to international immigration: the leading role of the environment confirmed. PLoS ONE. 2014;9:e105347.
24. Ostrom NK. Women with asthma: a review of potential variables and preferred medical management. Ann Allergy Asthma Immunol. 2006;96:655–65.
25. Tetrault JM, Crothers K, Moore BA, Mehra R, Concato J, Fiellin DA. Effects of marijuana smoking on pulmonary function and respiratory complications: a systematic review. Arch Intern Med. 2007;167:221–8.
26. Been JV, Nurmatov UB, Cox B, Nawrot TS, van Schayck CP, Sheikh A. Effect of smoke-free legislation on perinatal and child health: a systematic review and meta-analysis. Lancet. 2014;383:1549–60.
27. Nicholson PJ, Cullinan P, Taylor AJN, Burge PS, Boyle C. Evidence based guidelines for the prevention, identification, and management of occupational asthma. Occup Environ Med. 2005;62:290–9.
28. Malfertheiner MV, Kandulski A, Schreiber J, Malfertheiner P. Helicobacter pylori infection and the respiratory system: a systematic review of the literature. Digestion. 2011;84:212–20.
29. Wang Y, Bi Y, Zhang L, Wang C. Is Helicobacter pylori infection associated with asthma risk? A meta-analysis based on 770 cases and 785 controls. Int J Med Sci. 2012;9:603–10.

30. Zhou X, Wu J, Zhang G. Association between *Helicobacter pylori* and asthma: a meta-analysis. Eur J Gastroenterol Hepatol. 2013;25:460–8.

31. Wang Q, Yu C, Sun Y. The association between asthma and *Helicobacter pylori*: a meta-analysis. Helicobacter. 2013;18:41–53.

32. Mu M, Ye S, Bai M-J, Liu G-L, Tong Y, Wang S-F, et al. Birth weight and subsequent risk of asthma: a systematic review and meta-analysis. Heart Lung Circ. 2014;23:511–9.

33. Rodríguez E, Baurecht H, Herberich E, Wagenpfeil S, Brown SJ, Cordell HJ, et al. Meta-analysis of filaggrin polymorphisms in eczema and asthma: robust risk factors in atopic disease. J Allergy Clin Immunol. 2009;123(1361–1370):e7.

34. Van Wonderen KE, Van Der Mark LB, Mohrs J, Bindels PJE, Van Aalderen WMC, Ter Riet G. Different definitions in childhood asthma: how dependable is the dependent variable? Eur Respir J. 2009;36:48–56.

35. Sá-Sousa A, Jacinto T, Azevedo LF, Morais-Almeida M, Robalo-Cordeiro C, Bugalho-Almeida A, et al. Operational definitions of asthma in recent epidemiological studies are inconsistent. Clin Transl Allergy. 2014;4:24.

36. Pekkanen J, Lampi J, Genuneit J, Hartikainen A-L, Järvelin M-R. Analyzing atopic and non-atopic asthma. Eur J Epidemiol. 2012;27:281–6.

37. Fleming PS, Koletsi D, Seehra J, Pandis N. Systematic reviews published in higher impact clinical journals were of higher quality. J Clin Epidemiol. 2014;67:754–9.

11

Self-reported adverse reactions and IgE sensitization to common foods in adults with asthma

G. Rentzos[1*], L. Johanson[2], S. Sjölander[4], E. Telemo[3] and L. Ekerljung[2]

Abstract

Background: There is very few data available on the prevalence of food hypersensitivity among adults with asthma. The aim of this study was to explore the prevalence of self-reported adverse reactions and IgE sensitization to the different foods and to determine the spectrum and the prevalence of food-related gastrointestinal symptoms in adults with and with no asthma.

Methods: A cross sectional study based on interviews and questionnaire responses from 1527 subjects, aged 18–75 years of age, from Västra Götaland in Sweden, as part of the larger West Sweden Asthma Study. IgE analyses were performed in sera from all subjects.

Results: Fifty three percent of adults with asthma reported adverse reactions to foods compared to 30 % of non-asthmatics. Most asthmatics reported symptoms from eating hazelnut, followed by other nuts, birch-related foods, milk, peanut and shellfish. Furthermore, adults with asthma experienced significantly more often gastrointestinal symptoms from hazelnut, apple and milk and were found to significantly more often be sensitized to the most common foods compared to the non-asthmatic subjects. The asthmatics showed a significant correlation between IgE to both hazelnut and birch and self-reported symptoms after ingestion of hazelnut and to a lesser extent to almonds.

Conclusions: The prevalence of self-reported adverse reactions and sensitization to the most common foods was much higher among the asthmatic subjects. Hazelnut was the food that asthmatics most frequently experienced adverse reactions from, and the strong correlation between IgE to hazelnut and birch indicate that the observed adverse reactions are partly due to sensitization to allergens from the PR-10 family.

Keywords: Asthma, Food allergy, Epidemiology

Background

Determining the prevalence of food hypersensitivity and food allergy is a complex issue due to the different cultures, dietary habits, and geographical and regional differences of allergen distribution. It is still unclear if the prevalence of food allergy is continuously rising although many studies conclude that there is a rising trend at least in western and developing countries [1–3]. Most of the studies concerning the prevalence of food allergy are carried out in children, and therefore it is largely unknown as to what extent the adult population is affected.

The relationship between asthma and food allergy has also been discussed but the available data demonstrating a common pathogenetic mechanism are still few. In adults this relation was often denoted by case-reports, which claim that food hypersensitivity may trigger or affect asthma symptoms. It has been shown previously that having asthma might be a risk factor for a fatal food re-action and having food allergy might be a risk for complicated or poorly controlled asthma [4–6]. Oehling et al. has previously shown that one third of children with food allergy also have asthma [7] and about 4-8 % of children with asthma have food allergies [8], the prevalence though of food allergy in adults with asthma is still not known. However, it has been demonstrated that adult patients with one or more food allergies had

* Correspondence: grentzos@gmail.com
[1]Section of Allergology, University Hospital of Sahlgrenska, 413 45 Gothenburg, Sweden
Full list of author information is available at the end of the article

increased hospitalizations for asthma [4], and in a study from Woods et al., it was shown that adults with probable peanut and shrimp allergy often have more frequent asthma episodes and doctor's diagnosed asthma [9]. In addition, it has been also shown that inhalation of aerosolized food particles may lead to the development of asthma in adults [10–12]. The relation between asthma and gastrointestinal symptoms in adults is not extensively studied. A study on children by Cafarrelli et al. found a possible correlation between asthma and gastrointestinal symptoms [13]. In a previous study from Kivity et al., a relation between food allergy and concomitant asymptomatic bronchial hyper-reactivity could be shown [14]. It is still not fully explored though, if adults with asthma experience more often gastrointestinal adverse reactions to different food items in a greater frequency than non-asthmatics. The notion that there is a probable relation between asthma and gastrointestinal symptoms in adults was supported previously in a study by Powel et al. who confirmed that asthmatics generally experienced more gastrointestinal symptoms than the non-asthmatic population [15]. In a recent study, performed in the Netherlands, an association between gastrointestinal symptoms and asthma/COPD was found [16]. In addition, it has been shown that patients with irritable bowel syndrome (IBS) and inflammatory bowel disease (IBD) showed increased frequency of bronchial hyper-reactivity compared to control subjects [17, 18]. These results were further supported in a study on patients who suffered from asthma compared to asymptomatic atopic subjects [19].

The aim of this study was to explore the prevalence of self-reported adverse reactions to foods and to estimate the prevalence of IgE sensitization for the most common food among adults with asthma compared to non-asthmatics. We also wanted to describe the spectrum and the prevalence of gastrointestinal symptoms caused by the most common and different foods in both asthmatics and non-asthmatics.

Materials and methods

A postal questionnaire, which has been described in detail elsewhere [20], was mailed out to 30,000 randomly selected subjects, aged 18–75 years, living in the West of Sweden; 15,000 subjects lived in the urban area of Gothenburg and 15,000 in the remaining region of West Sweden. The total response rate was 62 %, and a non-response study showed no differences in prevalence of asthma symptoms or lung disease between responders and non-responders [20]. Of the responders to the postal questionnaire, 2000 were randomly selected for clinical examination and interviews. In addition, all responders that reported physician diagnosed asthma, or reported ever having asthma and used asthma medication or reported symptoms such as wheeze or attacks of shortness

of breath during the last year, were included. In total, 3524 subjects were invited, of which 2006 participated. All participants received a questionnaire containing detailed questions on food hypersensitivity as well as other hypersensitivity symptoms (Additional file 1: Hypersensitivity questionnaire). The questionnaire did not contain specific questions on gluten (coeliac disease) or lactose intolerance. Of the 2006 participants, 1725 responded to the food questionnaire of which 1527 were included in the analyses. A schematic flow chart of the study set up can be seen in Fig. 1. The clinical assessment of the subjects in the study included spirometry, blood samples for specific IgE-tests and a clinical interview performed by a specialist nurse. The clinical interview was used to assess whether the subjects currently suffered from asthma. This was defined as: a) asthma diagnosed by physician, and reported asthma symptoms or asthma medication during the last year, b) belief to have suffered from asthma, and currently report asthma symptoms and/or taking asthma medication, c) currently suffer from asthma symptoms and have either positive methacholine bronchial challenge test or positive reversibility test.

Specific IgE-tests included three allergen panel tests, Phadiatop Europe (cat, dog, horse, Dermatophagoides pteronyssinus, Dermatophagoides farinae Cladosporium herbarum, timothy grass, birch, mugwort, olive, wall pellitory), fx1 (peanut, hazel nut, brazil nut, almond, coconut) and fx5 (egg white, milk, fish, wheat, peanut, soy bean) (Thermofisher Scientific, Uppsala, Sweden). Subjects with a positive response to a panel were additionally tested specifically for the IgE of the allergens included in this positive panel, according to manufacturer's instructions. The foods tested in panels fx1 and fx5 were characterized as "common foods" since they comprise some of the most frequent food items consumed on a daily basis at least in Sweden and other Western countries.

Collection and encoding of data

The replies from food questionnaire (Additional file 1: Hypersensitivity questionnaire) regarding reactions to different foods were encoded for the different symptoms according to Table 1.

Then, encoded fields for milk, sour milk and cheese were added which were dissociated from the most relevant clinical symptoms for suspicious lactose intolerance as abdominal pain (abd), flatulence (gas) and diarrhea/loose stools (dia), or if lactose intolerance was specified in any free text field. Likewise, encoded fields were added for flour from wheat and flour from other cereal grains, in case of suspicious gluten intolerance (coeliac disease), that were dissociated from the clinical symptoms tiredness (tir), abdominal pain (abd), feeling of illness (gen), diarrhea/loose stools (dia), flatulence (gas) and/or hives, urticaria (urt), or if gluten intolerance was

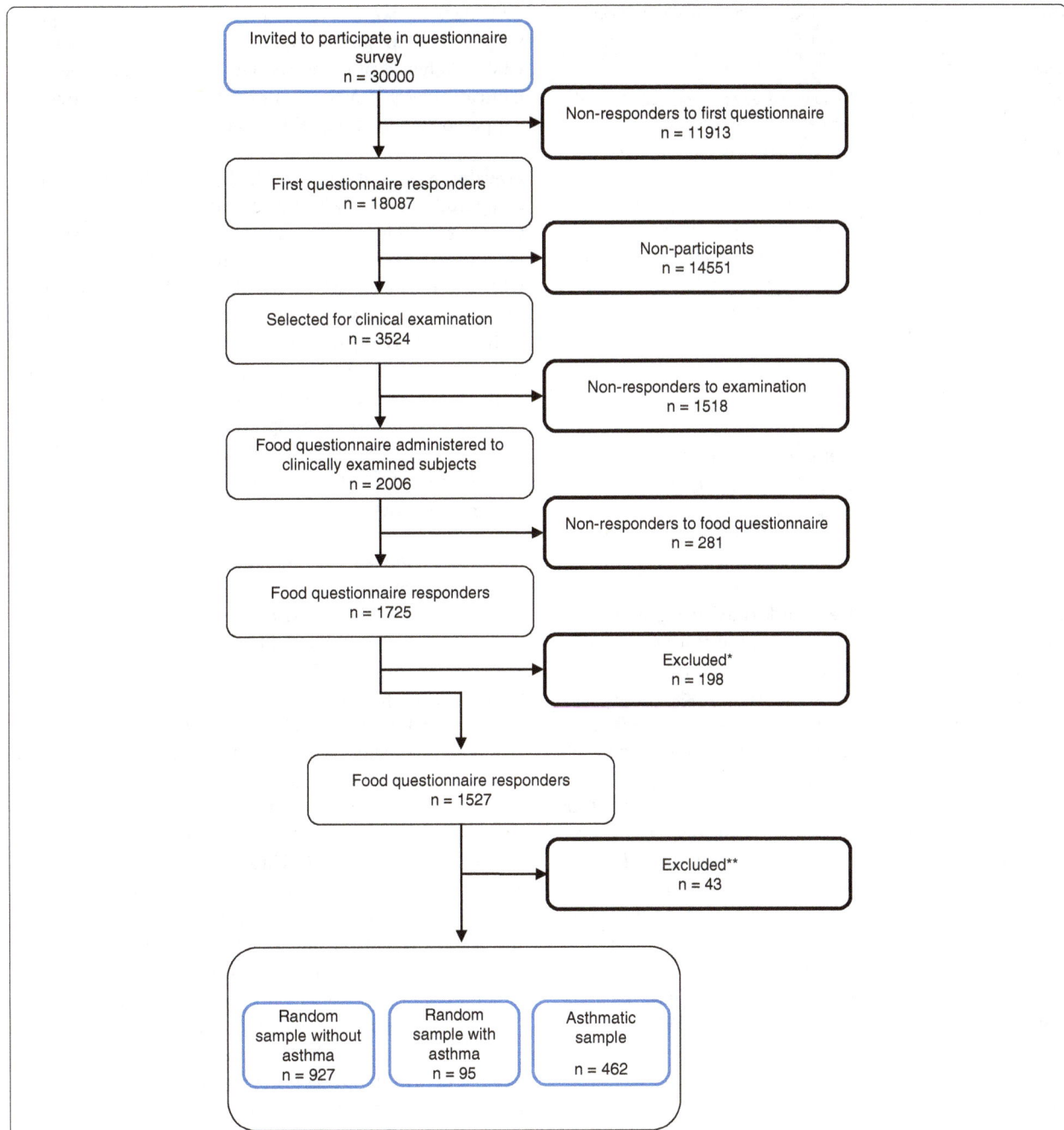

Fig. 1 Flow-chart of the subjects included or excluded from the study and the numbers of responders and non-responders of the selected participants. *198 subjects were excluded from the study since their initial categorization as asthmatics, while considered inappropriate, based on the questionnaire response and inclusion clinical criteria. **43 subjects were excluded from the study since they reported no symptoms from any food item, but did report that they avoided at least one food item in the food questionnaire

specified in any free text field. Three subjects reported that they suffered from gluten intolerance of which two avoided eating gluten strictly. Ten subjects reported that they suffered from lactose intolerance of which five avoided lactose strictly. In total thirty-two subjects suffered from symptoms that were interpreted as intolerance either to gluten or lactose.

Using the above described procedure, most cases of suspicious lactose and gluten intolerance could be excluded from the data of the analyses. Subjects with suspected asthma, based on the questionnaire, that could not be verified by the clinical examination as described in the previous section were also excluded from the analyses.

Table 1 Encoding for self-reported hypersensitivity reactions in food hypersensitivity questionnaire

Code	Meaning
Skin	Symptoms from the skin (urticaria, eczema, angioedema, flush, itching, tingling, skin pain, papules, redness etc.)
GI	Abdominal pain, oral symptoms, diarrhea, flatulence, reflux, vomiting, constipation
Airup	Symptoms from the upper airways –nose(rhinitis, nasal congestion, nasal itching, sneezing, red nasal papules), eyes
Airlo	Lower airways –respiratory symptoms(heavy breathing, difficulty getting air, wheezing, cough, chest pressure, bronchospasm, hoarseness, mucus/saliva in the throat)
Circ	Palpation, fainting, dizziness
CNS	Headache, confusion
Oth	Other(e.g., ear itching, gallstone)
Not	Do not eat
Unk	Unknown, uncertain whether intolerant or not
Ana	Anaphylactic reactions
Gen	General symptoms such as tiredness, feeling ill

Statistics

The statistical analyses were performed using SPSS 22.0 and Microsoft Excel 2007. Chi-squared test was used for the prevalence of self-reported symptoms as well as gastrointestinal symptoms to different foods among subjects with and without asthma. A p–value < 0.05 using Fischer's two tailed exact test was considered statistically significant. Correlations between different parameters within the same group were evaluated by using the Pearson's or Spearman's correlation coefficient. Tests were two-tailed and the level of significance was set to $P < 0.05$. Agreement between clinical objective asthma and self-reported asthma was analyzed by calculating the kappa coefficients (κ). κ < 0.00 was considered a poor strength of agreement, κ: 0.00–0.20 a slight strength, κ: 0.21–0.40 a fair strength, κ: 0.41–0.60 a moderate strength, κ: 0.61–0.80 a substantial strength, and κ: 0.81–1.00 an almost perfect agreement [21].

Ethical approval

The regional ethic committee in West Sweden (Central Ethical Review Board in Gothenburg) approved the study (Dnr 593–08).

Results

Of the total 1527 subjects that answered the food questionnaire, 43 reported no symptoms from any food item, but did report that they avoided at least one food item. These subjects were excluded from calculation of food hypersensitivity since the reason for their avoidance was unclear. From the 1527 subjects totally included in the study, 583 (38.2 %) had asthma while 944 (61.8 %) had no asthma ($p < 0.001$). Among the subjects with asthma

192 (32.9 %) were sensitized to birch pollen compared with 119 (12.6 %) among non-asthmatic subjects ($p < 0.001$). When evaluating the level of agreement between clinical objective asthma and self-reported asthma, the kappa-coefficient is equal to 0.94.

Prevalence of food hypersensitivity in adults with asthma compared to adults with no asthma

Of the remaining 1484, when excluding the 43 subjects reporting no symptoms from any food item, subjects with asthma reported a considerably higher prevalence of adverse reactions to food compared to those without asthma 53.1 % (49.0 % - 57.3 %, 95 % CI) vs. 29.8 % (26.8 % - 32.7 %, 95 % CI) with p < 0.001. When symptoms from suspicious lactose and gluten intolerance were excluded, asthmatics still reported more adverse reactions to food compared to non-asthmatics, 51.3 % (47.1 % - 55.4 %, 95 % CI) vs. 28.2 % (25.2 % - 31.1 %, 95 % CI) with $p < 0.001$ (Fig. 2).

Association between adverse reactions from specific foods and asthma

Subjects with asthma most commonly experienced adverse reactions (including all types of symptoms) to hazelnut (20.5 %), apple (17.5 %), kiwi (14.3 %), walnut (12.8 %), milk (11.5 %), peach (10.7 %), brazil nut (9.8 %), almond (9.5 %), nectarine (9.3 %), pear (8.9 %), plum (8.8 %), cherry (8.7 %), wine/beer (8.0 %), peanut (7.0 %), shellfish (6.5 %), carrot (6.4 %), strawberry (6.4 %), and apricot (6.3 %). Concerning the staple and dairy food items, subjects with asthma experienced adverse reactions most commonly against milk (including subjects with suspected lactose intolerance, 11.5 %), shellfish (6.5 %), sour milk/yogurt (6.25 %), cheese (4.5 %), egg (3.3 %), fish (2.9 %), soy (1.4 %), wheat (including subjects with suspected gluten intolerance, 3.23 %) while about 1.4 % to other flours. When excluding subjects with clinically suspected lactose intolerance, we observed that about 2.35 % of the asthmatics reacted to milk. When excluding subjects with suspicious gluten intolerance, as described previously, we observed that only 1.4 % of subjects reported adverse reactions to wheat. In addition 5.9 % of the asthmatics reported reactions to fried/fat food, and 1.6 % to food additives. More detailed data concerning the distribution of the self-reported adverse reactions to all the specific food items in asthmatics compared to non-asthmatics are presented in Table 2.

Association between self-reported food-related gastrointestinal symptoms and asthma

Subjects with asthma also report significantly more gastrointestinal symptom to hazelnut (13.0 % vs 5.2 %, $p < 0.001$), apple (11.4 % vs 6 %, $p < 0.001$), milk (10.4 % including subjects with suspicious lactose intolerance vs 5.7 %,

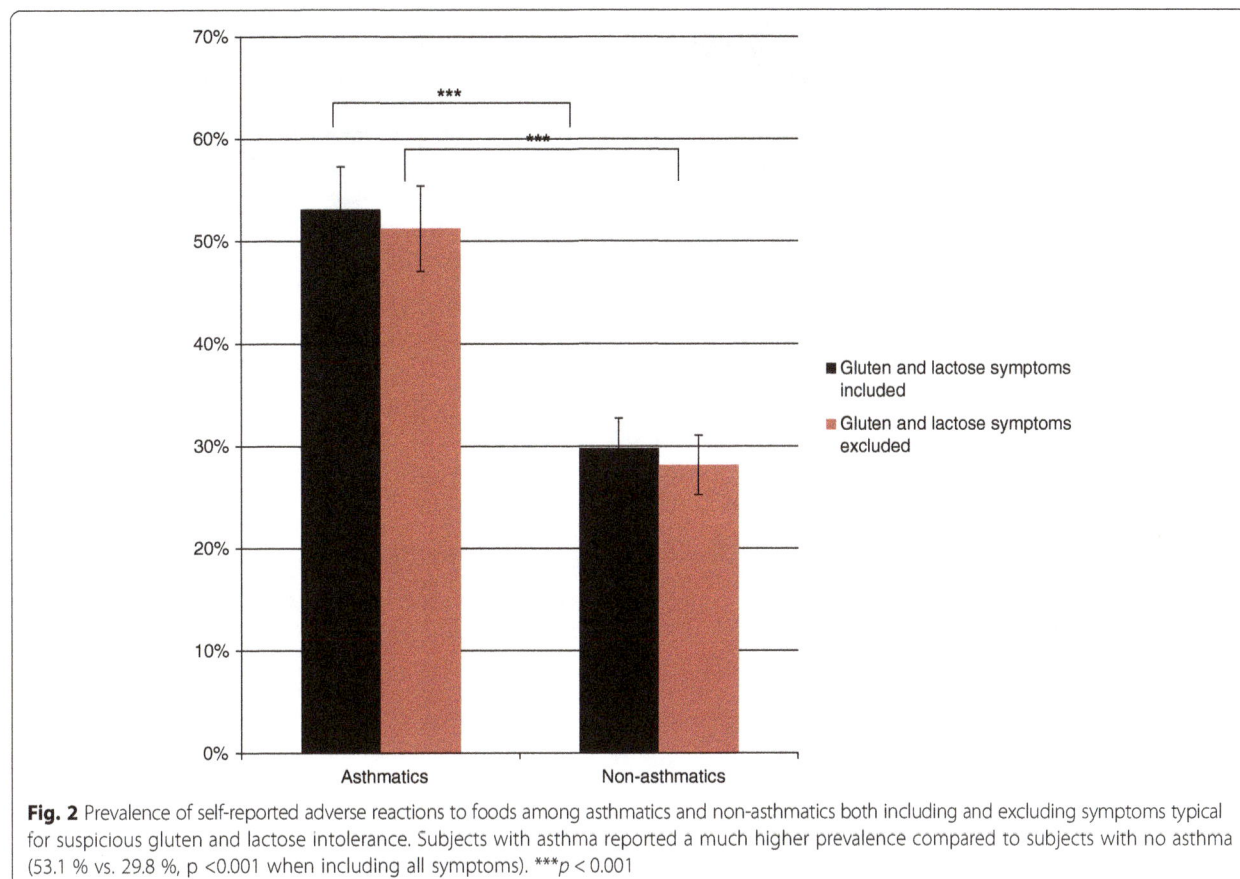

Fig. 2 Prevalence of self-reported adverse reactions to foods among asthmatics and non-asthmatics both including and excluding symptoms typical for suspicious gluten and lactose intolerance. Subjects with asthma reported a much higher prevalence compared to subjects with no asthma (53.1 % vs. 29.8 %, p <0.001 when including all symptoms). ***p < 0.001

$p < 0.01$), kiwi (9.7 % vs 5.3 %, $p < 0.01$), peach (8.3 % vs 2 %, $p < 0.001$), plum (6.75 % vs 2.2 %, $p < 0.001$), nectarine (6.7 % vs 1.3 %, $p < 0.001$), pear (6.4 % vs 2.4 %, $p < 0.001$), cherry (6.2 % vs 2.4 %, $p < 0.001$) followed by walnut (5.9 % vs 3.0 %, $p < 0.01$), fried/fat food (5.7 % vs 3.3 %, $p < 0.05$), sour milk/yoghurt (5.6 % vs 2.8 %, $p < 0.01$) and almond (5.45 % vs 2.3 %, $p < 0.01$) compared to non-asthmatics. Details concerning the prevalence of gastrointestinal symptoms between asthmatics and non-asthmatics for all foods are presented in Table 3.

IgE sensitization for the most common foods among asthmatics and non-asthmatics

When assessing the sIgE-sensitization profiles for the most-common foods in panels fx1 and fx5, we observed that subjects with asthma are generally more frequently sensitized to the food items tested compared to non-asthmatics (38.2 % vs 13.9 %, $p < 0.001$). More specifically, when comparing asthmatics with non-asthmatics, it was found that subjects with asthma were significantly more frequently sensitized to hazelnut (31.8 % vs 11.2 %, $p < 0.001$), peanut (9.1 % vs 4.3 %, $p < 0.001$), almond (6.6 % vs 2.4 %, $p < 0.001$), milk (6.0 % vs 1.6 %, $p < 0.001$), wheat

(5.5 % vs 1.8 %, $p < 0.001$), egg (5.3 % vs 1.4 %, $p < 0.001$), soy (3,5 % vs 1.1 %, $p = 0.003$), brazil nut (2.2 % vs 0.4 %, $p = 0.003$), fish (1.3 % vs 0.0 %, $p = 0.001$). All data are presented in Fig. 3a and b and in Table 4.

Hazelnut seems to be the most frequent food causing symptoms and is also the food item with the highest frequency of IgE-sensitization in asthmatics. Hazelnut is one of the birch pollen-related foods and IgE to hazelnut correlated strongly with IgE to birch in the asthmatic subjects ($r = 0.904$, $p < 0.001$) as well as in non-asthmatic subjects ($r = 0.920$, $p < 0.001$). A moderate correlation was observed between IgE to birch and IgE to peanut ($r = 0.357$, $p < 0.001$) in the asthmatic subjects as well as in non-asthmatic subjects (0.395, $p < 0.001$). When looking for possible correlations between IgE-sensitization and self-reported symptoms for the most common foods, we observed the highest correlation between IgE and self-reported symptoms for hazelnut ($r = 0.496$, $p < 0.001$) in the asthmatic group as well in the non-asthmatic adults ($r = 0.499$, $p < 0.001$). IgE-sensitization to birch also correlated with self-reported symptoms from hazelnut both in subjects with and without asthma, although slightly weaker ($r = 0.455$, $p < 0.001$ resp. $r = 0.472$, $p < 0.001$).

Table 2 Prevalence of adverse reactions (including GI symptoms) to the different foods among asthmatics (asthma), non-asthmatics (no asthma) and in the total sample (all)

Food	% asthma	% no asthma	% all	p	Risk ratio
Hazelnut	20.5	7.2	12.2	<0.001	2.83
Apple	17.5	7.15	11.1	< 0.001	2.45
Kiwi	14.3	6.3	9.3	< 0.001	2.27
Walnut	12.8	4.1	7.3	< 0.001	3.15
Milk	11.5	6.9	8.6	0.003	1.67
Peach	10.7	2.4	5.6	< 0.001	4.39
Brazil nut	9.8	3.5	5.9	< 0.001	2.78
Almond	9.5	2.9	5.4	< 0.001	3.30
Nectarine	9.3	1.8	4.7	< 0.001	5.15
Pear	8.85	2.9	5.1	< 0.001	3.09
Plum	8.8	2.45	4.9	< 0.001	3.61
Cherry	8.65	2.65	4.9	< 0.001	3.26
Wine/beer	8	3.8	5.4	< 0.001	2.08
Peanut	7	2.8	4.3	< 0.001	2.63
Shellfish	6.5	3.1	4.4	0.002	2.09
Carrot	6.4	2.3	3.9	< 0.001	2.73
Strawberry	6.4	1.8	3.5	< 0.001	3.53
Apricot	6.3	1.4	3.3	< 0.001	4.52
Sourmilk/yogurt	6.25	3.5	4.55	0.015	1.78
Fried/fat food	5.9	3.3	4.3	0.018	1.79
Potato	5.5	1.2	2.8	< 0.001	4.70
Cheese	4.5	1.7	2.8	0.001	2.65
Others	4.5	3.1	3.6	0.16	1.46
Sweet pepper	4.4	1.9	2.8	0.006	2.28
Chili/tabasco	4.3	1.8	2.8	0.004	2.40
Tomato	4.15	1.9	2.8	0.011	2.18
Orange	3.8	2.8	3.1	0.26	1.38
Banana	3.8	1.1	2.1	< 0.001	3.56
Bean	3.3	1.6	2.2	0.033	2.06
Egg	3.3	1.1	1.9	0.002	3.09
Flour (wheat)	3.3	1.6	2.2	0.033	2.05
Avocado	3.1	0.5	1.5	< 0.001	5.84
Fish	2.9	0.2	1.25	< 0.001	13.80
Cheese[a]	2.8	0.6	1.5	< 0.001	4.37
Cayenne/red pepper	2.8	1.4	1.9	0.056	2.01
Chocolate	2.8	1.5	2	0.084	1.86
Milk[a]	2.35	1	1.6	0.063	2.15
Pea	2.2	0.4	1.1	0.001	5.27
Additives	1.6	0.4	0.9	0.021	3.66
Curry	1.55	1	1.25	0.41	1.46
Sour milk/yogurt[a]	1.4	0.5	0.9	0.076	2.64
Flour (wheat)[b]	1.4	0.1	0.6	0.002	12.94

Table 2 Prevalence of adverse reactions (including GI symptoms) to the different foods among asthmatics (asthma), non-asthmatics (no asthma) and in the total sample (all) *(Continued)*

Celery	1.4	0.2	0.7	0.006	6.49
Soy	1.4	0.2	0.7	0.006	6.49
Melon	1.4	0.2	0.65	0.006	6.48
Flour (non wheat)	1.4	0.5	0.85	0.083	2.59
Dried fruit	1.2	0.2	0.6	0.014	5.71
Salami	1	0.4	0.7	0.15	2.44
Pork	1	0.5	0.7	0.26	1.94
Sunflower seed	0.9	0	0.3	0.004	-
Chestnut	0.7	0.4	0.5	0.47	1.65
Flour (non wheat)[b]	0.7	0	0.3	0.011	-
Chicken	0.7	0.1	0.3	0.054	6.48
Camomile	0.7	0.5	0.6	0.69	1.30
Sesame seed	0.7	0.1	0.3	0.054	6.49
Anise/caraway	0.5	0.1	0.3	0.13	4.86
Beef	0.35	0.3	0.3	0.93	1.08
Lingonberry	0.3	0.1	0.2	0.31	3.25
Coriander	0.2	0.1	0.1	0.73	1.62
Poppy seed	0.2	0	0.1	0.20	-
Parsley	0.2	0.2	0.2	0.86	0.81

P-value was considered significant when <0.05 comparing the self-reported intolerance for the different foods between asthmatics to non-asthmatics
[a]lactose intolerance symptoms excluded
[b]gluten intolerance symptoms excluded

Seasonal variation of gastrointestinal symptoms in subject with and without asthma

Asthmatics experienced more symptoms from the gastrointestinal tract during the spring (6.7 % vs 2.2 %, $p < 0.001$), summer (5.1 % vs 1.9 %, $p = 0.001$) and autumn (5.9 % vs 3.2 %, $p = 0.013$), but not during the winter compared to non-asthmatics. In addition, asthmatic subjects with IgE reactivity to birch pollen more frequently report gastrointestinal symptoms compared to birch pollen sensitized subjects without asthma during the spring (5.7 % vs 0.8 %, $p = 0.034$), summer (4.2 % vs 0.0 %, $p = 0.026$) and autumn (3.7 % vs 0.0 %, $p = 0.046$) (Fig. 4 and Additional file 2: Table S1).

Discussion

In the present study, subjects with asthma more frequently reported adverse reactions to foods compared to non-asthmatics (53 % vs 30 %), and patients with asthma more frequently showed IgE reactivity to the most common foods. These results are in line with data from a previous study by Woods et al. in which it was suggested a positive association between IgE sensitization to foods and asthma or allergic disease [22]. The data was supported also by the sensitisation patterns of specific-IgE

Table 3 Prevalence of self-reported gastrointestinal symptoms for the different foods among asthmatics (asthma), non-asthmatics (no asthma) and in the total sample (all)

Food	% asthma	% no asthma	p	Ratio
Hazelnut	13	5.2	< 0.001	2.51
Apple	11.4	6	< 0.001	1.91
Milk	10.4	5.7	0.001	1.84
Kiwi	9.7	5.3	0.002	1.82
Peach	8.3	2	< 0.001	4.11
Plum	6.75	2.2	< 0.001	3.02
Nectarine	6.7	1.3	< 0.001	5.27
Pear	6.4	2.4	< 0.001	2.63
Cherry	6.2	2.4	< 0.001	2.55
Walnut	5.9	3	0.006	1.99
Fried/fat food	5.7	3.3	0.026	1.73
Sour milk/yogurt	5.6	2.8	0.007	2.01
Almond	5.45	2.3	0.002	2.33
Brazil nut	5.3	2.6	0.008	2.06
Apricot	3.8	1.3	0.001	2.99
Sweet pepper	3.7	1.7	0.018	2.15
Cheese	3.5	1	0.001	3.27
Tomato	3.5	1.4	0.007	2.51
Strawberry	3.4	0.95	< 0.001	3.61
Peanut	3.3	1.7	0.045	1.95
Carrot	3.3	1.6	0.033	2.06
Others	3.1	1.7	0.074	1.83
Shellfish	3	1.2	0.013	2.53
Chili/tabasco	2.8	1	0.0075	2.90
Egg	2.8	1	0.008	2.89
Banana	2.7	0.95	0.008	2.88
Wine/beer	2.6	1.4	0.090	1.88
Bean	2.6	1.6	0.18	1.62
Potato	2.4	0.5	0.0015	4.52
Flour (wheat)	2.2	1.4	0.21	1.62
Avocado	2.2	0.4	0.001	5.27
Chocolate	1.9	0.85	0.074	2.24
Orange	1.9	1.4	0.43	1.38
Pea	1.9	0.3	0.002	5.95
Cheese[a]	1.6	0	< 0.001	-
Fish	1.55	0.1	< 0.001	14.61
Cayenne/red pepper	1.4	0.7	0.22	1.87
Soy	1.4	0.2	0.006	6.49
Milk[a]	1.3	0.2	0.013	5.78
Melon	1.2	0.2	0.014	5.67
Flour (non wheat)	1.2	0.4	0.083	2.83
Sour milk/yogurt[a]	0.9	0.1	0.021	8.26

Table 3 Prevalence of self-reported gastrointestinal symptoms for the different foods among asthmatics (asthma), non-asthmatics (no asthma) and in the total sample (all) *(Continued)*

Pork	0.9	0.4	0.28	2.02
Salami	0.7	0.2	0.15	3.25
Flour (wheat)[b]	0.7	0	0.011	-
Dried fruit	0.7	0.1	0.053	6.53
Celery	0.7	0.1	0.054	6.49
Curry	0.7	0.4	0.49	1.62
Sunflower seed	0.7	0	0.011	-
Chestnut	0.5	0.3	0.54	1.65
Additives	0.5	0.3	0.55	1.63
Flour (non wheat)[b]	0.5	0	0.027	-
Chicken	0.5	0	0.027	-
Anise/caraway	0.5	0	0.027	-
Beef	0.35	0.3	0.93	1.08
Camomile	0.3	0.1	0.31	3.25
Lingonberry	0.3	0.1	0.31	3.25
Sesame seed	0.3	0.1	0.31	3.24
Coriander	0.2	0.1	0.73	1.62
Parsley	0.2	0	0.20	-
Poppy seed	0.2	0	0.20	-

P-value was considered significant when <0.05 comparing the self-reported intolerance for the different foods between asthmatics to non-asthmatics
[a]lactose intolerance symptoms excluded
[b]gluten intolerance symptoms excluded

for the most common foods found in the present study. We also show that asthmatics reported symptoms from the GI-tract in a greater frequency compared to non-asthmatics and the most common foods causing self-reported symptoms were nuts, fruits, milk dairy products, alcohol, peanuts and shellfish. The non-asthmatic subjects seem to report adverse reaction to the same food items as asthmatics but at a significantly lower frequency. These data are in the line with previous reports that show a clear relation between food sensitization/allergy and asthma [23, 24]. Here, we demonstrate that the most common foods causing self-reported adverse reactions in subjects with asthma, when excluding those with suspected lactose- and gluten-intolerance, are fruits (as apple, kiwi, peach, nectarine), nuts (hazelnut, walnut, brazil nut), almond, peanut, followed by shellfish, milk dairy products, fried/fat food, potato, tomato, egg, flour and fish. The main allergens found in the reported fruits and nuts, carry allergens with known cross-reactivity with PR-10 allergens which are related to birch pollen. This, may explain the high prevalence of adverse reactions to these foods, since birch pollen sensitization is very common in Sweden [25]. These findings are confirmed in the present study, in which, 32.9 % of the asthmatics and 12.6 % of the non-asthmatics were sensitized to birch pollen. Thus, birch

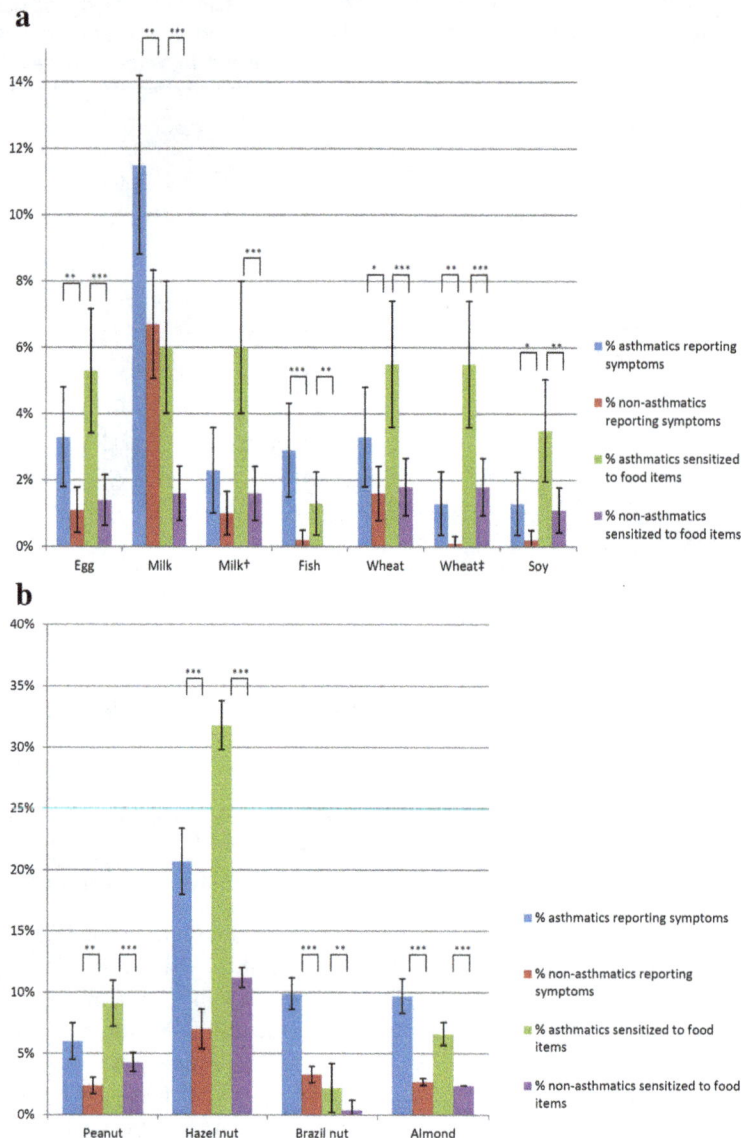

Fig. 3 Prevalence of self-reported symptoms and IgE sensitization for the most common foods among asthmatics and non-asthmatics (95 % CI). **a** staple foods **b** birch-related foods. †: lactose intolerance symptoms excluded. ‡: gluten intolerance symptoms excluded. *$p < 0.05$. **$p < 0.01$. ***$p < 0.001$

sensitization could explain the frequent adverse reactions observed following ingestion of birch related foods [26]. When testing the subjects included, with the allergen panels for the most common staple foods and nuts (fx1 and fx5), we observe interesting differences between asthmatics and non-asthmatics. Generally, adults with asthma are significantly more sensitized to any food, compared to non-asthmatics (38.2 % vs 13.9 %, $p < 0.001$) which may be a result of a general atopic phenotype in asthmatics. Subjects with asthma are more frequently sensitized to hazelnut, peanut, almond and milk compared to non-asthmatics which is mainly in accordance with the results from self-reported symptoms in this study. However, the correlation between

IgE sensitization to specific food items and the symptoms they cause are rather low, but significant.

Concerning the staple foods, we show that asthmatic subjects more frequently report symptoms from egg, fish, milk, and wheat as well as soy compared to non-asthmatics and when we exclude subjects with suspected lactose- and gluten-intolerance, we notice an important difference in the results for milk and wheat (Table 2). When excluding subjects with suspicious intolerance to gluten and/or lactose though, the risk of losing some subjects with true allergy is inevitable, however the difference between asthmatics and non-asthmatics still remains. These results are in the line with previous reports

Table 4 Prevalence for self-reported symptoms with 95 % CI and IgE-sensitization profile for the most common foods among asthmatics and non-asthmatics

Food	Self-reported symptoms of the food among asthmatics (95 % CI)	Self-reported symptoms of the food among non-asthmatics (95 % CI)	IgEsensitization to food among asthmatics (95 % CI)	IgEsensitization to food among non-asthmatics (95 % CI)
Egg	3.30 % (1.80 % -4.80 %)	1.10 % (0.42 % -1.78 %)	5.30 % (3.42 % -7.18 %)	1.40 % (0.64 % -2.16 %)
Milk	11.50 % (8.81 % -14.19 %)	6.70 % (5.07 % -8.33 %)	6.00 % (4.01 % -7.99 %)	1.60 % (0.79 % -2.41 %)
Milk[a]	2.30 % (1.01 % -3.59 %)	1.00 % (0.34 % -1.66 %)	6.00 % (4.01 % -7.99 %)	1.60 % (0.79 % -2.41 %)
Fish	2.90 % (1.49 % -4.31 %)	0.20 % (-0.09 % -0.49 %)	1.30 % (0.35 % -2.25 %)	0.00 % (0.00 % -0.00 %)
Wheat	3.30 % (1.80 % -4.80 %)	1.60 % (0.78 % -2.42 %)	5.50 % (3.59 % -7.41 %)	1.80 % (0.94 % -2.66 %)
Wheat[b]	1.30 % (0.35 % -2.25 %)	0.10 % (-0.11 % -0.31 %)	5.50 % (3.59 % -7.41 %)	1.80 % (0.94 % -2.66 %)
Soy	1.30 % (0.35 % -2.25 %)	0.20 % (-0.09 % -0.49 %)	3.50 % (1.96 % -5.04 %)	1.10 % (0.42 % -1.78 %)
Peanut	6.00 % (3.99 % -8.01 %)	2.40 % (1.41 % -3.39 %)	9.10 % (6.69 % -11.51 %)	4.30 % (2.98 % -5.62 %)
Hazel nut	20.70 % (17.26 % -24.14 %)	7.00 % (5.34 % -8.66 %)	31.80 % (27.90 % -35.70 %)	11.20 % (9.15 % -13.25 %)
Brazil nut	9.90 % (7.32 % -12.48 %)	3.30 % (2.14 % -4.46 %)	2.20 % (0.97 % -3.43 %)	0.40 % (-0.01 % -0.81 %)
Almond	9.70 % (7.19 % -12.21 %)	2.70 % (1.65 % -3.75 %)	6.60 % (4.52 % -8.68 %)	2.40 % (1.41 % -3.39 %)
Any of the above	37.00 % (32.90 % -41.10 %)	15.40 % (13.04 % -17.76 %)	38.20 % (34.13 % -42.27 %)	13.90 % (11.66 % -16.14 %)

[a]lactose intolerance symptoms excluded
[b]gluten intolerance symptoms excluded

from a Swedish epidemiological survey by Eriksson et al. concerning self-reported food hypersensitivity in north Europe [27]. Interestingly subjects with asthma report significantly more symptoms in high rates after alcohol ingestion as from wine/beer compared to non-asthmatics (7.97 % vs 5.41 %, $p < 0.001$), which is supported by results from previous reports [28–30].

When the IgE sensitization to birch pollen is taken into consideration, we observe that among both asthmatics and non-asthmatics, birch-related foods are the most common causatives for adverse reactions with hazelnut in the first place (20.5 % and 7.2 % respectively) followed by apple (17.5 % and 7.15 % respectively) and other birch related fruits and nuts (Table 2). IgE reactivity

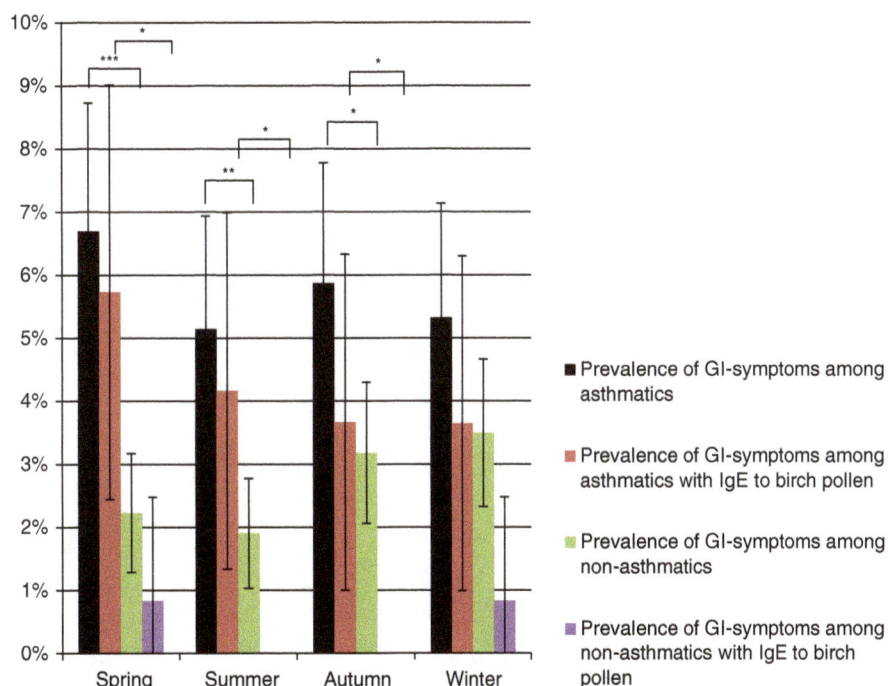

Fig. 4 Prevalence of self-reported gastrointestinal symptoms (GI) among asthmatics and non-asthmatics, and among subjects sensitized to IgE for birch pollen for the different seasons of the year (95 % CI). *$p < 0.05$. **$p < 0.01$. ***$p < 0.001$

to hazelnut and birch were also correlated to self-reported symptoms evoked by hazelnut, which is supported by the reported strong correlation between IgE for birch and IgE for hazelnut in both asthmatic and non-asthmatic subjects.

It is worth to comment that the prevalence of allergic asthma is much higher in the paediatric and adolescent population [31] and at about 40 years of age the prevalence of allergic and non-allergic asthma is approximately the same, and thereafter the non-allergic asthma dominates [32–35]. IgE-sensitization to the different foods and even other allergens may be more strongly connected to allergic asthma in the paediatric population [36] and less so in adults, which is supported by several recent studies, that show remission of the allergic disease before adulthood [37], and a decrease in the prevalence of IgE sensitization to foods among adults [38]. However, as shown in the present study adult asthmatics also have a high frequency of adverse reactions to foods that correlate with their IgE sensitization profile.

In this study, asthmatics reported more gastrointestinal symptoms during spring, summer and autumn compared to non-asthmatics. It is still not clear if increased asthma symptoms can be related to the increased frequency of gastrointestinal symptoms observed in the present study. The possible seasonal variation in gastrointestinal symptoms may be related to the pollen season where exposure to pollen may increase the reactivity after the ingestion of pollen related food items [25], which could be aggravated by the increased intestinal permeability seen in asthmatic patients [39] as well as in patients with atopy and IBS [40]. In two other studies, it was demonstrated that asthmatics with allergy to birch pollen experience more symptoms from the gastrointestinal tract, which resemble irritable bowel syndrome (IBS)-like symptoms, during the pollen season [41, 42]. It has also been shown that atopic subjects with IBS and self–reported food hypersensitivity had more severe gastrointestinal symptoms when compared to non-atopic subjects with IBS [40]. Interestingly, besides the reported symptoms from the birch-pollen related foods, asthmatics reported more gastrointestinal symptoms to fried/fat food, rich in carbohydrate, wine/beer, legumes and spices which would signify that these patients may more frequently suffer from IBS [43, 44].

The present study has some limitations that should be taken into consideration. It is well known that self-reported food intolerance yield a much higher prevalence compared to prevalence from performed food challenges and IgE data for food allergies [45]. However, the comparison between asthmatics and non-asthmatics should still be valid, since we have no reason to believe that the self-reporting accuracy differs between these two groups. It would also have been of great value to have asked specifically for lactose and gluten intolerance, and not only get input from the free text fields. Nevertheless, the reported symptoms do affect the subjects, whether it is a true allergy or not. The large number of participants in the study makes the findings reliable and fascinating as there are very few studies to date having examined the relation between food hypersensitivity and IgE sensitization to the most common foods in adults.

Conclusions

The novelty of this study, as one of the largest epidemiological studies in the adult population, is that it examines the relation between self-reported adverse reactions and IgE-sensitization for the most common foods and in adult asthmatic and non-asthmatic subjects as well as the relation between asthma and gastrointestinal symptoms caused by various foods in adults, for which the existing data are still very scarce.

In conclusion, the prevalence of both self-reported symptoms and IgE sensitization to various foods were much higher among asthmatics compared to non-asthmatic Swedish adults, both in total and for most individual food items studied. Hazelnut and other birch pollen related foods most commonly induced gastrointestinal symptoms in asthmatics and we propose that one important factor that may explain these findings is the high frequency of sensitization to birch pollen in asthmatic patients in Northern Europe.

Competing interests
The authors declare that they have no competing interests.

Authors' contributions
All authors were involved in the discussions and contributed to writing the manuscript. All authors read, revised and approved the final version of the manuscript to be published.

Acknowledgements
We would like to thank Ass Prof Ulf Bengtsson for making the questionnaire for the adverse reactions to different foods available to be used in this study. We would also like to thank the research nurses in Krefting Research Centre for their help in collecting all data and interviewing all subjects who participated in this study.

Author details
[1]Section of Allergology, University Hospital of Sahlgrenska, 413 45 Gothenburg, Sweden. [2]Krefting Research Centre, Department of Internal Medicine and Clinical Nutrition, University of Gothenburg, Gothenburg, Sweden. [3]Department for Rheumatology and Inflammation Research, Sahlgrenska Academy, University of Gothenburg, Gothenburg, Sweden. [4]R&D, ImmunoDiagnostics, Thermofischer Scientific, Uppsala, Sweden.

References

1. Chafen JJ, Newberry SJ, Riedl MA, Bravata DM, Maglione M, Suttorp MJ, et al. Diagnosing and managing common food allergies: a systematic review. JAMA. 2010;303(18):1848–56.
2. Nwaru BI, Hickstein L, Panesar SS, Muraro A, Werfel T, Cardona V, et al. The epidemiology of food allergy in Europe: a systematic review and meta-analysis. Allergy. 2014;69(1):62–75.
3. Sicherer SH, Sampson HA. Food allergy: epidemiology, pathogenesis, diagnosis, and treatment. J Allergy Clin Immunol. 2014;133(2):291–307. 2.
4. Berns SH, Halm EA, Sampson HA, Sicherer SH, Busse PJ, Wisnivesky JP. Food allergy as a risk factor for asthma morbidity in adults. J Asthma. 2007;44(5):377–81.
5. Roberts G, Patel N, Levi-Schaffer F, Habibi P, Lack G. Food allergy as a risk factor for life-threatening asthma in childhood: a case-controlled study. J Allergy Clin Immunol. 2003;112(1):168–74.
6. Bock SA, Munoz-Furlong A, Sampson HA. Fatalities due to anaphylactic reactions to foods. J Allergy Clin Immunol. 2001;107(1):191–3.
7. Oehling A, Baena Cagnani CE. Food allergy and child asthma. Allergol Immunopathol (Madr). 1980;8(1):7–14.
8. Roberts G, Lack G. Food allergy and asthma–what is the link? Paediatr Respir Rev. 2003;4(3):205–12.
9. Woods RK, Thien F, Raven J, Walters EH, Abramson M. Prevalence of food allergies in young adults and their relationship to asthma, nasal allergies, and eczema. Ann Allergy Asthma Immunol. 2002;88(2):183–9.
10. Blanco Carmona JG, Juste Picon S, Garces Sotillos M, Rodriguez GP. Occupational asthma in the confectionary industry caused by sensitivity to egg. Allergy. 1992;47(2 Pt 2):190–1.
11. Boulet LP, Laberge F. Occupational asthma to fish. Occup Environ Med. 2014;71(11):804.
12. James JM, Crespo JF. Allergic reactions to foods by inhalation. Curr Allergy Asthma Rep. 2007;7(3):167–74.
13. Caffarelli C, Deriu FM, Terzi V, Perrone F, De Angelis G, Atherton DJ. Gastrointestinal symptoms in patients with asthma. Arch Dis Child. 2000;82(2):131–5.
14. Kivity S, Fireman E, Sade K. Bronchial hyperactivity, sputum analysis and skin prick test to inhalant allergens in patients with symptomatic food hypersensitivity. Isr Med Assoc J. 2005;7(12):781–4.
15. Powell N, Huntley B, Beech T, Knight W, Knight H, Corrigan CJ. Increased prevalence of gastrointestinal symptoms in patients with allergic disease. Postgrad Med J. 2007;83(977):182–6.
16. Tielemans MM, Jaspers Focks J, van Rossum LG, Eikendal T, Jansen JB, Laheij RJ, et al. Gastrointestinal symptoms are still prevalent and negatively impact health-related quality of life: a large cross-sectional population based study in The Netherlands. PLoS One. 2013;8(7):e69876.
17. Louis E, Louis R, Drion V, Bonnet V, Lamproye A, Radermecker M, et al. Increased frequency of bronchial hyperresponsiveness in patients with inflammatory bowel disease. Allergy. 1995;50(9):729–33.
18. White AM, Stevens WH, Upton AR, O'Byrne PM, Collins SM. Airway responsiveness to inhaled methacholine in patients with irritable bowel syndrome. Gastroenterology. 1991;100(1):68–74.
19. Wallaert B, Desreumaux P, Copin MC, Tillie I, Benard A, Colombel JF, et al. Immunoreactivity for interleukin 3 and 5 and granulocyte/macrophage colony-stimulating factor of intestinal mucosa in bronchial asthma. J Exp Med. 1995;182(6):1897–904.
20. Ronmark EP, Ekerljung L, Lotvall J, Toren K, Ronmark E, Lundback B. Large scale questionnaire survey on respiratory health in Sweden: effects of late- and non-response. Respir Med. 2009;103(12):1807–15.
21. Landis JR, Koch GG. The measurement of observer agreement for categorical data. Biometrics. 1977;33(1):159–74.
22. Woods RK, Stoney RM, Raven J, Walters EH, Abramson M, Thien FC. Reported adverse food reactions overestimate true food allergy in the community. Eur J Clin Nutr. 2002;56(1):31–6.
23. Liu AH, Jaramillo R, Sicherer SH, Wood RA, Bock SA, Burks AW, et al. National prevalence and risk factors for food allergy and relationship to asthma: results from the National Health and Nutrition Examination Survey 2005–2006. J Allergy Clin Immunol. 2010;126(4):798–806. 4.
24. Patelis A, Gunnbjornsdottir M, Malinovschi A, Matsson P, Onell A, Hogman M, et al. Population-based study of multiplexed IgE sensitization in relation to asthma, exhaled nitric oxide, and bronchial responsiveness. J Allergy Clin Immunol. 2012;130(2):397–402. 2.
25. Vieths S, Scheurer S, Ballmer-Weber B. Current understanding of cross-reactivity of food allergens and pollen. Ann N Y Acad Sci. 2002;964:47–68.
26. Eriksson NE, Holmen A. Skin prick tests with standardized extracts of inhalant allergens in 7099 adult patients with asthma or rhinitis: cross-sensitizations and relationships to age, sex, month of birth and year of testing. J Investig Allergol Clin Immunol. 1996;6(1):36–46.
27. Eriksson NE, Moller C, Werner S, Magnusson J, Bengtsson U, Zolubas M. Self-reported food hypersensitivity in Sweden, Denmark, Estonia, Lithuania, and Russia. J Investig Allergol Clin Immunol. 2004;14(1):70–9.
28. Lieberoth S, Backer V, Kyvik KO, Skadhauge LR, Tolstrup JS, Gronbaek M, et al. Intake of alcohol and risk of adult-onset asthma. Respir Med. 2012;106(2):184–8.
29. Linneberg A, Berg ND, Gonzalez-Quintela A, Vidal C, Elberling J. Prevalence of self-reported hypersensitivity symptoms following intake of alcoholic drinks. Clin Exp Allergy. 2008;38(1):145–51.
30. Vally H, Thompson PJ. Allergic and asthmatic reactions to alcoholic drinks. Addict Biol. 2003;8(1):3–11.
31. Ronmark E, Bjerg A, Perzanowski M, Platts-Mills T, Lundback B. Major increase in allergic sensitization in schoolchildren from 1996 to 2006 in northern Sweden. J Allergy Clin Immunol. 2009;124(2):357–63. 63.e1-15.
32. Ekerljung L, Bossios A, Lotvall J, Olin AC, Ronmark E, Wennergren G, et al. Multi-symptom asthma as an indication of disease severity in epidemiology. Eur Respir J. 2011;38(4):825–32.
33. Kamdar TA, Peterson S, Lau CH, Saltoun CA, Gupta RS, Bryce PJ. Prevalence and characteristics of adult-onset food allergy. J Allergy Clin Immunol Pract. 2015;3(1):114. 5.e1.
34. Pallasaho P, Juusela M, Lindqvist A, Sovijarvi A, Lundback B, Ronmark E. Allergic rhinoconjunctivitis doubles the risk for incident asthma–results from a population study in Helsinki. Finland Respir Med. 2011;105(10):1449–56.
35. Warm K, Backman H, Lindberg A, Lundback B, Ronmark E. Low incidence and high remission of allergic sensitization among adults. J Allergy Clin Immunol. 2012;129(1):136–42.
36. Strinnholm A, Winberg A, West C, Hedman L, Ronmark E. Food hypersensitivity is common in Swedish schoolchildren, especially oral reactions to fruit and gastrointestinal reactions to milk. Acta Paediatr. 2014;103(12):1290–6.
37. Winberg A, Strinnholm A, Hedman L, West C, Perzanowski M, Ronmark E. High incidence and remission of reported food hypersensitivity in Swedish children followed from 8 to 12years of age - a population based cohort study. Clin Trans Allergy. 2014;4(1):32.
38. Patelis A, Gunnbjornsdottir M, Borres MP, Burney P, Gislason T, Toren K, et al. Natural history of perceived food hypersensitivity and IgE sensitisation to food allergens in a cohort of adults. PLoS One. 2014;9(1):e85333.
39. Benard A, Desreumeaux P, Huglo D, Hoorelbeke A, Tonnel AB, Wallaert B. Increased intestinal permeability in bronchial asthma. J Allergy Clin Immunol. 1996;97(6):1173–8.
40. Lillestol K, Helgeland L, Arslan Lied G, Florvaag E, Valeur J, Lind R, Berstad, A. Indications of 'atopic bowel' in patients with self-reported food hypersensitivity. Aliment Pharmacol Ther. 2010;31(10):1112–22.
41. Magnusson J, Lin XP, Dahlman-Hoglund A, Hanson LL, Telemo E, Magnusson O, et al. Seasonal intestinal inflammation in patients with birch pollen allergy. J Allergy Clin Immunol. 2003;112(1):45–50.
42. Rentzos G, Lundberg V, Stotzer PO, Pullerits T, Telemo E. Intestinal allergic inflammation in birch pollen allergic patients in relation to pollen season, IgE sensitization profile and gastrointestinal symptoms. Clin Trans Allergy. 2014;4:19.
43. Bohn L, Storsrud S, Tornblom H, Bengtsson U, Simren M. Self-reported food-related gastrointestinal symptoms in IBS are common and associated with more severe symptoms and reduced quality of life. Am J Gastroenterol. 2013;108(5):634–41.
44. Simren M, Mansson A, Langkilde AM, Svedlund J, Abrahamsson H, Bengtsson U, et al. Food-related gastrointestinal symptoms in the irritable bowel syndrome. Digestion. 2001;63(2):108–15.
45. O'Keefe AW, De Schryver S, Mill J, Mill C, Dery A, Ben-Shoshan M. Diagnosis and management of food allergies: new and emerging options: a systematic review. J Asthma Allergy. 2014;7:141–64.

12

POLLAR: Impact of air POLLution on Asthma and Rhinitis; a European Institute of Innovation and Technology Health (EIT Health) project

Jean Bousquet[1,2,3,4,5,6]*[iD], Josep M. Anto[7,8,9,10], Isabella Annesi-Maesano[11], Toni Dedeu[12], Eve Dupas[13], Jean-Louis Pépin[14,15], Landry Stephane Zeng Eyindanga[16], Sylvie Arnavielhe[13], Julia Ayache[17,18], Xavier Basagana[7], Samuel Benveniste[17,19], Nuria Calves Venturos[20], Hing Kin Chan[13], Mehdi Cheraitia[21], Yves Dauvilliers[22], Judith Garcia-Aymerich[7], Ingrid Jullian-Desayes[14,15], Chitra Dinesh[21], Daniel Laune[13], Jade Lu Dac[21], Ismael Nujurally[21], Giovanni Pau[23], Robert Picard[24], Xavier Rodo[25], Renaud Tamisier[14,15], Michael Bewick[26], Nils E. Billo[27], Wienczyslawa Czarlewski[28], Joao Fonseca[29,30], Ludger Klimek[31], Oliver Pfaar[31,32] and Jean-Marc Bourez[33]

Abstract

Allergic rhinitis (AR) is impacted by allergens and air pollution but interactions between air pollution, sleep and allergic diseases are insufficiently understood. POLLAR (Impact of air POLLution on sleep, Asthma and Rhinitis) is a project of the European Institute of Innovation and Technology (EIT Health). It will use a freely-existing application for AR monitoring that has been tested in 23 countries (the *Allergy Diary*, iOS and Android, 17,000 users, TLR8). The Allergy Diary will be combined with a new tool allowing queries on allergen, pollen (TLR2), sleep quality and disorders (TRL2) as well as existing longitudinal and geolocalized pollution data. Machine learning will be used to assess the relationship between air pollution, sleep and AR comparing polluted and non-polluted areas in 6 EU countries. Data generated in 2018 will be confirmed in 2019 and extended by the individual prospective assessment of pollution (portable sensor, TLR7) in AR. Sleep apnea patients will be used as a demonstrator of sleep disorder that can be modulated in terms of symptoms and severity by air pollution and AR. The geographic information system GIS will map the results. Consequences on quality of life (EQ-5D), asthma, school, work and sleep will be monitored and disseminated towards the population. The impacts of POLLAR will be (1) to propose novel care pathways integrating pollution, sleep and patients' literacy, (2) to study sleep consequences of pollution and its impact on frequent chronic diseases, (3) to improve work productivity, (4) to propose the basis for a sentinel network at the EU level for pollution and allergy, (5) to assess the societal implications of the interaction. MASK paper N°32.

Keywords: Asthma, Pollen, Pollution, Rhinitis, mHealth, Climate change

*Correspondence: jean.bousquet@orange.fr
[6] CHU Montpellier, 371 Avenue du Doyen Gaston Giraud, 34295 Montpellier Cedex 5, France
Full list of author information is available at the end of the article

Background

Exposure to ambient air pollution increases morbidity and mortality. It is a leading contributor to global disease burden [1, 2]. The role of air pollution on cardiovascular events [3], COPD [4], sleep apnea [5] and asthma exacerbations [6] is clear. In allergic rhinitis (AR), air pollution is one of the risk factors that induces allergic sensitization and deteriorates the AR condition, but data are sometimes conflicting [7]. Moreover, data on the impact of air pollution on AR multimorbidity [8] or severity are scarce [9] and not always conclusive, probably due to methodological problems.

Meteorological factors such as temperature, sunlight and humidity as well as air pollution can affect pollen emission and allergenic concentration [10–12]. Traffic-related pollutants [13] and diesel exhaust particles can disrupt pollen, leading to the release of pauci-micronic particles which can penetrate in the bronchi [14]. Asthma due to pollen may be associated to peaks of air pollution [15–19]. These data suggest an important interaction between pollens and pollution, inducing asthma in AR patients during the pollen season. However, more data should be collected and mobile technology may be interesting.

MASK-rhinitis (Mobile Airways Sentinel NetworK for allergic rhinitis) is a patient centred ICT system [20]. A mobile phone app (*Allergy Diary*) central to MASK has been launched in 23 countries and has been validated [21–24].

Many different methods are used to monitor pollen exposure [25–28]. Pollen counts can assess the exposure of pollen-allergic patients [29]. The assessment of allergen content in the air is feasible [30] but requires sophisticated methods that may not account for all of the pollen species in the ambient air. Meteorological data may, in the future, be of interest for predicting the onset of the season, but more data are required [31]. Combining several sources using advanced data engineering may also be important but these data are still complex and, in many different areas, not yet available for all pollen species [25–28, 32]. Google Trends (GT) is a Web-based surveillance tool that uses Google to explore the searching trends of specific queries. Recent studies have suggested the utility of GT for assessing the seasonality of allergic diseases [33–37]. GT reflects the real-world AR epidemiology and could potentially be used as a monitoring tool for allergic rhinitis [38, 39].

Interactions between air pollution, sleep quality, sleep disorders [40] and allergic diseases are clear but insufficiently understood. POLLAR (Impact of Air POLLution on sleep, Asthma and Rhinitis) is a new project of the EIT Health that will embed environmental data into the *Allergy Diary*. POLLAR aims at combining emerging technologies (search engine Technology Readiness level TLR2; sleep assessment, pollution sampler TLR6, *Allergy Diary* TLR9) with machine learning to (1) understand the effects of air pollution in allergic rhinitis and its impact on sleep, work and asthma, (2) assess societal consequences, shared with citizens, corporate citizens and professionals (3) propose preventive strategies and (4) develop participative policies.

EIT health

European Institute of Innovation and Technology (EIT) and Knowledge and Innovation Communities (KICs)

The European Institute of Innovation and Technology (EIT), the research and technological agency of the EU, was set up in 2008. It aims to spur innovation and entrepreneurship across Europe in order to overcome some of its greatest challenges. The EIT strengthens cooperation among its partners to form dynamic pan-European partnerships and to develop favorable environments for creative thought processes and innovations. Real sustainable products, services, entrepreneurs, engineers, scientists, companies, revenue, profit and jobs are emerging from the Innovation Communities making this innovation network the largest in Europe, if not in the world.

The Knowledge and Innovation Communities (KICs) represent a unique feature of the EIT for the integration of education, research and innovation (the so-called *Knowledge Triangle*) in a common organization. The KICs carry out activities that cover the entire innovation chain: training and education programmes, reinforcing the journey from research to the market, innovation projects, as well as business incubators and accelerators.

There are currently six Innovation Communities and each one focuses on a different societal challenge (https://eit.europa.eu/activities/innovation-communities): EIT Climate-KIC (climate change mitigation and adaptation), EIT Digital (Information and Communication Technologies), EIT InnoEnergy (sustainable energy), EIT Health (healthy living and active ageing), EIT Raw Materials (sustainable exploration, extraction, processing, recycling and substitution) and EIT Food (putting Europe at the centre of a global revolution in food innovation and production).

EIT health

EIT Health (European Institute of Innovation and Technology-Health) is a consortium of over 50 core partners and 90 associate partners from leading businesses, research centres and universities across 14 EU countries. EIT Health works to give EU citizens greater opportunities to enjoy a healthier and active life for longer, and to postpone dependency on others, by leveraging big data and new technologies, identifying and removing barriers to innovation, and building on education and talent creation (https://www.eithealth.eu). EIT Health allows:

- Innovative products and services to be developed in every area imaginable, including climate change, healthy living and active and healthy ageing (AHA).
- New companies to be started.
- A new generation of entrepreneurs to be trained.

The EIT's role is to guide the process and set the strategies, but the KICs should put these into practice and provide results.

Three pillars have been defined:

- Promote healthy living, self-management of health and life style interventions.
- Support active ageing.
- Improve healthcare with innovations and a patient-centric approach, in particular for chronic diseases.

EIT Health brings together the three sides of the knowledge triangle through three programmes:

- Campus (education) provides up-to-date knowledge, skills and attitudes to help turn the brightest learners into healthcare leaders and entrepreneurs to shape the future of Europe's health. Campus educational offerings are intended to increase industry knowledge and deliver novel skills, as EIT seeks to inject an entrepreneurial approach into European healthcare education (https://www.eithealth.eu/campus).
- Accelerator (business creation) supports the best and brightest health industry entrepreneurs, creating a favorable environment for innovation and providing skills and services to get promising business ideas into the market.
- Innovation Projects provide comprehensive support for innovations that show the potential to have a positive impact on healthcare for a societal challenge. The most promising ideas are developed into commercially-viable products through a multi-disciplinary approach.

The Allergy Diary
MASK (Mobile Airways Sentinel NetworK)
In 2012, the European Commission launched the European Innovation Partnership on Active and Healthy Ageing (DG Santé and DG CONNECT) [41]. The B3 Action Plan devoted to innovative integrated care models for chronic diseases has selected Integrated care pathways for airway diseases (AIRWAYS ICPs) [42, 43] with a life cycle approach [44] as the model for chronic diseases. The Action Plan of AIRWAYS ICPs has been devised

[42], implemented [45] and scaled up [46, 47]. AIRWAYS ICPs is a GARD (WHO Global Alliance for Chronic Respiratory Diseases) [48] research demonstration project (Fig. 1).

MASK (Mobile Airways Sentinel NetworK) represents Phase 3 of ARIA and is an AIRWAYS ICPs tool [20, 49]. It represents a Good Practice focusing on the implementation of multi-sectoral care pathways using emerging technologies with real life data in rhinitis and asthma multi-morbidity. MASK follows the JA-CHRODIS (Joint Action on Chronic Diseases and Promoting Healthy Ageing across the Life Cycle, 2nd EU Health Programme 2008-2013 [50]) recommendations for good practices [51].

MASK was initiated to reduce the global burden of rhinitis and asthma, by giving the patient a simple tool to better prevent and manage respiratory allergic diseases. More specifically, MASK should help to (i) understand the disease mechanisms and the effects of air pollution in allergic diseases, (ii) better appraise the burden incurred by medical needs but also the indirect costs, (iii) propose novel multidisciplinary care pathways integrating pollution and patients' literacy, (iv) improve work productivity, (v) propose the basis for a sentinel network at the EU level for pollution and allergy and (vi) assess the societal implications of the project to reduce health and social inequalities globally.

The *Allergy Diary*
The mobile technology of MASK is the *Allergy Diary*, an App (Android and iOS) which is freely available for AR and asthma sufferers in 23 countries (16 EU countries, Argentina, Australia, Brazil, Canada, Mexico, Switzerland and Turkey) and 17 languages (translated and back-translated, culturally adapted and legally compliant) [20]. Users fill in a simple questionnaire on asthma and rhinitis upon registration and daily assess the impact of their disease using a visual analogue scale (VAS) [52] for global allergy symptoms, rhinitis, conjunctivitis, asthma and for work. Moreover, two specific questionnaires are applied every week to assess disease impact on patients' QoL (EQ-5D) [24] and productivity at work (WPAI-AS) [53]. The *Allergy Diary* is associated with an inter-operable tablet with a CDSS for physicians and other health care professionals [54].

Pilot studies in up to 17,000 users and over 95,000 days are available. The *Allergy Diary* has been validated [23] and has shown that (1) totally anonymized geolocation can be used in 22 countries (in preparation), (2) the *Allergy Diary* data can be analyzed in 22 countries and 16 languages, (3) sleep, work productivity and daily activities are impaired in AR [22, 24], (4) daily work productivity is associated with AR severity [21], (5) everyday use of

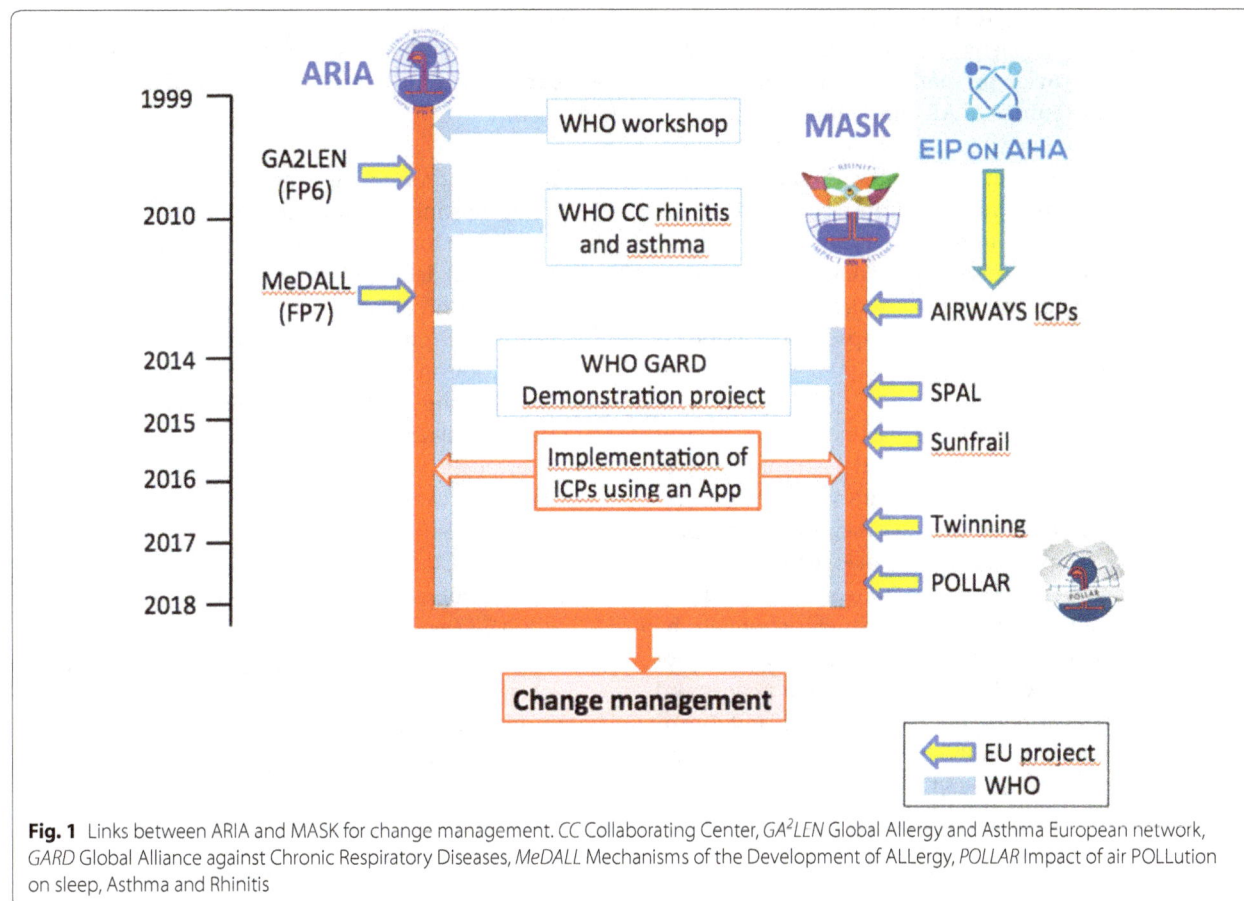

Fig. 1 Links between ARIA and MASK for change management. *CC* Collaborating Center, *GA²LEN* Global Allergy and Asthma European network, *GARD* Global Alliance against Chronic Respiratory Diseases, *MeDALL* Mechanisms of the Development of ALLergy, *POLLAR* Impact of air POLLution on sleep, Asthma and Rhinitis

medications can be monitored proposing a novel assessement of treatment patterns (in press), (6) novel patterns of multimorbidity have been identified [55] and confirmed in epidemiological studies [56, 57] and (7) over 80% of AR patients self-medicate and are non-observant (Menditto, in preparation).

The *Allergy Diary* (TLR 9, Technology Readiness level) represents a validated mHealth tool for the management of AR. Asthma has also been monitored but data have not yet been analysed. Economic impact can be monitored using work productivity. The results of the Allergy Diary have made innovative approaches of AR possible and are directly strengthening the Change Management (CM) strategies in ARIA.

Transfer of innovation of MASK

A Transfer of Innovation (Twinning) project has been funded by the European Innovation Partnership on Active and Healthy Ageing using MASK in 22 Reference Sites or regions across Europe, Australia, Brazil and Mexico [58]. This will improve the understanding, assessment of burden, diagnosis and management of rhinitis in old age by comparison with an adult population. Specific

objectives are: (1) to assess the percentage of adults and elderly who are able to use the Allergy Diary, (2) to study phenotypic characteristics and treatment over a period of one year of rhinitis and asthma multimorbidity at baseline (cross-sectional study) (3) to provide some insight into the differences between elderly people and adults in terms of response to treatment and practice.

The Twinning has been tested in Germany (Region Kohl-Bohn) in a pilot study that has now been extended to the other countries of the Twinning project.

Pollar

Goals

AR and asthma impact the social life, school and work [59] of dozens of millions of EU citizens [21]. Their impact on work productivity is estimated to cost 30–50 billion € per year in the EU. AR affects sleep quality and the severity of sleep disorders, namely sleep apnea, and is associated with asthma. AR and asthma induce health and social inequalities across the life cycle. Air pollution has a significant impact on AR severity and its consequences. The cost of inaction is unacceptable.

POLLAR's mission is to better understand the links between AR, asthma allergen exposure, sleep and pollution in order to provide preventive and treatment strategies to reduce the burden of AR and asthma.

POLLAR's ambition is to deliver an integrated solution tailored to the needs of EU citizens, employers and healthcare systems (including insurance companies).

POLLAR's objective is to better manage health societal consequences of the disease by providing assistance during peaks of allergens and air pollution.

POLLAR is user-designed with specific functionalities adapted to patients, employers, policy makers and clinicians.

POLLAR's aims are (1) to deliver a medical device/treatment with high eligibility for the stratification of patients who need to be treated with OTC drugs, prescribed drugs or allergen immunotherapy, (2) to provide a sentinel for air pollution and allergen exposure for municipalities or regions that can be relayed by media or social networks, (3) to help reimbursement strategies by health care systems or insurances, (4) to improve work productivity in the workplace, (5) to better understand the reciprocal links between AR, pollution and sleep/sleep disorders and (6) in the end, to reduce health and social inequalities between and within countries.

Consortium

The consortium is led by BULL and includes EIT Health members from France and Spain as well as two SMEs (Figs. 2, 3).

- BULL is responsible for the platform. The physician of the hosting platform provider (Santeos) will be responsible for ethical issues, privacy preservation in general and data mining.
- UPMC (Université Pierre et Marie Curie, Paris, France) will provide the personal pollution sampler, medication analyses and the prediction model.
- Grenoble University and Kyomed (France) will be in charge of sleep, data analysis of sleep and patients' inclusion in year 2. Grenoble University will make innovative capabilities available for complex and big data analysis [60, 61].
- ISGlobal (Global Health Institute, Barcelona, Spain) will be responsible for data analysis.
- AQuAS (*Agencia de Qualitat i Avaluacio Sanitaries de Catalunya*, Barcelona, Spain) will be dedicated to policies.
- Kyomed (SME, Montpellier, France) will provide integrated solutions (Allergy Diary) and business

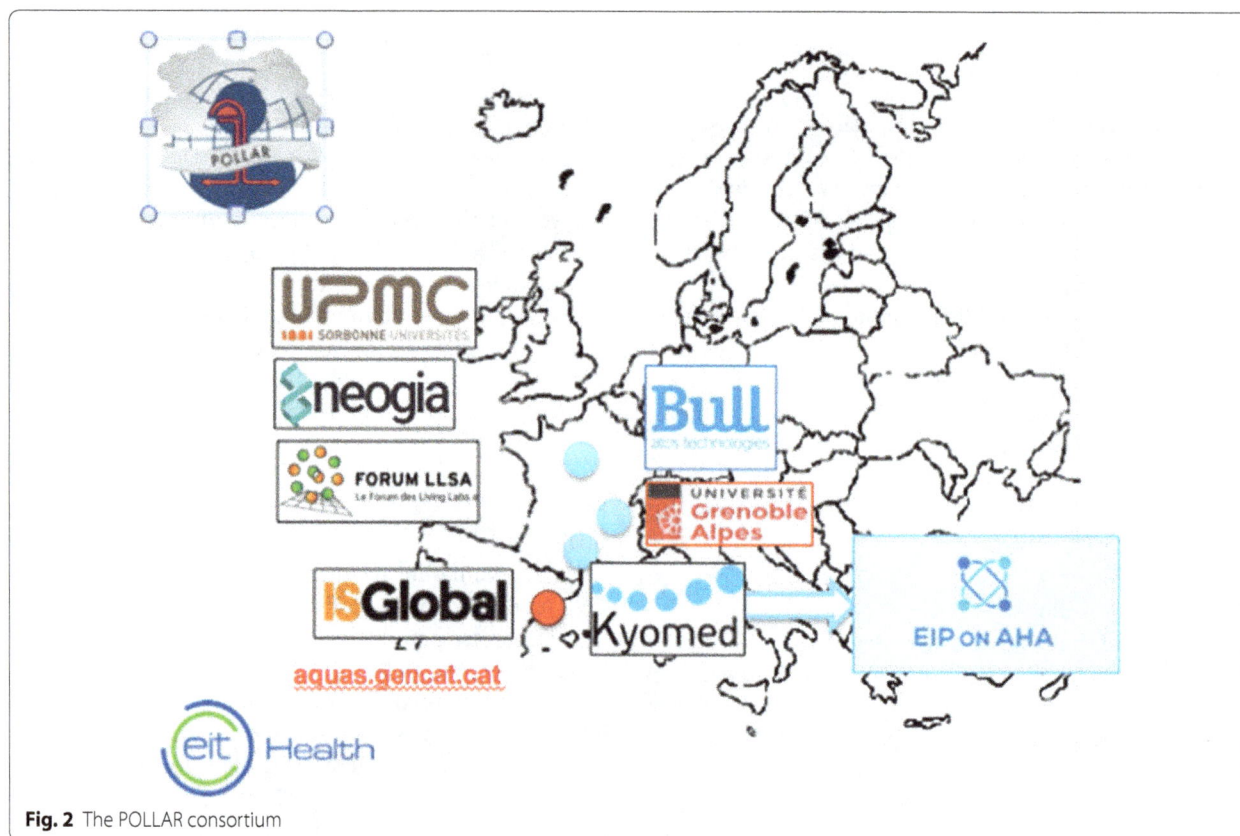

Fig. 2 The POLLAR consortium

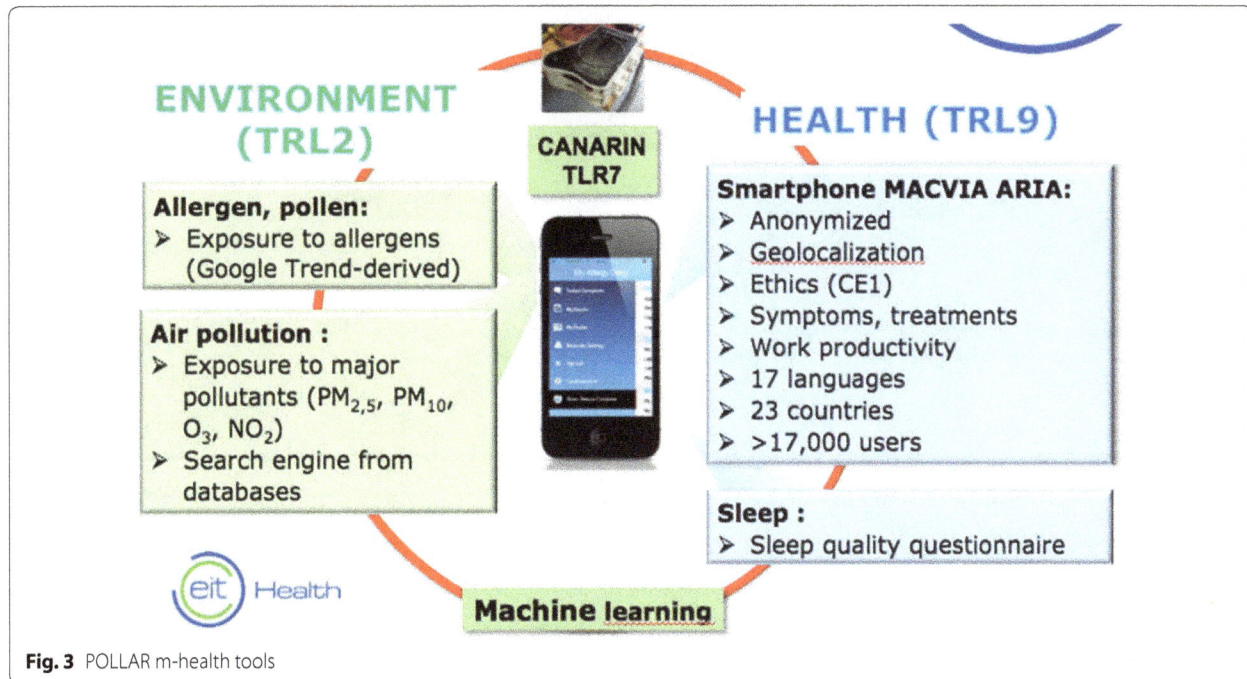

Fig. 3 POLLAR m-health tools

models, as well as support to product design, sales and marketing activities for the project.

- Forum of Living Labs (Paris, France) will prepare and analyze the qualitative data collection of population awareness on air pollution and literacy.
- The National Center of Expertise in Cognitive Stimulation (CEN STIMCO, NGO, Paris, France), as a founding member of the Forum of Living Labs for Health and Independent Living (Forum LLSA, NGO, Paris, France), will prepare and analyze the qualitative data collection of population awareness on air pollution and literacy.
- Neogia (SME, Paris, France) will provide the database of daily trends in air pollution and allergen queries.
- In 2019, the Alfred Health hospital will lead studies in Australia.

m-Health tools and platform

POLLAR combines TRL2, TLR7 and TLR9 m-health tools (Fig. 3).

Allergy Diary

The existing *Allergy Diary* App (Android and iOS) has been tested in 23 countries and 17 languages. The tool has now been deployed to 22 Reference Sites of the European Innovation Partnership on Active and Healthy Ageing (Transfer of Innovation).

Sleep is an important component of the social consequences of AR. The *Allergy Diary* has shown that sleep is impaired by some of the components of AR [22, 53].

A new sleep questionnaire is being added to the *Allergy Diary* (Fig. 4).

Monitoring of pollen exposure and air pollution

Monitoring of the allergy season will be carried out with an improved Google Trends (GT) method. However, GT has some defects [36, 37], in particular, the lack of quantitative data and the non-exhaustivity of internet. We have developed a new tool derived from GT (TLR2) that will analyze all trends and that will be quantitative for allergen and pollution. A similar method will be used for the assessment of air pollution levels.

Set up of the platform, secure storage database and tools for machine and deep learning

The analytic technologies have shown their limits in delivering accurate results and insights. The introduction of artificial intelligence and cognitive computing is bridging the gap. Artificial intelligence and cognitive computing provide technologies and capabilities to solve the challenge of ingesting large amounts of diverse data and to deliver more accurate and timely results and insights.

Thus, main technological challenges focus on delivering a multi-usage and agile cognitive and integrated software suite, leveraging artificial intelligence to enable deep learning capabilities and fast deployments of accurate use cases on multiple environments.

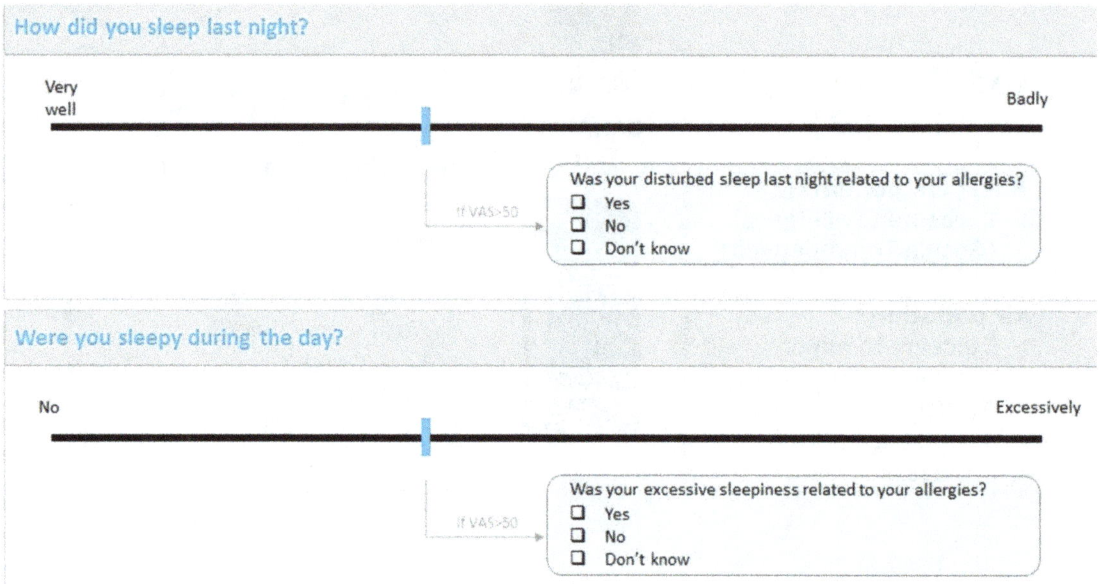

Fig. 4 MASK questions on sleep

Canarin®

To assess the individual's exposure to air pollution in real-time, we will use a remote sensor named CANARIN®. The CANARIN® device is intended to provide the user with a cost-efficient means of determining air quality exposure in real-time in the different places the user is located. CANARIN focuses on particulate matter (PM) of 3 sizes (0.1 μm, 2.5 μm and 10 μm). Furthermore, it includes a temperature and humidity sensor as these parameters can affect the performance of the PM sensors. It also allows the geolocalization of the carrier. All the data are stored via WIFI in an ad hoc cloud. CANARIN has been validated.

Ethical considerations

The Allergy Diary is a CE1 application for which an ethical committee is not necessary. The Terms of Use and Privacy Policy of the App have been reviewed and adapted by lawyers in each of the 23 countries in order to account for differences between countries.

POLLAR will need ethical approval and new regulations in some of the countries (e.g. Loi Jardé in France [62, 63]). We are currently deploying the App to 25 Reference Sites of the EIP on AHA and we have obtained ethical approval from the Köhln-Bohn Region.

The Allergy Diary is completely anonymized except for the geolocation aspect that has been pseudo-anonymized. We have now used k-anonymity [64] to fully anonymize geolocation [65]. We are updating the ethical approval for POLLAR in order to comply with the GDPR [66].

Test case implementation (Mo 1–12)

We shall use the data from 4 countries with 20,000 users during the pollen season and analyse the interactions between air pollution, sleep and allergens.

1. Data collection

Collection of *Allergy Diary* data over one year during the pollen season (March-July or September in areas with ragweed pollen) and outside the pollen season (September–October in areas without ragweed pollen).

2. Data analysis using the Allergy Diary

- Interactive data analysis during the pollen season.
- Interactive data analysis outside of the pollen season.
- Specific analyses on sleep. We will analyze the trajectories of symptoms reflecting sleep quality and daytime sleepiness along with exposure to air pollution and allergic rhinitis. We will take advantage of the knowledge gained from the two existing cross disciplinary programmes of IDEX Grenoble (Life is made of Choice (https://life.univ-grenoble-alpes.fr/)) and of the Grenoble data institute (https://data-institute.univ-greno

ble-alpes.fr). We will use innovative visualization tools for these trajectories that will be included in the Allergy Diary.

- Interactive maps with GIS (geographic information system) technology: GIS is one of many information technologies that have transformed the way geographers conduct research and contribute to society. GIS can be viewed as an integrating technology. With GIS, it is possible to map, model, query and analyze large quantities of data all held together within a single database.

3. Impact of allergy/pollution interactions on prescribed medications in France

Epidemiological studies have suggested a potential causal relationship between air pollution and exacerbations of asthma and allergies. In particular, air pollution exposure is associated with increased medication use and need for rescue medication for asthma and allergies. The potential exaggerating effects of the interaction between pollen and air pollution on asthma and allergic diseases are of serious concern. The collection of data from pharmacy databases for both prescribed and over-the-counter medications for asthma and allergies constitutes an appropriate method for studying the impact of the interaction between air pollution and pollen on asthma and allergy aggravation.

4. Establishment of the business plan

It is expected that POLLAR will generate substantial and highly valuable scientific data as well as information correlating the biological phenomena with the highlighted environmental factors. It is also highly possible that novel technologies or platforms may be developed as a result of the project. Both aspects are not only of scientific but also of commercial value. To capitalize on the value generated both from the data/information and potential novel technology, Kyomed will establish a business plan towards the monetization of these assets. The business plan will include analyses of (1) the properties, functionalities, uniqueness and potential of the data/information or technology generated, (2) the market trends and needs, (3) the competitive landscape; the competitive advantages of the POLLAR offer. It will make further recommendations on the commercial positioning, product placement, pricing and promotional activities for the offer. Financial forecasts and budgeting will also be provided.

5. Education (CEN STIMCO)

Citizens and patients participating in the programme will gain awareness regarding the risk associated with air pollution. This effect will be estimated and results will help disseminate key messages together with the application.

Test case validation (Mo 12–24)

In year 2, we shall validate the results of year 1 in all EU countries where pollution data are available. We will also provide policies. The test-case implementation will be deployed to account for different climates (allergen exposure) and pollution (low and high levels and different pollutants). We shall use the existing EIP on AHA transfer of innovation network (25 Reference Sites across Europe in 16 languages).

Moreover, Canarin®, a personal pollution sampler, will be tested in AR patients with multimorbid sleep disorders (1) to confirm the data obtained using the Allergy Diary and (2) to check the effect of air pollution on sleep and sleep apnea severity [67]. It is well documented that nasal obstruction associated with AR is increasing pharyngeal collapsibility and modulating the severity of moderate to severe sleep apnea. This has been suggested by single night sleep studies and small intervention trails. However, the dynamic of the night after night evolution of OSA severity in relationship with air pollution and AR is poorly documented by repeated objective measurements. The test case validation will address this issue by combining simplified diagnosis methods for assessing the night after night evolution of OSA severity and a synchronization with the Allergy Diary and the Canarin personal pollution sampler. The impact will be huge for patients and the society as some OSA phenotypes might benefit from a better AR management and improve sleep apnea conditions.

Impact of POLLAR

The innovative aspect of POLLAR lies in the integration of existing hardware and software blocks (BULL) with newly-developed methods in a patient-centric designed set of easy-learning functionalities (Kyomed, CEN STIMCO). These will be embedded in a solution for all stakeholders including patients, clinicians and policy makers. The Allergy Diary represents an innovation that is creating a new market and value network and that will eventually disrupt the existing market and value network.

Reduction of social and health inequalities

By integrating risk perception analysis and increasing stakeholder engagement, POLLAR aims at (1) bringing more attention to the links between AR and air pollution,

(2) educating the public about the threat of air pollution, and (3) efficiently using financial resources to implement a more sustainable solution. POLLAR should reduce health and social inequalities within and between countries, in particular in vulnerable populations (children and old age people).

Gender dimension

Gender is an important aspect of allergic diseases. Before puberty, there is a male predominance of allergy whereas, after puberty, there is a female predominance [68]. Women may be more susceptible to the effects of air pollution. A specific gender analysis will be carried out in POLLAR to account for gender differences and, if needed, policies will be proposed.

Economic impact

The *Allergy Diary* can accurately measure loss of work productivity. It is expected that POLLAR will reduce these indirect costs. For industries, the demonstration of the link between AR incidence/severity and productivity underpins the importance of prevention, timely diagnosis, adequate treatment and patient compliance. For public healthcare organizations and private health insurance companies, prevention, timely diagnosis and effective treatments are primordial to healthcare cost management.

Interactions with EIT Health

EIT Health resources needed for POLLAR

EIT Health fosters cross-disciplinal collaborations to tackle major healthcare challenges, such as the growing allergy epidemic and air pollution effects. It provides a privileged frame for validating a comprehensive solution by paving the roads between all stakeholders. It also provides an integrated use of knowledge in medical device development, data management and analytics, and clinical conditions. EIT Health will interconnect POLLAR with its innovation project portfolio and with its CAMPUS (link to "Patient-centred and personalized healthcare description and main outcomes") and ACCELERATOR programmes, thereby catalyzing both.

Relevance of POLLAR for the core mission of EIT Health

The proposed POLLAR solution is aligned with EIT Health core missions: (1) Promote healthy living, lifestyle intervention and self-management of health, (2) Improve healthcare systems, treat and manage chronic diseases and (3) Improve work productivity.

Knowledge triangle integration

POLLAR follows the KIC knowledge triangle closely (Fig. 5).

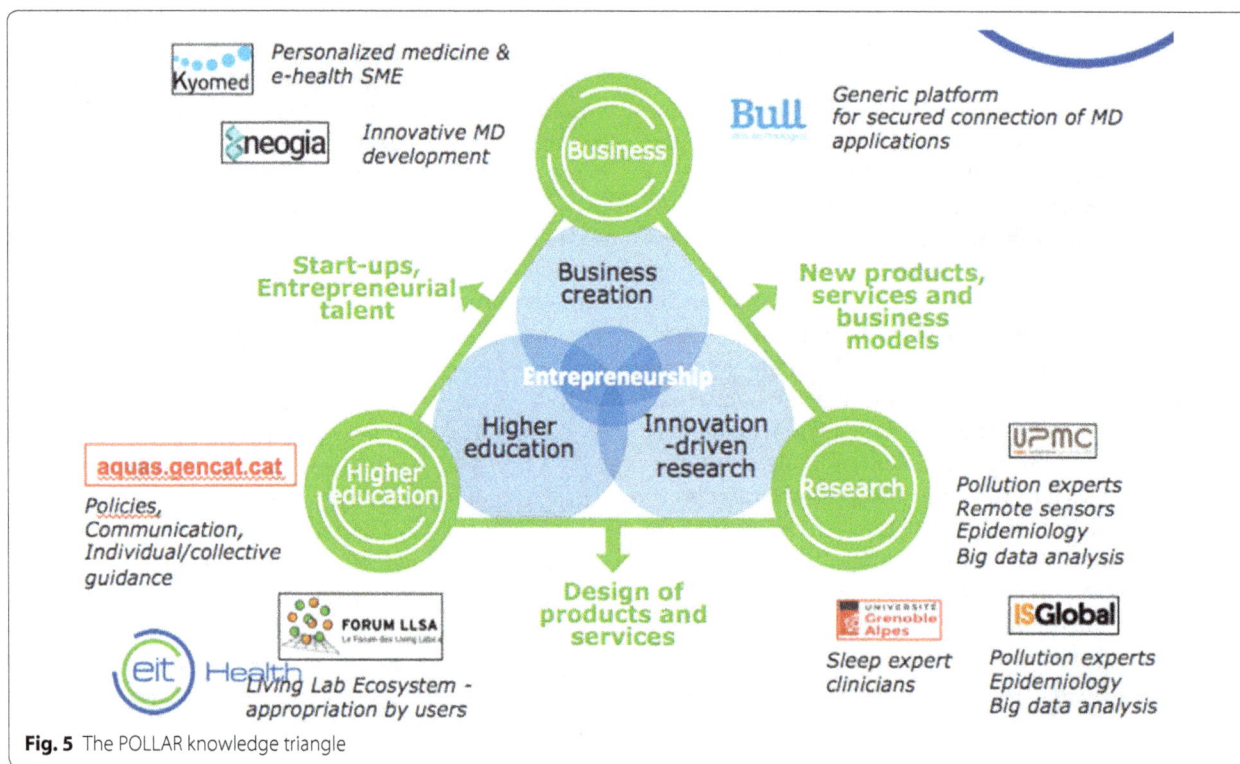

Fig. 5 The POLLAR knowledge triangle

- *Business and entrepreneurship* POLLAR is typically designing, launching and running a new business, which began as a small business, such as a startup company (Kyomed, Neogia). It is offering a validated product (Allergy Diary, TLR9) which will be embedded with other tools (TLR2) and scaled up. The prevalence of AR and asthma, and the levels of pollution in Europe, represent a huge business opportunity. Being part of the EIP on AHA, goals are an acceleration of time-to-market.
- *Link to accelerator* BULL is a major company which will help to develop new and startup companies (Kyomed, Neogia). It will use the business accelerator effect of the Forum LLSA and will provide services as a catalyst tool for regional and national economic development. It will help to scale the business of several inter-related projects and to catapult promising ideas already working and tested (*Allergy Diary*) onto the market. This will support Europe's premier innovations that tackle today's healthcare challenges (air pollution and allergy).
- *Research and technology* The MASK pilot study has shown that guidelines in AR should be revised to account for patients' self-management which was found to be unexpectedly high [21, 22, 24, 53]. The pilot study suggested several novel pathways for AR treatment. The inclusion of air pollution data is needed to alert patients (Allegy Diary, media, social networks) and to provide new recommendations for a better AR control [45, 69].

  - The patient's centric approach is essential and will be brought by the CEN STIMCO.
  - A personalized approach targeted to each patient is needed and the *Allergy Diary* can be of great help [70, 71].
  - Sleep is an important component of AR and asthma. It should be better understood and embedded into guidelines.
  - The societal approach is a research project that will bring a novel approach to this complex disease allowing a holistic approach.
  - POLLAR will allow machine learning but also deep learning. The analytical expertise raised in MeDALL (Mechanisms of the Development of ALLergy, a success story of FP7 devoted to systems biology in allergy [57, 72]), with the technologic capabilities of BULL, will make a success story out of POLLAR.

- *Higher education* Higher education will be provided by major teaching groups of Europe (UPMC, Grenoble University and ISGlobal) but also by the Forum LLA and CEN STIMCO. Some modern approaches will be combined with classical education. Integrated training modules are needed. Because of the expected trends in AR, it is of paramount importance to train physicians, other health care professionals, health scientists, lawyers and socio-economic professionals. Transversal training is needed.
- *Health, chronic diseases and society* POLLAR will combine teaching and will cover the relationship between chronic illnesses, chronicity, health and health education, ethics and the assistance relationship, chronicity policies, life with a chronic illness and research methods in the field of human or soft science [73].
- *Management education* The overall care of people suffering from chronic illness requires the coordination of people who will help them throughout life. The *case manager* is a unique correspondent in charge of coordinating care.
- *Patient therapeutic education* will also be provided in collaboration with patients' organizations (involved in the *Allergy Diary*).

Benefits for the citizens and the patients

Guidelines have improved the knowledge on rhinitis and made a significant impact on AR management. However, many patients are insufficiently controlled and the costs for society are enormous. Allergic Rhinitis and its Impact on Asthma (ARIA) has evolved from a guideline to care pathways using mobile technology in AR and asthma multimorbidity. ARIA appears to be close to the patient's needs but real-life data obtained using an App in 22 countries have shown that very few patients use guidelines and that they often self-medicate. Moreover, patients largely use OTC medications dispensed in pharmacies. Self-medication and shared decision making (SDM) centered around the patient should be used more often. The knowledge by patients of peaks of air pollution and allergens will help them to better control their disease. In POLLAR, self-medication strategies and a sentinel network will be integrated in care pathways to optimize the treatment of AR and asthma multimorbidity. These changes should prepare and support individuals, teams and organizations in making organizational change centered around the patient.

Political agenda

POLLAR is supported by several national and international scientific societies (including EAACI, ERS, IPCRG) and patients' organizations (EFA and ELF).

One of the POLLAR members is AQuaS (Agencia de Qualitat i Avaluacio Sanitaries de Catalunya, Barcelona, Spain).

The EIP on AHA is involved in POLLAR through the Reference Site Collaborative Network (J Bousquet, M Illario).

POLLAR is a WHO GARD (Global Alliance against Chronic Respiratory Diseases) demonstration project.

Conclusion

POLLAR aims to propose novel care pathways integrating pollution, sleep and patients' literacy. It also aims to study the sleep consequences of pollution and its impact on frequent chronic diseases, to improve work productivity, to propose the basis for a sentinel network at the EU level for pollution and allergy, and to assess the societal implications of the interaction.

Abbreviations

AHA: active and healthy aging; AIRWAYS ICPs: integrated care pathways for airway diseases; AR: allergic rhinitis; ARIA: Allergic Rhinitis and its Impact on Asthma; CDSS: clinical decision support system; CEN STIMCO: Centre d'Expertise National en Stimulation Cognitive; CHRODIS: Joint Action on Chronic Diseases and Promoting Healthy Ageing across the Life Cycle; COPD: chronic obstructive pulmonary disease; DG CONNECT: Directorate General for Communications Networks, Content & Technology; DG Santé: Directorate General for Health and Food Safety; DG: Directorate General; EAACI: European Academy of Allergy and Clinical Immunology; EFA: European Federation of Allergy and Airways Diseases Patients' Associations; EIP: European Innovation Partnership; EIT Health: European Institute of Innovation and Technology-Health; ELF: European Lung Foundation; EQ-5D: Euroquol; ERS: European Respiratory Society; EU: European Union; EUFOREA: European Forum for Research and Education in Allergy; GARD: WHO Global Alliance against Chronic Respiratory Diseases; GT: Google Trends; HIT: health information technology; ICP: integrated care pathway; ICT: information and communications technology; IT: information technology; JA-CHRODIS: Joint Action on Chronic Diseases and Promoting Healthy Ageing across the Life Cycle; KIC: Knowledge Innovation Community; LLSA: living lab; MACVIA: contre les MAladies Chroniques pour un VIeillissement Actif; MASK: Mobile Airways Sentinel NetworK; mHealth: mobile health; OSA: obstructive sleep apnea; POLLAR: Impact of Air POLLution on sleep, Asthma and Rhinitis; SDM: shared decision making; TLR: technology readiness level; VAS: visual analogue scale.

Authors' contributions

JB wrote the paper which was revised by all members of the consortium and the experts (MB, NB, WC, JF, LK and OP). All authors read and approved the final manuscript.

Author details

[1] MACVIA-France, Fondation partenariale FMC VIA-LR, Montpellier, France. [2] INSERM U 1168, VIMA : Ageing and Chronic Diseases Epidemiological and Public Health Approaches, Villejuif, France. [3] Université Versailles St-Quentin-en-Yvelines, UMR-S 1168, Montigny le Bretonneux, France. [4] Euforea, Brussels, Belgium. [5] Charité, Berlin, Germany. [6] CHU Montpellier, 371 Avenue du Doyen Gaston Giraud, 34295 Montpellier Cedex 5, France. [7] ISGlobal, Centre for Research in Environmental Epidemiology (CREAL), Barcelona, Spain. [8] IMIM (Hospital del Mar Research Institute), Barcelona, Spain. [9] Universitat Pompeu Fabra (UPF), Barcelona, Spain. [10] CIBER Epidemiología y Salud Pública (CIBERESP), Barcelona, Spain. [11] Epidemiology of Allergic and Respiratory Diseases, Department Institute Pierre Louis of Epidemiology and Public Health, INSERM and UPMC Sorbonne Universités, Medical School Saint Antoine, Paris, France. [12] AQuAS, Barcelona, Spain. [13] Kyomed

INNOV, Montpellier, France. [14] Université Grenoble Alpes, Laboratoire HP2, INSERM, U1042 Grenoble, France. [15] CHU de Grenoble, Grenoble, France. [16] Bull SAS, Échirolles, France. [17] National Center of Expertise in Cognitive Stimulation (CEN STIMCO), Broca Hospital, Paris, France. [18] Memory and Cognition Laboratory, Institute of Psychology, Paris Descartes University, Sorbonne Paris Cité, Boulogne Billancourt, France. [19] Mines ParisTech CRI - PSL Research University, Fontainebleau, France. [20] Direction de la Recherche, Innovation et Valorisation, Université Grenoble Alpes, Grenoble, France. [21] Neogia, Paris, France. [22] Centre National de Référence Narcolepsie Hypersomnies, Département de Neurologie, Hôpital Gui-de-Chauliac Inserm U1061, Unité des Troubles du Sommeil, Montpellier, France. [23] LIP6 SU, Place Jussieu, Paris, France. [24] Conseil Général de l'Economie Ministère de l'Economie, de l'Industrie et du Numérique, Paris, France. [25] Climate and Health Program and ISGlobal and ICREA, Barcelona, Spain. [26] iQ4U Consultants Ltd, London, UK. [27] Joensuu, Finland. [28] Medical Consulting Czarlewski, Levallois, France. [29] Center for Health Technology and Services Research- CINTESIS, Faculdade de Medicina, Universidade do Porto, Porto, Portugal. [30] MEDIDA, Lda, Porto, Portugal. [31] Center for Rhinology and Allergology, Wiesbaden, Germany. [32] Department of Otorhinolaryngology, Head and Neck Surgery, Universitätsmedizin Mannheim, Medical Faculty Mannheim, Heidelberg University, Mannheim, Germany. [33] Managing Director, EIT Health France, Paris, France.

Acknowledgements

Not applicable.

Competing interests

JB reports personal fees and other from Chiesi, Cipla, Hikma, Menarini, Mundipharma, Mylan, Novartis, Sanofi-Aventis, Takeda, Teva, Uriach, other from Kyomed, outside the submitted work. JB is co-Editor-in-Chief of Clinical and Translational Allergy and was excluded from the editorial and peer review processes for this article. OP reports grants and personal fees from ALK-Abelló, Allergopharma, Stallergenes Greer, HAL Allergy Holding B.V./HAL Allergie GmbH, Bencard Allergie GmbH/Allergy Therapeutics, Lofarma, Biotech Tools S.A, Laboratorios LETI/LETI Pharma, Anergis S.A.; grants from Biomay, Nuvo, Circassia, Glaxo Smith Kline; personal fees from Novartis Pharma, MEDA Pharma, Mobile Chamber Experts (a GA²LEN Partner), Pohl-Boskamp, Indoor Biotechnologies, grants from, outside the submitted work.

Funding

EIT Health (European Union).

References

1. Lim SS, Vos T, Flaxman AD, Danaei G, Shibuya K, Adair-Rohani H, et al. A comparative risk assessment of burden of disease and injury attributable to 67 risk factors and risk factor clusters in 21 regions, 1990–2010: a systematic analysis for the Global Burden of Disease Study 2010. Lancet. 2012;380(9859):2224–60.

2. Cohen AJ, Brauer M, Burnett R, Anderson HR, Frostad J, Estep K, et al. Estimates and 25-year trends of the global burden of disease attributable to ambient air pollution: an analysis of data from the Global Burden of Diseases Study 2015. Lancet. 2017;389(10082):1907–18.

3. Gorr MW, Falvo MJ, Wold LE. Air Pollution and other environmental modulators of cardiac function. Compr Physiol. 2017;7(4):1479–95.

4. Li J, Sun S, Tang R, Qiu H, Huang Q, Mason TG, et al. Major air pollutants and risk of COPD exacerbations: a systematic review and meta-analysis. Int J Chron Obstruct Pulmon Dis. 2016;11:3079–91.

5. Weinreich G, Wessendorf TE, Pundt N, Weinmayr G, Hennig F, Moebus S, et al. Association of short-term ozone and temperature with sleep disordered breathing. Eur Respir J. 2015;46(5):1361–9.

6. Orellano P, Quaranta N, Reynoso J, Balbi B, Vasquez J. Effect of outdoor air pollution on asthma exacerbations in children and adults: systematic review and multilevel meta-analysis. PLoS ONE. 2017;12(3):e0174050.

7. Behrendt H, Alessandrini F, Buters J, Kramer U, Koren H, Ring J. Environmental pollution and allergy: historical aspects. Chem Immunol Allergy. 2014;100:268–77.

8. Cingi C, Gevaert P, Mosges R, Rondon C, Hox V, Rudenko M, et al. Multi-morbidities of allergic rhinitis in adults: European Academy of Allergy and Clinical Immunology Task Force Report. Clin Transl Allergy. 2017;7:17.

9. Konishi S, Ng CF, Stickley A, Nishihata S, Shinsugi C, Ueda K, et al. Particulate matter modifies the association between airborne pollen and daily medical consultations for pollinosis in Tokyo. Sci Total Environ. 2014;499:125–32.

10. D'Amato G, Holgate ST, Pawankar R, Ledford DK, Cecchi L, Al-Ahmad M, et al. Meteorological conditions, climate change, new emerging factors, and asthma and related allergic disorders. A statement of the World Allergy Organization. World Allergy Organ J. 2015;8(1):25.

11. Schiavoni G, D'Amato G, Afferni C. The dangerous liaison between pollens and pollution in respiratory allergy. Ann Allergy Asthma Immunol. 2017;118(3):269–75.

12. Kanter U, Heller W, Durner J, Winkler JB, Engel M, Behrendt H, et al. Molecular and immunological characterization of ragweed (Ambrosia artemisiifolia L.) pollen after exposure of the plants to elevated ozone over a whole growing season. PLoS ONE. 2013;8(4):e61518.

13. Motta AC, Marliere M, Peltre G, Sterenberg PA, Lacroix G. Traffic-related air pollutants induce the release of allergen-containing cytoplasmic granules from grass pollen. Int Arch Allergy Immunol. 2006;139(4):294–8.

14. Bartra J, Mullol J, del Cuvillo A, Davila I, Ferrer M, Jauregui I, et al. Air pollution and allergens. J Investig Allergol Clin Immunol. 2007;17(Suppl 2):3–8.

15. Braat JP, Mulder PG, Duivenvoorden HJ, Gerth Van Wijk R, Rijntjes E, Fokkens WJ. Pollutional and meteorological factors are closely related to complaints of non-allergic, non-infectious perennial rhinitis patients: a time series model. Clin Exp Allergy. 2002;32(5):690–7.

16. Steerenberg PA, Bischoff EW, de Klerk A, Verlaan AP, Jongbloets LM, van Loveren H, et al. Acute effect of air pollution on respiratory complaints, exhaled NO and biomarkers in nasal lavages of allergic children during the pollen season. Int Arch Allergy Immunol. 2003;131(2):127–37.

17. Feo Brito F, Mur Gimeno P, Martinez C, Tobias A, Suarez L, Guerra F, et al. Air pollution and seasonal asthma during the pollen season. A cohort study in Puertollano and Ciudad Real (Spain). Allergy. 2007;62(10):1152–7.

18. Heguy L, Garneau M, Goldberg MS, Raphoz M, Guay F, Valois MF. Associations between grass and weed pollen and emergency department visits for asthma among children in Montreal. Environ Res. 2008;106(2):203–11.

19. Jariwala SP, Kurada S, Moday H, Thanjan A, Bastone L, Khananashvili M, et al. Association between tree pollen counts and asthma ED visits in a high-density urban center. J Asthma. 2011;48(5):442–8.

20. Bousquet J, Hellings PW, Agache I, Bedbrook A, Bachert C, Bergmann KC, et al. ARIA 2016: care pathways implementing emerging technologies for predictive medicine in rhinitis and asthma across the life cycle. Clin Transl Allergy. 2016;6:47.

21. Bousquet J, Bewick M, Arnavielhe S, Mathieu-Dupas E, Murray R, Bedbrook A, et al. Work productivity in rhinitis using cell phones: the MASK pilot study. Allergy. 2017;72(10):1475–84.

22. Bousquet J, Caimmi DP, Bedbrook A, Bewick M, Hellings PW, Devillier P, et al. Pilot study of mobile phone technology in allergic rhinitis in European countries: the MASK-rhinitis study. Allergy. 2017;72(6):857–65.

23. Caimmi D, Baiz N, Tanno LK, Demoly P, Arnavielhe S, Murray R, et al. Validation of the MASK-rhinitis visual analogue scale on smartphone screens to assess allergic rhinitis control. Clin Exp Allergy. 2017;47:1526–33.

24. Bousquet J, Arnavielhe S, Bedbrook A, Fonseca J, Morais Almeida M, Todo Bom A, et al. The ARIA score of allergic rhinitis using mobile technology correlates with quality-of-life: the MASK study. Allergy. 2018;73(2):505–10.

25. Csepe Z, Makra L, Voukantsis D, Matyasovszky I, Tusnady G, Karatzas K, et al. Predicting daily ragweed pollen concentrations using Computational Intelligence techniques over two heavily polluted areas in Europe. Sci Total Environ. 2014;476–477:542–52.

26. Khwarahm NR, Dash J, Skjoth CA, Newnham RM, Adams-Groom B, Head K, et al. Mapping the birch and grass pollen seasons in the UK using satellite sensor time-series. Sci Total Environ. 2017;578:586–600.

27. Navares R, Aznarte JL. Predicting the Poaceae pollen season: six month-ahead forecasting and identification of relevant features. Int J Biometeorol. 2017;61(4):647–56.

28. Silva-Palacios I, Fernandez-Rodriguez S, Duran-Barroso P, Tormo-Molina R, Maya-Manzano JM, Gonzalo-Garijo A. Temporal modelling and forecasting of the airborne pollen of Cupressaceae on the southwestern Iberian Peninsula. Int J Biometeorol. 2016;60(2):297–306.

29. Bastl K, Kmenta M, Pessi AM, Prank M, Saarto A, Sofiev M, et al. First comparison of symptom data with allergen content (Bet v 1 and Phl p 5 measurements) and pollen data from four European regions during 2009–2011. Sci Total Environ. 2016;548–549:229–35.

30. Buters JT, Weichenmeier I, Ochs S, Pusch G, Kreyling W, Boere AJ, et al. The allergen Bet v 1 in fractions of ambient air deviates from birch pollen counts. Allergy. 2010;65(7):850–8.

31. Myszkowska D, Majewska R. Pollen grains as allergenic environmental factors–new approach to the forecasting of the pollen concentration during the season. Ann Agric Environ Med. 2014;21(4):681–8.

32. de Weger LA, Beerthuizen T, Hiemstra PS, Sont JK. Development and validation of a 5-day-ahead hay fever forecast for patients with grass-pollen-induced allergic rhinitis. Int J Biometeorol. 2014;58(6):1047–55.

33. Konig V, Mosges R. A model for the determination of pollen count using google search queries for patients suffering from allergic rhinitis. J Allergy (Cairo). 2014;2014:381983.

34. Willson TJ, Lospinoso J, Weitzel E, McMains K. Correlating regional aeroallergen effects on internet search activity. Otolaryngol Head Neck Surg. 2015;152(2):228–32.

35. Zuckerman O, Luster SH, Bielory L. Internet searches and allergy: temporal variation in regional pollen counts correlates with Google searches for pollen allergy related terms. Ann Allergy Asthma Immunol. 2014;113(4):486–8.

36. Bousquet J, Agache I, Anto JM, Bergmann KC, Bachert C, Annesi-Maesano I, et al. Google Trends terms reporting rhinitis and related topics differ in European countries. Allergy. 2017;72:1261–6.

37. Bousquet J, O'Hehir RE, Anto JM, D'Amato G, Mosges R, Hellings PW, et al. Assessment of thunderstorm-induced asthma using Google Trends. J Allergy Clin Immunol. 2017;140(3):891–3.

38. Kang MG, Song WJ, Choi S, Kim H, Ha H, Kim SH, et al. Google unveils a glimpse of allergic rhinitis in the real world. Allergy. 2015;70(1):124–8.

39. Bousquet J, Agache I, Anto J, Bergmann K, Bachert C, Annesi-Maesano I, et al. Google Trends terms reporting rhinitis and related topics differ in European countries. Allergy. 2017;72(8):1261–6.

40. Leger D, Annesi-Maesano I, Carat F, Rugina M, Chanal I, Pribil C, et al. Allergic rhinitis and its consequences on quality of sleep: an unexplored area. Arch Intern Med. 2006;166(16):1744–8.

41. Bousquet J, Michel J, Standberg T, Crooks G, Iakovidis I, Gomez M. The European Innovation Partnership on Active and Healthy Ageing: the European geriatric medicine introduces the EIP on AHA column. Eur Geriatr Med. 2014;5(6):361–2.

42. Bousquet J, Addis A, Adcock I, Agache I, Agusti A, Alonso A, et al. Integrated care pathways for airway diseases (AIRWAYS-ICPs). Eur Respir J. 2014;44(2):304–23.

43. Bousquet J, Barbara C, Bateman E, Bel E, Bewick M, Chavannes N, et al. AIRWAYS ICPs (European Innovation Partnership on Active and Healthy Ageing) from concept to implementation. Eur Respir J. 2016;47(4):1028–33.

44. Bousquet J, Anto JM, Berkouk K, Gergen P, Antunes JP, Auge P, et al. Developmental determinants in non-communicable chronic diseases and ageing. Thorax. 2015;70(6):595–7.

45. Bousquet J, Barbara C, Bateman E, Bel E, Bewick M, Chavannes NH, et al. AIRWAYS-ICPs (European Innovation Partnership on Active and Healthy Ageing) from concept to implementation. Eur Respir J. 2016;47(4):1028–33.

46. Bousquet J, Farrell J, Crooks G, Hellings P, Bel EH, Bewick M, et al. Scaling up strategies of the chronic respiratory disease programme of the European Innovation Partnership on Active and Healthy Ageing (Action Plan B3: area 5). Clin Transl Allergy. 2016;6:29.

47. Bousquet J, Bewick M, Cano A, Eklund P, Fico G, Goswami N, et al. Building bridges for innovation in ageing: synergies between action groups of the EIP on AHA. J Nutr Health Aging. 2017;21(1):92–104.

48. Bousquet J, Dahl R, Khaltaev N. Global alliance against chronic respiratory diseases. Allergy. 2007;62(3):216–23.

49. Bousquet J, Schunemann HJ, Fonseca J, Samolinski B, Bachert C, Canonica GW, et al. MACVIA-ARIA Sentinel NetworK for allergic rhinitis (MASK-rhinitis): the new generation guideline implementation. Allergy. 2015;70(11):1372–92.

50. Onder G, Palmer K, Navickas R, Jureviciene E, Mammarella F, Strandzheva M, et al. Time to face the challenge of multimorbidity. A European perspective from the joint action on chronic diseases and promoting healthy ageing across the life cycle (JA-CHRODIS). Eur J Intern Med. 2015;26(3):157–9.

51. Bousquet J, Onorato GL, Bachert C, Barbolini M, Bedbrook A, Bjermer L, et al. CHRODIS criteria applied to the MASK (MACVIA-ARIA Sentinel NetworK) Good Practice in allergic rhinitis: a SUNFRAIL report. Clin Transl Allergy. 2017;7:37.

52. Klimek L, Bergmann K, Biederman T, Bousquet J, Hellings P, et al. Visual analogue scales (VAS): measuring instruments for the documentation of symptoms and therapy monitoring in allergic rhinitis in everyday health care. Position paper of the German Society of Allergology. Allergo J Int. 2017;26(1):16–24.

53. Bousquet J, VandenPlas O, Bewick M, Arnavielhe S, Bedbrook A, Murray R, et al. Work productivity and activity impairment allergic specific (WPAI-AS) Questionnaire using mobile technology: the MASK study. J Investig Allergol Clin Immunol. 2018;28(1):42–4.

54. Bourret R, Bousquet J, Mercier J, Camuzat T, Bedbrook A, Demoly P, et al. MASK rhinitis, a single tool for integrated care pathways in allergic rhinitis. World Hosp Health Serv. 2015;51(3):36–9.

55. Bousquet J, Arnavielhe S, Bedbrook A, Alexis-Alexandre G, Mv Eerd, Murray R, et al. Treatment of allergic rhinitis using mobile technology with real world data: the MASK observational pilot study. Allergy. 2018. https://doi.org/10.1111/all.13406.

56. Burte E, Bousquet J, Siroux V, Just J, Jacquemin B, Nadif R. The sensitization pattern differs according to rhinitis and asthma multimorbidity in adults: the EGEA study. Clin Exp Allergy. 2017;47(4):520–9.

57. Anto JM, Bousquet J, Akdis M, Auffray C, Keil T, Momas I, et al. Mechanisms of the development of allergy (MeDALL): introducing novel concepts in allergy phenotypes. J Allergy Clin Immunol. 2017;139(2):388–99.

58. Bousquet J, Agache I, Aliberti MR, Angles R, Annesi-Maesano I, Anto JM, et al. Transfer of innovation on allergic rhinitis and asthma multimorbidity in the elderly (MACVIA-ARIA)—EIP on AHA Twinning Reference Site (GARD research demonstration project). Allergy. 2018;73(1):77–92.

59. Vandenplas O, Vinnikov D, Blanc PD, Agache I, Bachert C, Bewick M, et al. Impact of Rhinitis on work productivity: a systematic review. J Allergy Clin Immunol Pract. 2017 Oct 7. pii: S2213-2198(17)30725-0. https://doi.org/10.1016/j.jaip.2017.09.002. [Epub ahead of print].

60. Liu D, Armitstead J, Benjafield A, Shao S, Malhotra A, Cistulli PA, et al. Trajectories of emergent central sleep apnea during CPAP therapy. Chest. 2017;152(4):751–60.

61. Bailly S, Destors M, Grillet Y, Richard P, Stach B, Vivodtzev I, et al. Obstructive sleep apnea: a cluster analysis at time of diagnosis. PLoS ONE. 2016;11(6):e0157318.

62. Mamzer MF. Regulation of French research: how to use it? Rev Med Interne. 2017;38(7):427–9.

63. Bernhard JC, Latxague C. Impact of the Jarde's law on research management. Prog Urol. 2017;27(6):334–6.

64. Aristodimou A, Antoniades A, Pattichis CS. Privacy preserving data publishing of categorical data through k-anonymity and feature selection. Healthc Technol Lett. 2016;3(1):16–21.

65. REGULATION (EU) 2016/679 OF THE EUROPEAN PARLIAMENT AND OF THE COUNCIL of 27 April 2016 on the protection of natural persons with regard to the processing of personal data and on the free movement of such data, and repealing Directive 95/46/EC (General Data Protection Regulation). Official Organ of the European Union. 2016(http://eur-lex.europa.eu/legal-content/EN/TXT/PDF/?uri=CELEX:32016R0679&from=EN).

66. Article 28 EU General Data Protection Regulation (EU-GDPR). https://www.eugdp.rorg/. 2018.

67. Bousquet J, Cruz A, Robalo-Cordeiro C. Obstructive sleep apnoea syndrome is an under-recognized cause of uncontrolled asthma across the life cycle. Rev Port Pneumol. 2016;22:1–3.

68. Frohlich M, Pinart M, Keller T, Reich A, Cabieses B, Hohmann C, et al. Is there a sex-shift in prevalence of allergic rhinitis and comorbid asthma from childhood to adulthood? A meta-analysis. Clin Transl Allergy. 2017;7:44.

69. Bousquet J, Bourret R, Camuzat T, Auge P, Bringer J, Nogues M, et al. MACVIA-LR (Fighting Chronic Diseases for Active and Healthy Ageing in Languedoc-Roussillon): a Success Story of the European Innovation Partnership on Active and Healthy Ageing. J Frailty Aging. 2016;5(4):233–41.

70. Muraro A, Fokkens WJ, Pietikainen S, Borrelli D, Agache I, Bousquet J, et al. European symposium on precision medicine in allergy and airways diseases: report of the European Union parliament symposium (October 14, 2015). Allergy. 2016;71(5):583–7.

71. De Greve G, Hellings PW, Fokkens WJ, Pugin B, Steelant B, Seys SF. Endotype-driven treatment in chronic upper airway diseases. Clin Transl Allergy. 2017;7:22.

72. Bousquet J, Anto JM, Akdis M, Auffray C, Keil T, Momas I, et al. Paving the way of systems biology and precision medicine in allergic diseases: the MeDALL success story. Allergy. 2016;71(11):1513–25.

73. Bousquet J, Jorgensen C, Dauzat M, Cesario A, Camuzat T, Bourret R, et al. Systems medicine approaches for the definition of complex phenotypes in chronic diseases and ageing. From concept to implementation and policies. Curr Pharm Des. 2014;20(38):5928–44.

13

Allergic respiratory disease (ARD), setting forth the basics: proposals of an expert consensus report

Ana M. Navarro[1]* [ID], Julio Delgado[2], Rosa M. Muñoz-Cano[3], M. Teresa Dordal[4,5], Antonio Valero[3], Santiago Quirce[6] and Behalf of the ARD Study Group

Abstract

Background: The variability of symptoms observed in patients with respiratory allergy often hampers classification based on the criteria proposed in guidelines on rhinitis and asthma.

Objectives: We assessed specific aspects of allergic respiratory disease (ARD) that are not explicitly addressed in the guidelines in order to issue specific recommendations and thus optimize clinical practice.

Methods: Using the Delphi technique, 40 Spanish allergists were surveyed to reach consensus on 71 items related to ARD.

Results: Consensus was achieved for 95.7% of the items. These included the following: the clinical manifestations of ARD are heterogeneous and individual airborne allergens can be related to specific clinical profiles; the optimal approach in patients with ARD is based on the global assessment of rhinoconjunctivitis and asthma; aeroallergens are largely responsible for the clinical features and severity of the disease; and clinical expression is associated with the period of environmental exposure to the allergen. Pharmacological treatment of ARD is often based on the intensity of symptoms recorded during previous allergen exposures and cannot always be administered following a step-up approach, as recommended in clinical practice guidelines. Allergen immunotherapy (AIT) is the only option for overall treatment of respiratory symptoms using an etiological approach. AIT can modify the prognosis of ARD and should therefore be considered a valuable first-line treatment.

Conclusions: The present study highlights gaps in current asthma and rhinitis guidelines and addresses specific aspects of ARD, such as global assessment of both asthma and rhinitis or the specific role of variable allergen exposure in the clinical expression of the disease.

Keywords: Consensus, Delphi method, Allergic respiratory disease, One airway, Aeroallergens, Allergic asthma, Allergic rhinitis, Allergic rhinoconjunctivitis, Allergen immunotherapy

Background

Since the publication of the ARIA document in 2001 [1], the "one airway" concept has been accepted almost unanimously by the medical community to describe specific aspects of patients diagnosed with rhinoconjunctivitis with or without asthma. This concept reflects the obvious epidemiological, pathophysiological, diagnostic, and therapeutic relationship between both disorders. In fact, rhinoconjunctivitis and asthma are considered different manifestations of the same disease, and this observation determines clinical management.

It is therefore surprising that consensus guidelines do not usually consider asthma and rhinoconjunctivitis as one disease that should be managed using a comprehensive approach. Furthermore, the focus of current guidelines is mostly on the pathophysiological, clinical, and therapeutic aspects of rhinoconjunctivitis and asthma,

*Correspondence: anam.navarro.sspa@juntadeandalucia.es

[1] UGC of Allergy, Hospital El Tomillar , Carretera Alcalá - Dos Hermanas km 6, 41700 Dos Hermanas, Seville, Spain

Full list of author information is available at the end of the article

with no emphasis on the etiological factors [2–10]. Nevertheless, allergens play a decisive role in the onset of symptoms and influence the clinical manifestations and progress of both rhinoconjunctivitis and allergic asthma. Current classifications of asthma and/or allergic rhinitis by consensus guidelines cannot be universally applied to patients with allergic respiratory disease owing to their high heterogeneity. Therefore, a comprehensive understanding of patients with allergic respiratory disease (ARD) requires that specific aspects of the etiological agent be addressed in the guidelines.

The present consensus defines the characteristics of ARD and reflects on the peculiarities of the disease as a single entity. This document is based on available evidence and the experience of clinical experts. It provides advice to professionals treating patients whose peculiarities are not explicitly included in guidelines and makes a series of recommendations to address this unmet need.

Methods

A scientific committee formed by the authors of this manuscript reviewed the relevant medical literature and developed a structured questionnaire to include specific aspects of ARD from routine practice that are poorly covered by current guidelines. Using a modified Delphi methodology [11], 40 expert allergists who were members of the Committees of Asthma and rhinoconjunctivitis of the Spanish Society of Allergy and Clinical Immunology (SEAIC) between 2010 and 2014 (see "Acknowledgements" section) anonymously assessed the 71 statements in 2 consecutive rounds between September and December 2014. The 71 items were divided into 4 blocks as follows: (1) Definition and Epidemiology, (2) Physiopathology and Etiology, (3) Symptoms, Classification, and Diagnosis; and (4) Treatment: Avoidance, Drug Treatment, and Allergen Immunotherapy (AIT).

After analyzing the results of the first round, one of the facilitators provided an anonymous summary of the results, as well as the reasons allergists provided for their judgements. Thus, allergists were encouraged to revise their earlier answers in light of the replies of other members of the panel, and a second round was held to address the remaining questions. A 9-point, single, ordinal, Likert-type scale was used to grade opinion on each item. Following the Delphi categorization, responses were classified into 3 groups: "disagreement" (1–3), "neither agreement nor disagreement" (4–6), and "agreement" (7–9). The survey also offered the possibility of adding individual explanatory observations for each answer. Once the second round was finished, the results were analyzed. The median position of the scores and the level of agreement or disagreement [12] achieved were measured according to the following criterion: consensus was considered to

have been reached for an item when no more than a third of the scores were outside the region of three points (1–3, 4–6, 7–9) from where the median was located. In this case, the value of the median score determined the group consensus reached, as follows: "agreement", majority with medians ≥ 7; "disagreement", majority with medians ≤ 3; "no consensus", items with medians in the region 4–6 and when the scores of a third or more of the participants were in the region 1–3, and another third or more in the region 7–9. The items for which dispersion of opinions was high (interquartile range ≥ 4 points) were also considered for assessment.

Results

In the literature review carried out, we found that most guidelines and position papers on rhinitis [2–6] emphasize the relationship between asthma and rhinitis (Table 1), and specific sections of some asthma guidelines discuss the relationship between asthma and rhinitis [7–10] (Table 2). However, no guidelines consider both asthma and rhinoconjunctivitis as one disease and offer a comprehensive approach.

With respect to the issues addressed in this study, consensus was achieved for 95.7% (68/71) of the items (agreement, 67; disagreement, 1) (Tables 3, 4, 5, 6). In the first round, consensus was achieved in all but 7. Among the items for which consensus was achieved, it is especially interesting that experts consider that individual aeroallergens may be related to specific clinical profiles and should be taken into account for patient management. In addition, pharmacological treatment of ARD in routine practice is often based on the intensity of symptoms during previous exposures and may not always be established using a step-up approach, as recommended by clinical practice guidelines. As for AIT, the experts think that this approach can modify the prognosis of ARD and should therefore be considered a valuable first-line treatment. No agreement was reached for item 46 ("Patients with ARD sensitized to pollens present symptoms only during the pollen season").

Consensus was not reached on 3 items in the diagnosis and treatment blocks, as follows: "The diagnosis of ARD with lower respiratory tract involvement can be assumed in patients with allergic rhinoconjunctivitis and symptoms of bronchial asthma (even if asthma has not been confirmed by lung function tests)" (item 48); "The doses used in the pharmacological treatment of ARD patients may be greater than those commonly used in non-allergic patients" (item 59); and "AIT decreases the occurrence of new sensitizations in ARD patients" (item 67).

Detailed results for each item (mean, median, percentage of distribution of respondents located outside the

Table 1 Asthma in guidelines on rhinitis

Guideline	Author, year	Chapter	Diagnostic or therapeutic considerations
Clinical practice guideline: allergic rhinitis [6]	Seidman, 2015	Statement 5. Chronic Conditions and Comorbidities: Clinicians should assess patients with a clinical diagnosis of allergic rhinitis for, and document in the medical record, the presence of associated conditions such as asthma, atopic dermatitis, sleep-disordered breathing, conjunctivitis, rhinosinusitis, and otitis media	Evaluation of allergic rhinitis must always include the assessment of asthma. The clinician should inquire about typical symptoms such as dyspnea, cough, wheezing, and exercise-related symptoms. A physical examination should be performed, and the evaluation must be repeated at the follow-up visits, particularly in children. Spirometry must be performed whenever asthma is suspected
Allergic Rhinitis and its Impact on Asthma (ARIA) guidelines: 2010 Revision [5]	Brozek, 2010	VI. Treatment of allergic rhinitis and asthma in the same patient	Recommendations about medical treatment and immunotherapy: subcutaneous immunotherapy (SCIT) and sublingual immunotherapy (SLIT)
The diagnosis and management of rhinitis. An updated practice parameter [4]	Wallace, 2008	Major comorbid conditions Asthma	Lung function tests must be considered in patients with rhinitis Treatment of allergic rhinitis may improve asthma control in patients with coexisting allergic rhinitis and asthma Treatment of allergic rhinitis with intranasal corticosteroids and certain second-generation antihistamines may improve asthma control when both diseases coexist Allergen immunotherapy may prevent the development of new allergen sensitizations and reduce the risk for the future development of asthma in patients with allergic rhinitis
BSACI (British Society for Allergy and Clinical Immunology) guidelines for the management of allergic and non-allergic rhinitis [3]	Scadding, 2008	Co morbid association Rhinitis and asthma–the link	Treatment of rhinitis is associated with improvement of asthma (Grade of recommendation, A) Patients with comorbid asthma and rhinitis receiving treatment for allergic rhinitis have a significantly lower risk of hospitalization or emergency department visits for asthma
Allergic Rhinitis and its Impact on Asthma (ARIA) 2008 Update [2]	Bousquet, 2008	9. Link between rhinitis and asthma	Allergic rhinitis should be considered a risk factor for asthma along with other known risk factors Patients with persistent allergic rhinitis must be evaluated for asthma based on symptoms, physical examination, and, if possible lung function tests (spirometry pre- and post-bronchodilator). Patients with asthma must be appropriately evaluated (history and physical examination) for rhinitis A combined strategy for the treatment of both upper and lower airway diseases is strongly recommended

region of the median, interquartile range, and consensus result) are shown in Tables 3, 4, 5 and 6.

Discussion

The "one airway, one disease" concept [13] has successfully taken root in the medical community, although it is far from being a reality in clinical practice. In fact, there are currently no consensus guidelines for ARD patients. Thus, management is not based on homogeneous criteria and requires the use of 2 separate guidelines, 1 for asthma and 1 for rhinoconjunctivitis.

This consensus study aimed to collect expert opinions from Spanish allergologists about the symptoms, classification, diagnosis, and treatment of ARD to provide a comprehensive approach for clinical practice. A major

goal was to address the importance of the allergen as the modulator of individual variability in clinical expression based on the duration and intensity of exposure.

ARD: Definition

Given the publication of the ARIA guidelines in 2001 [1], the panel agreed that "there is abundant evidence confirming the notion of *one airway, one disease* as the conceptual basis of the management of patients diagnosed with rhinoconjunctivitis and/or asthma" (item 1). Therefore, it follows that "the definition of ARD as a single entity that includes rhinoconjunctivitis and asthma would facilitate its management" (item 2), especially when allergy is its main cause. Finally, the experts of this consensus agreed on the definition that "ARD is

Table 2 Rhinitis in asthma: guidelines

Guideline	Author, year	Chapter	Diagnostic or therapeutic considerations
GEMA 4.0 [7], Spanish Guideline on the Management of Asthma	Executive Committee of the GEMA, 2015	6. Rhinitis and nasal polyposis	Treatment of rhinitis is indicated in the treatment of asthma Inter-relationships between treatments (anti-leukotrienes, intranasal corticosteroids, immunotherapy) and epidemiological aspects are addressed
GINA 2016, Global Strategy for Asthma Management and Prevention [8]	2016 GINA Report	Part D. Managing asthma with comorbidities and in special populations Rhinitis, sinusitis and nasal polyps	Refers to ARIA
British guideline on the Management of Asthma [9]	British Thoracic Society, 2014	No	Studies confirm that atopic dermatitis and atopic rhinitis are amongst the factors most strongly associated with asthma persisting into teenage years
NAEPP [10], National Asthma Education and Prevention Program	Expert Panel Report 3, 2007	Section 3, Component 3: Control of Environmental Factors and Comorbid Conditions That Affect Asthma Comorbid conditions Rhinitis/sinusitis	It is important for clinicians to appreciate the association between upper and lower airway conditions and the part this association plays in asthma management

an altered state of health caused by the generation of IgE antibodies to airborne allergens leading to various clinical manifestations in the upper and/or lower airway" (item 3).

Allergic inflammation is present in both the upper airway and the lower airway [14, 15], although it may be of locally different intensity (items 4, 17, 18). Therefore, a unified assessment of the airway is necessary, irrespective of whether symptoms of both asthma and rhinoconjunctivitis are present at a given time in a patient (item 9).

The concept of ARD is based on the allergic origin of the disease, and its clinical spectrum includes conjunctivitis, rhinitis, and/or asthma. Not all clinical manifestations must occur simultaneously in ARD patients, although the risk of developing the other clinical manifestations of ARD in the future is greater than in the general population [16].

The allergen as a key factor in ARD

In ARD patients, allergens and clinical exacerbations are the main triggers of inflammation (acute and chronic). The ARD consensus highlights the importance of considering allergic sensitization in diagnostic and therapeutic decisions.

Various airborne allergens can induce a variety of respiratory symptoms with a wide spectrum of severity [17]. Furthermore, sensitization to several agents (polysensitization) can also substantially modify the clinical features and prognosis of ARD patients [18]. As shown by several studies, specific allergens more frequently induce symptoms in the upper respiratory tract than in the lower respiratory tract (item 27) [19]. In addition, some airborne allergens are related to the most severe

forms of asthma (item 28) [20] or persistent forms of asthma [21], and some allergens can lead to worse quality of life than others owing to the characteristics of their exposure (item 29) [22]. Age at sensitization and allergen involved have even been linked to the appearance of specific symptoms [23]. Sensitization to certain allergens, for instance *Alternaria* species, has also been noted as a risk factor for exacerbations [24], severe exacerbations, and even death from asthma [25]. Furthermore, recent studies have linked specific allergens to various late reactions in asthma: whereas house dust mites induce more severe late reactions than pollens, animal dander allergens are related to reactions of intermediate intensity [26].

Other factors modulate the clinical response to the allergen. These include "allergenic pressure", which is the combination of both intensity and duration of exposure to an airborne allergen. The experts agreed that "a patient with ARD can manifest allergic rhinoconjunctivitis after being exposed to a specific allergen and asthma after exposure to a different one" (item 32) and "in the same patient, the presence of rhinoconjunctivitis and/or asthma at a particular time may depend on the intensity and duration of exposure to the allergen" (item 33).

For the experts consulted, unlike non-allergic asthma or rhinitis, "control of ARD varies significantly depending on the intensity of exposure to the responsible allergen" (item 41).

Contact with an allergen causes pathophysiological changes that affect the development of symptoms triggered not only by allergens, but also by other agents, such as infectious microorganisms (item 23). These symptoms are more intense when patients are exposed to both an allergen and an infectious agent [27]. Recent studies have

Table 3 Items included in the questionnaire and results

		Mean	Median	Interquartile range	Above the median	Result
1	There is abundant evidence confirming the notion of *one airway, one disease*, which is the conceptual basis of the management of patients diagnosed with rhinoconjunctivitis and/or asthma	8.13	8	1	10	Agreement
2	The definition of allergic respiratory disease (ARD) as a single entity that includes rhinoconjunctivitis and asthma would facilitate its management	7.38	8	2.5	25	Agreement
3	ARD is an altered state of health caused by the generation of IgE antibodies to airborne allergens leading to various clinical manifestations in the upper and/or lower airway	7.85	8	2	10	Agreement
4	The ARD endotype is characterized by the presence of allergic airway inflammation that constitutes the etiological basis of the disease and its exacerbations	7.98	8.5	1.5	12.5	Agreement
5	The clinical manifestations of ARD include nasal (or naso-ocular) symptoms and/or bronchial symptoms	8.55	9	1	0	Agreement
6	The clinical manifestations of ARD may be present perennially or seasonally	8.08	9	1	15	Agreement
7	The clinical manifestations of ARD may be present intermittently or persistently	8.3	9	1	7.5	Agreement
8	The clinical manifestations of ARD may be variable at different times in the patient's life	8.55	9	1	0	Agreement
9	A comprehensive approach to rhinoconjunctivitis and allergic asthma includes the assessment of both entities, irrespective of whether they are present at a given time in a patient	8.15	9	1	7.5	Agreement
10	The prevalence of ARD depends on the age of the patient	7.93	8	2	7.5	Agreement
11	The prevalence of ARD depends on the clinical manifestations analyzed (rhinoconjunctivitis, asthma, or both)	7.6	8	2	12.5	Agreement
12	The prevalence of ARD has geographic variability.	7.43	8	2	20	Agreement
13	Allergic rhinitis usually precedes the development of asthma in adults	7.7	8	1	7.5	Agreement
14	The probability of developing symptoms affecting the lower airway is increased by up to 3-5 times in patients with ARD expressed as persistent allergic rhinitis	7.83	8	1.5	5	Agreement
15	Rhinoconjunctivitis and asthma may appear consecutively or simultaneously in ARD patients	8.3	8	1	0	Agreement
16	An early assessment of ARD should be in made children with food allergy and/or atopic dermatitis	8	8	1	7.5	Agreement

Definition and Epidemiology

linked the persistence of asthma after removing the allergenic trigger in individuals with ARD with the activation of Th2-mediated myeloid dendritic cells [28]. The experts agreed that the allergic nature/substrate of ARD might also influence the persistence of respiratory symptoms during periods of no exposure to an allergen (item 46).

Specific aspects of the diagnosis of ARD
The expert panel agreed that control of ARD depends on a comprehensive diagnosis, including identification of the causative allergen/s and its/their clinical relevance (item 41).

It is well known that "patients with ARD may not meet functional and inflammatory criteria for rhinitis and/or asthma when allergen exposure is not present" (item 47), as occurs in individuals sensitized to pollens out of season [29].

Allergen exposure can influence the results of the diagnostic tests most commonly used in rhinoconjunctivitis and asthma. Whereas allergy tests (skin prick test, specific IgE, allergen challenge) are still useful when patients have no symptoms (item 49), lung function tests may fail to detect bronchial involvement (item 50). Thus, the diagnosis of allergic rhinitis can be made independently of the allergenic exposure. However, according to guidelines, diagnosis of asthma requires the objective demonstration of lower respiratory tract involvement (reversible obstruction, hyperresponsiveness) [7].

Specific aspects of treatment of ARD: drug therapy
The expert panel agreed that the therapeutic and diagnostic approach to ARD patients cannot be solely and strictly based on the recommendations of current guidelines. Adjustment of drugs and doses is based on the

Table 4 Items included in the questionnaire and results

		Mean	Median	Interquartile range	Above the median	Result
17	ARD is characterized as an inflammatory process with a characteristic Th2-mediated response profile	8.08	8	1.5	5	Agreement
18	ARD is characterized by inflammation of both the upper and the lower respiratory tract, which may be of different intensity	8.35	8.5	1	0	Agreement
19	Bronchial hyperresponsiveness is observed in more than one-third of ARD patients who have clinical manifestations in the upper airway	8.13	8	1	2.5	Agreement
20	Although no single mechanism fully explains rhinitis-asthma inter-relationships, systemic spread of allergic inflammatory mediators is the most widely accepted pathway	6.55	7	1	30	Agreement
21	Functional impairment of the bronchial epithelium leads to increased susceptibility to infections and facilitates new allergic sensitizations in ARD patients	7.45	8	2	17.5	Agreement
22	The underlying pathophysiological changes are present all year long in ARD patients with only seasonal clinical manifestations, as a result of infections or exposure to environmental irritants	7.5	8	1	20	Agreement
23	Respiratory infections are usually more severe and last longer in ARD patients	7.05	8	1	22.5	Agreement
24	Clinical manifestations are determined mainly by environmental factors but also by genetic factors	6.7	7	3	30	Agreement
25	The presence and persistence of allergens account for the characteristics of clinical manifestations in ARD patients	7.15	7	1	22.5	Agreement
26	Allergen characteristics and type of exposure can partially determine whether rhinoconjunctivitis precedes asthma or both entities develop simultaneously	7.1	7	1	17.5	Agreement
27	Some allergens induce symptoms more frequently in the upper airway than in the lower airway	7.5	8	2	17.5	Agreement
28	Some airborne allergens are related to more severe forms of asthma	7.98	8.5	2	12.5	Agreement
29	In ARD patients, some allergens can cause worse quality of life than others owing to the characteristics of their exposure	7.85	8	2	10	Agreement

Pathophysiology and Etiology

severity of symptoms in previous allergen exposures and does not follow the frequently recommended "step-up" strategy (item 58), especially in patients with seasonal manifestations.

Although a personalized treatment plan is recommended, we may use the "maximum severity of symptoms recorded in previous exposures" as a guide to establishing future treatments (item 57). This must be registered in the medical history (Items 34 and 35) and is particularly important if therapeutic recommendations are given when patients are not exposed to the allergens.

In the opinion of the expert panel, unlike non-allergic rhinitis and asthma, maintenance therapy may only be administered to ARD patients during allergen exposure (item 55) [9]. However, maintenance therapy may also be used over longer periods to ensure good control (item 56).

Specific aspects of treatment of ARD: AIT
As suggested previously [30], there is a common underlying pathogenic mechanism in all patients with ARD,

despite differences in clinical manifestations and types of allergic sensitization. Identification of the causative allergen and prescription of an allergen-oriented treatment improve disease control and prognosis, irrespective of whether asthma and rhinoconjunctivitis appear simultaneously or sequentially. Allergen immunotherapy (AIT) is an etiology-based treatment and should be considered a first-line option in ARD based on the clinical relevance of allergen sensitization, in which exposure to an allergen elicits allergic symptoms with significant intensity or duration.

However, contrary to published evidence [31] and the opinion of the expert panel, some guidelines [8, 9] do not consider AIT to be first-line treatment. The experts agreed that "failure of drug therapy is not a prerequisite for AIT in patients with ARD" (item 62), and that "most of these patients will benefit from treatment with AIT to slow disease progression" (item 64). This consensus advocates for early indication of AIT under the premise that immunotherapy is most effective in the early stages of ARD (item 63) when the optimal dose is applied, thus combining efficacy and safety.

Table 5 Items included in the questionnaire and results

		Mean	Median	Interquartile range	Above the median	Result
30	Ocular itching and sneezing (upper respiratory tract) and recurrent wheezing (lower respiratory tract) are the symptoms that best correlate with the diagnosis of ARD	7.33	7	2	25	Agreement
31	The presence of asthma must be evaluated in all patients with allergic rhinoconjunctivitis	8.58	9	1	2.5	Agreement
32	A patient with ARD can manifest allergic rhinoconjunctivitis after being exposed to a specific allergen and asthma after exposure to a different one	7.88	8	1.5	12.5	Agreement
33	In the same patient, the presence of rhinoconjunctivitis and/or asthma at a particular time may depend on the intensity and duration of exposure to the allergen	8.2	8	1	0	Agreement
34	We define the concept of "maximum severity" as the highest intensity of symptoms achieved in previous allergen exposures	7.4	7.5	1	17.5	Agreement
35	Due to the variability of symptoms in ARD patients, it is important to record the "most severe" episodes as well as the symptom-free periods	7.98	8	1.5	10	Agreement
36	The variability of symptoms in ARD patients hampers their classification using the criteria proposed by consensus guidelines	7.85	8	2	12.5	Agreement
37	The current classification used by guidelines is based on the assessment of the intensity and frequency of symptoms of rhinoconjunctivitis and asthma separately and does not assess specific aspects of the causative allergens	8.18	8	1	10	Agreement
38	Besides the intensity and duration, the description of ARD symptoms should consider other aspects such as the frequency of the episodes, seasonality, and recurrence of symptoms at specific times	8.35	8.5	1	0	Agreement
39	A specific classification emphasizing the role of the causative allergen is required for patients with ARD	7.55	8	2	12.5	Agreement
40	A classification considering severity, control level, and clinical characteristics of the airborne allergens is required for diagnosis of ARD and treatment	7.63	8	2	12.5	Agreement
41	Control of ARD varies significantly depending on the intensity of the exposure to the responsible allergen	8.08	8	1	5	Agreement
42	ARD must be suspected on the basis of a compatible history and allergy workup	8.43	9	1	2.5	Agreement
43	Diagnosis of ARD is based on compatible clinical manifestations, the allergological study, and environmental exposure	8.35	9	1	2.5	Agreement
44	An allergological study must be indicated when symptoms of ARD have an impact on a patient's quality of life	7.03	8	2	22.5	Agreement
45	Precise information regarding the characteristics of a pollen seasons is required for a proper diagnosis	8.23	8	1	5	Agreement
46	Patients with ARD sensitized to pollens present symptoms only during the pollen season	3.08	3	1	17.5	Disagreement
47	Patients with ARD may not meet functional and inflammatory criteria for rhinitis and/or asthma when allergen exposure is not present	7.93	8	2	2.5	Agreement
48	The diagnosis of ARD with lower respiratory tract involvement can be assumed in patients with allergic rhinoconjunctivitis and symptoms of bronchial asthma (even if asthma has not been confirmed by lung function tests)	5.63	7	4	42.5	No consensus
49	Allergy tests (prick tests, specific IgE, specific challenge) are reliable both in and out of the pollen season	8.55	9	1	0	Agreement
50	Lung function tests may be normal out of the pollen season in patients with upper and lower ARD during the pollen season	7.73	8	2	10	Agreement

Symptoms, Classification, and Diagnosis

Table 6 Items included in the questionnaire and results

		Mean	Median	Interquartile range	Above the median	Result
51	Treatment of rhinitis in patients with asthma contributes to the improvement of bronchial symptoms	7.7	8	2	7.5	Agreement
52	Treatment of rhinitis in patients with asthma reduces socio-economic costs	7.93	8	1.5	12.5	Agreement
53	Treatment of rhinitis in patients with asthma improves their quality of life	8.33	8.5	1	2.5	Agreement
54	Allergen avoidance in ARD is the first line of treatment for all patients, regardless of severity	7.8	8	2	12.5	Agreement
55	Maintenance drug therapy must be recommended, at least as long as the patient is exposed to the causative airborne allergen	7.35	8	2	22.5	Agreement
56	Maintenance drug therapy can be extended for as long as is necessary to achieve good control of the disease	8.38	9	1	0	Agreement
57	Adjustment of treatment in ARD patients must consider the "maximum severity reached in previous allergenic exposures"	7.28	8	1	15	Agreement
58	Treatment of patients who experienced severe symptoms in previous allergenic exposures may not follow the step-up strategy recommended by consensus guidelines and can begin with a higher therapeutic step	7.85	8	2	7.5	Agreement
59	The doses used in the pharmacological treatment of ARD patients may be greater than those commonly used in non-allergic patients	6.23	7	3	42.5	No consensus
60	The prognosis of ARD depends on the presence of polysensitization	6.6	7	2	30	Agreement
61	The treatment strategy in polysensitized patients consists of adapting maintenance treatment to the relevant allergen	6.95	7	1	22.5	Agreement
62	Failure of drug therapy is not a prerequisite for AIT in patients with ARD	8.35	9	1	2.5	Agreement
63	AIT is most effective in early stages of ARD	7.95	8	1.5	10	Agreement
64	Most patients will benefit from treatment with AIT to slow disease progression	7.75	8	2	15	Agreement
65	Most patients with ARD will benefit from treatment with AIT to reduce the severity of symptoms and use of medication and to improve quality of life	7.95	8	1.5	7.5	Agreement
66	Unlike pharmacological treatment, AIT improves the prognosis of ARD	8.08	8	1	5	Agreement
67	AIT decreases the occurrence of new sensitizations in ARD patients	6.53	7	3	37.5	No consensus
68	AIT can prevent the development of bronchial symptoms in patients with rhinoconjunctivitis	7.85	8	2	10	Agreement
69	In ARD patients, identification of the airborne allergen that is clinically responsible for symptoms is essential when attempting to establish the indication of AIT	8.7	9	0.5	0	Agreement
70	The composition of immunotherapy in polysensitized ARD patients must be based on a selection of the relevant allergen(s) according to the patient's clinical and sensitization profile	8.3	9	1	2.5	Agreement
71	A sufficient dose of each allergen must be ensured in AIT with mixtures of allergens in polysensitized ARD patients	8.23	8.5	1	5	Agreement

Treatment–avoidance, drug treatment and allergen immunotherapy (AIT)

ARD allergic respiratory disease, *AIT* allergen immunotherapy

"Unlike pharmacological treatment, AIT improves the prognosis of ARD" (item 66), mostly in monosensitized patients and when an adequate immune response is observed [32]. There is sufficient evidence to support the observation that "most patients with ARD will benefit from treatment with AIT to reduce the severity of symptoms and the use of medication and to improve quality of life" (item 65) [33–35]. Likewise, substantial evidence indicates a preventive effect in the progression from allergic rhinitis to asthma [36] (item 68), especially in children [37].

Some of the authors on the panel agreed that "AIT decreases the occurrence of new sensitizations in ARD patients" (item 67) [38, 39], although consensus was not reached. The experts considered that only some studies in children treated with pollen AIT have demonstrated the development of fewer new sensitizations when compared with those not treated with AIT. Furthermore, this has not been demonstrated for every allergen or in adults treated with AIT.

Polysensitization is an important factor when determining the prognosis of ARD and the indication for AIT (item 70). In polysensitized patients, both maintenance treatment strategies (item 61) and AIT composition (item 69) must be tailored after taking into consideration the most clinically relevant allergen. Therefore, AIT has proven to alleviate patients' overall symptoms owing to its effect on reducing the most relevant allergen-related symptoms [40].

However, polysensitization does not necessarily mean polyallergy [41]. Molecular diagnosis and knowledge of the predominant allergen are very useful for selecting genuinely polyallergic patients to receive AIT. It has been shown that the final composition of the AIT prescribed may need to be modified in up to 50% of patients when molecular diagnosis is used instead of the classic approach [42].

The inclusion of more than 1 allergen in AIT must be considered when there is more than 1 relevant allergen. The authors of this consensus advocate administration of the complete doses of each allergen to ensure the effectiveness of AIT, although this issue warrants further research (item 71).

Classification of patients with ARD

ARD is not reflected in the main clinical practice guidelines. Consequently, given that allergy is the most important cause of persistent rhinoconjunctivitis and asthma, the absence of specific references to patients with ARD [9] is remarkable. It is also interesting that the defining characteristics of ARD, such as the clinical variability conditioned by allergen exposure, have not been assessed. Therefore it is difficult to classify ARD patients according to the criteria currently proposed by guidelines (item 36).

The difficulty in fitting patients diagnosed with ARD with the guidelines lies in the fact that "the current classification is based on the assessment of the intensity and frequency of symptoms of rhinoconjunctivitis and asthma separately and does not assess the specific aspects of the causative allergens" (item 37). However, the expert panel agreed that "besides the intensity and duration, the description of ARD symptoms should also consider other aspects such as the frequency of the episodes, seasonality, and recurrence of symptoms at certain times" (item 38). The assessment of these aspects would enable a better approach in ARD patients.

The dynamic nature of allergic diseases has previously been described [37]. Indeed, "the clinical manifestations of ARD may be variable at different times in the patient's life" (item 8), with variation in the preponderance of nasal over bronchial symptoms [43]. Therefore, appropriate control of these patients requires the evaluation of the whole airway, even though symptoms may not be present at a given time.

The panel of experts highlighted the existence of several unmet needs. 1) Patients diagnosed with ARD require a specific classification that gives prominence to the causative agent (item 39). 2) It is necessary to propose a classification for diagnosis and treatment of ARD that simultaneously takes into account the severity, control, and clinical characteristics of the airborne allergens involved (Item 40). 3) The development of diagnostic and therapeutic approaches that take allergen exposure and the patient's environment into account would be useful in daily clinical practice. Multiple allergens are frequently implicated in ARD, making it very difficult to identify the most important one. Furthermore, we must bear in mind the existence of other factors not related to the allergen that might contribute to the onset of symptoms. 4) Rhinitis and asthma are currently classified, treated, and evaluated using different guidelines. However, the expert panel recommends a holistic approach to ARD patients, taking into account the clinical expression of respiratory disease at different levels and including its severity and level of control after treatment (Figs. 1, 2). It would be desirable to use questionnaires on disease control [44] and quality of life [45] to provide a global evaluation of ARD.

Conclusions

Despite the almost unanimous acceptance of the "one airway, one disease" concept, the current consensus guidelines apply two different standards for the management of patients with ARD. As far as we know, no one has previously addressed the need for a global approach to ARD. Therefore, the expert panel proposes a series of recommendations based on the specific aspects of allergic patients with rhinitis and asthma that can be useful in daily clinical practice (Table 7).

ARD patients are characterized by the presence of allergic rhinoconjunctivitis and/or asthma. The most suitable approach to these patients involves the assessment of all clinical manifestations of the disease, including both rhinoconjunctivitis and asthma, irrespective of whether they are present at a given time.

The clinical manifestations of ARD are variable and related to allergen exposure. Different airborne allergens can be related to specific clinical profiles in patients with

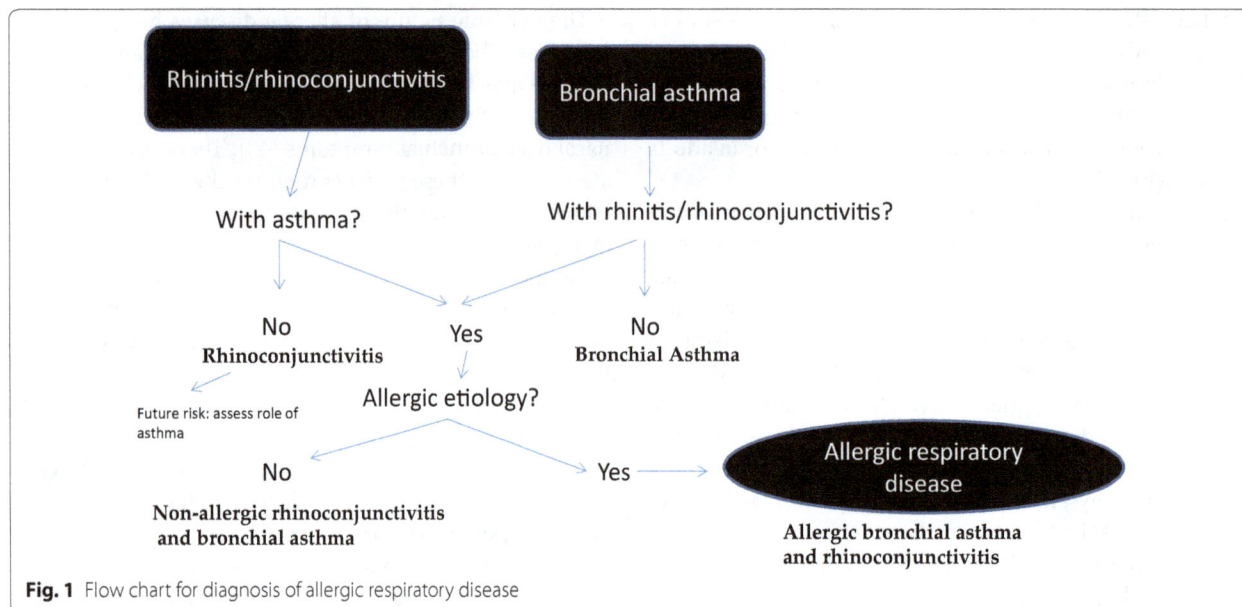

Fig. 1 Flow chart for diagnosis of allergic respiratory disease

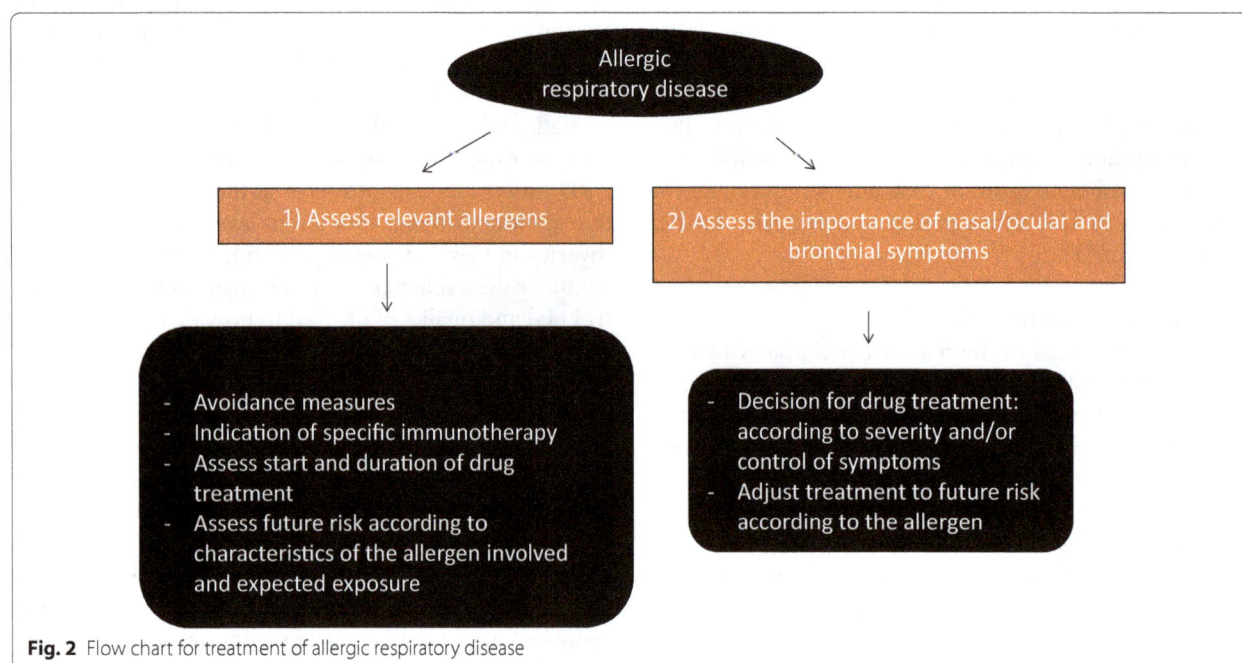

Fig. 2 Flow chart for treatment of allergic respiratory disease

ARD. Thus, the causative allergen must play a greater role in decisions on diagnosis and therapy, since the duration and severity of the disease are determined to a large extent by the allergen.

Pharmacological treatment is often chosen based on the severity of symptoms reached in previous allergenic exposures. Treatment with AIT is a comprehensive and etiological approach to the "one airway" disease. Therefore, AIT must be considered a first-line treatment and indicated in the early phases because, unlike pharmacological treatment, it can modify the prognosis of the disease.

Unmet needs

The peculiarities of ARD are not adequately reflected in the classifications of rhinitis and/or asthma proposed in current guidelines. Therefore, the expert panel considers the development of guidelines that recommend a comprehensive approach to patients with respiratory allergy to be an unmet need.

Table 7 Allergic respiratory disease (ARD): key points

Allergic respiratory disease (ARD) includes patients with clinical manifestations of rhinoconjunctivitis and/or bronchial asthma of allergic etiology

The optimal approach to ARD involves the simultaneous assessment of the upper and lower respiratory tract, irrespective of whether there are symptoms at a given time in a given patient

The clinical features of patients with ARD depend (in part) on the allergen that caused the symptoms and the characteristics of the exposure

The causative allergens of ARD must play a greater role in the choice of treatment

Decisions on drug treatment in patients with ARD may be affected by the clinical severity of previous allergen exposures and not follow the phased strategy suggested by guidelines

Allergen immunotherapy is a comprehensive etiological approach that can modify ARD. Failure of drug therapy is not a prerequisite for allergen immunotherapy in ARD patients

Abbreviations
ARD: allergic respiratory disease; AIT: allergen immunotherapy; SEAIC: Spanish Society of Allergology and Clinical Immunology.

Authors' information
All authors took part in the study as members of Asthma and Rhinoconjunctivitis Committees of the Spanish Society of Allergology and Clinical Immunology (SEAIC).

Author details
[1] UGC of Allergy, Hospital El Tomillar , Carretera Alcalá - Dos Hermanas km 6, 41700 Dos Hermanas, Seville, Spain. [2] UGC of Allergy, Hospital Universitario Virgen Macarena, Seville, Spain. [3] Allergy Unit, Pneumology Department, Hospital Clinic, Institut d'Investigacions Biomèdiques August Pi Sunyer (IDIBAPS), Barcelona, Spain. [4] Allergy Service, Hospital Municipal, Badalona Serveis Assistencials, Badalona, Spain. [5] Allergy Service, Sant Pere Claver Fundació Sanitària, Barcelona, Spain. [6] Department of Allergy, Hospital La Paz Institute for Health Research (IdiPAZ), Madrid, Spain.

Authors' contributions
AN, JD, RM, TD, AV, and SQ designed the study, reviewed the medical literature on the topic, and discussed the main items to be included in the structured questionnaire. All of the members of the Asthma and Rhinoconjunctivitis Committees SEAIC 2010-2014 took part in the study. AN, JD, RM, TD, AV, and SQ analyzed the results, discussed the main conclusions, and drafted the manuscript. All authors read and approved the final manuscript.

Acknowledgements
ARD Study Group: M José Álvarez, Complejo Hospitalario de Navarra, Pamplona; Encarnación Antón, Hospital Universitario Marqués de Valdecilla, Santander; Pilar Barranco, Hospital La Paz, Madrid; Paloma Campo, Hospital Regional Universitario, Málaga; Remedios Cárdenas, Hospital Universitario de Guadalajara; Carlos Colás, Hospital Clínico Universitario, Instituto de Investigación Sanitaria de Aragón, Zaragoza; Ignacio Dávila, Hospital Universitario, IBSAL Departamento de Ciencias Biomédicas y del Diagnóstico, Salamanca; Alfonso del Cuvillo, Hospital de Especialidades de Jerez, Cádiz; Javier Domínguez-Ortega, Hospital La Paz, Madrid; Beatriz Fernández, Hospital El Bierzo, Ponferrada, León; M José Giménez, Área Vigilancia de La Salud CPRL, Málaga; Elisa Gómez, Hospital General Universitario de Ciudad Real; M Luisa González, Hospital Clínico San Carlos, Madrid; Ruperto González, Hospital Universitario Nuestra Señora de Candelaria, Tenerife; Valentina Gutiérrez, Hospital Dr. Peset, Valencia; F. Javier Iglesias-Souto, Hospital Universitario Nuestra Señora de Candelaria, Tenerife; Magdalena Lluch, Hospital La Paz, Madrid; M Aránzazu Martín, Hospital Santa Bárbara de Puertollano, Ciudad Real; Víctor Matheu, Hospital Universitario Nuestra Señora de Candelaria, Tenerife; Javier Montoro, Hospital Arnau de Vilanova, Valencia; José M Olaguibel, Complejo Hospitalario de Navarra; M Carmen Panizo, Hospital Nuestra Señora del Prado, Toledo; Antonio Parra, Complexo Hospitalario Universitario A Coruña; M José Pascual, Centro de Alergia y Asma Balear, Palma de Mallorca; Carmen Pérez, Hospital Dr. Peset, Valencia; Fernando Rodríguez, Hospital Universitario Marqués de Valdecilla, Santander; Mercedes Rodríguez, Hospital Universitario Príncipe de Asturias, Alcalá de Henares, Madrid; Carmen Rondón, Hospital Regional Universitario, Málaga; M Cesárea Sánchez, Hospital Juan Ramón Jiménez, Huelva; Silvia Sánchez-García, Hospital Infantil Universitario Niño Jesús, Madrid; Joaquín Sastre, Hospital Universitario Fundación Jiménez Díaz, Madrid; Francisco Vega, Hospital de la Princesa, Madrid; Jose M Vega, Hospital Regional Universitario, Málaga; M Esther Velázquez; Hospital Quirón Sagrado Corazón, Sevilla. The authors thank Laboratorios LETI SLU (Spain) for logistic support for in the Delphi meetings and SEAIC by its endorsed.

Competing interests
All of the authors took part in the study as members of the Asthma and Rhinoconjunctivitis Committees of the Spanish Society of Allergology and Clinical Immunology (SEAIC). This study was endorsed by SEAIC. The authors declare that they have no competing interests.

References
1. Bousquet J, Van Cauwenberge P, Khaltaev N, Aria Workshop Group, World Health Organization. Allergic rhinitis and its impact on asthma. J Allergy Clin Immunol. 2001;108(Suppl 5):147–334.
2. Bousquet J, Khaltaev N, Cruz AA, Denburg J, Fokkens WJ, Togias A, et al. Allergic Rhinitis and its Impact on Asthma (ARIA) 2008 update (in collaboration with the World Health Organization, GA(2)LEN and AllerGen). Allergy. 2008;63(Suppl 86):8–160.
3. Scadding GK, Durham SR, Mirakian R, Jones NS, Leech SC, Farooque S, et al. BSACI guidelines for the management of allergic and non-allergic rhinitis. Clin Exp Allergy. 2008;38:19–42.
4. Wallace DV, Dykewicz MS, Bernstein DI, Blessing-Moore J, Cox L, Khan DA, et al. The diagnosis and management of rhinitis: an updated practice parameter. J Allergy Clin Immunol. 2008;122(Suppl 2):1–84.
5. Brozek JL, Bousquet J, Baena-Cagnani CE, Bonini S, Canonica GW, Casale TB, et al. Allergic Rhinitis and its Impact on Asthma (ARIA) guidelines: 2010 revision. J Allergy Clin Immunol. 2010;126:466–76.
6. Seidman MD, Gurgel RK, Lin SY, Schwartz SR, Baroody FM, Bonner JR, et al. Clinical practice guideline: allergic rhinitis. Otolaryngol Head Neck Surg. 2015;152(Suppl 1):S1–43.
7. Plaza V, Alonso S, Alvarez C, Gomez-Outes A, Gómez F, López A, et al. Spanish Guideline on the Management of Asthma. J Investig Allergol Clin Immunol. 2016;26(Suppl 1):S1–92.
8. 2016 GINA Report, Global Strategy for Asthma Management and Prevention. http://www.ginasthma.org. Accessed 23 Jan 2016.
9. British Thoracic Society; Scottish Intercollegiate Guidelines Network. British guideline on the Management of Asthma. Thorax. 2014;69(Suppl 1):1–192. https://www.brit-thoracic.org.uk/document-library/clinical-information/asthma/btssign-asthma-guideline-2014/. Accessed 23 Jan 2016.
10. National Asthma Education and Prevention Program. Expert panel report 3 (EPR-3): guidelines for the Diagnosis and Management of Asthma-Summary Report 2007. J Allergy Clin Immunol. 2007;120(Suppl 5):S94–138.
11. Paul CL. A modified Delphi approach to a new card sorting methodology.

J Usability Stud. 2008; 4:7–30. http://uxpajournal.org/a-modified-delphi-approach-to-a-new-cardsorting-methodology/ Accessed 23 Jan 2016.

12. Holey EA, Feeley JL, Dixon J, Whittaker VJ. An exploration of the use of simple statistics to measure consensus and stability in Delphi studies. BMC Med Res Methodol. 2007;7:52.

13. Grossman J. One airway, one disease. Chest. 1997;111:11–6.

14. Braunsthal GJ, Kleinjan A, Overbeek SE, Prins JB, Hoogsteden HC, Fokkens WJ. Segmental bronchial provocation induces nasal inflammation in allergic rhinitis patients. Am J Respir Crit Care Med. 2000;161:2051–7.

15. Panzner P, Malkusová I, Vachová M, Liška M, Brodská P, Růžičková O, et al. Bronchial inflammation in seasonal allergic rhinitis with or without asthma in relation to natural exposure to pollen allergens. Allergol Immunopathol (Madr). 2015;43:3–9.

16. Bousquet J, Vignola AM, Demoly P. Links between rhinitis and asthma. Allergy. 2003;58:691–706.

17. Domínguez-Ortega J, Quirce S, Delgado J, Dávila I, Martí-Guadaño E, Valero A. Diagnostic and therapeutic approaches in respiratory allergy are different depending on the profile of aeroallergen sensitisation. Allergol Immunopathol (Madr). 2014;42:11–8.

18. Li J, Huang Y, Lin X, Zhao D, Tan G, Wu J, et al. China alliance of research on respiratory allergic disease (CARRAD). Influence of degree of specific allergic sensitivity on severity of rhinitis and asthma in Chinese allergic patients. Respir Res. 2011;12:95.

19. Ramirez DA. The natural history of mountain cedar pollinosis. J Allergy Clin Immunol. 1984;73:88–93.

20. Knutsen AP, Bush RK, Demain JG, Denning DW, Dixit A, Fairs A, et al. Fungi and allergic lower respiratory tract diseases. J Allergy Clin Immunol. 2012;129:280–91.

21. Kidon MI, Chiang WC, Liew WK, Ong TC, Tiong YS, Wong KN, et al. Mite component-specific IgE repertoire and phenotypes of allergic disease in childhood: the tropical perspective. Pediatr Allergy Immunol. 2011;22:202–10.

22. Delgado J, Dávila I, Domínguez-Ortega J, Quirce S, Martí-Guadaño E, Valero A. Quality of life in patients with respiratory allergy is influenced by the causative allergen. J Investig Allergol Clin Immunol. 2013;23:309–14.

23. Warm K, Hedman L, Lindberg A, Lötvall J, Lundbäck B, Rönmark E. Allergic sensitization is age-dependently associated with rhinitis, but less so with asthma. J Allergy Clin Immunol. 2005;136:1559–65.

24. ten Brinke A, Sterk PJ, Masclee AA, Spinhoven P, Schmidt JT, Zwinderman AH, et al. Risk factors of frequent exacerbations in difficult-to-treat asthma. Eur Respir J. 2005;26:812–8.

25. Twaroch TE, Curin M, Valenta R, Swoboda I. Mold allergens in respiratory allergy: from structure to therapy. Allergy Asthma Immunol Res. 2015;7:205–20.

26. Boulet LP, Gauvreau G, Boulay ME, O'Byrne PM, Cockcrof DW. Allergen-induced early and late asthmatic responses to inhaled seasonal and perennial allergens. Clin Exp Allergy. 2015;45:1647–53.

27. Murray CS, Poletti G, Kebadze T, Morris J, Woodcock A, Johnston SL, et al. Study of modifiable risk factors for asthma exacerbations: virus infection and allergen exposure increase the risk of asthma hospital admissions in children. Thorax. 2006;61:376–82.

28. Froidure A, Vandenplas O, D'Alpaos V, Evrard G, Pilette C. Persistence of asthma following allergen avoidance is associated with proTh2 myeloid dendritic cell activation. Thorax. 2015;70:967–73.

29. Canova C, Heinrich J, Anto JM, Leynaert B, Smith M, Kuenzli N, et al. The influence of sensitisation to pollens and moulds on seasonal variations in asthma attacks. Eur Respir J. 2013;42:935–45.

30. Calderón MA, Linneberg A, Kleine-Tebbe J, De Bley F, Fernandez Hernandez, de Rojas D, Virchow JC, et al. Respiratory allergy caused by house dust mites: what do we really know? J Allergy Clin Immunol. 2015;136:38–48.

31. Canonica GW, Cox L, Pawankar R, Baena-Cagnani CE, Blaiss M, Bonini S, et al. Sublingual immunotherapy: world Allergy Organization position paper 2013 update. World Allergy Organ J. 2014;7:6.

32. Jutel M, Agache I, Bonini S, Burks AW, Calderon M, Canonica W, et al. International consensus on allergy immunotherapy. J Allergy Clin Immunol. 2015;136:556–68.

33. Lin SY, Erekosima N, Kim JM, Ramanathan M, Suarez-Cuervo C, Chelladurai Y, et al. Sublingual immunotherapy for the treatment of allergic rhinoconjunctivitis and asthma: a systematic review. JAMA. 2013;309:1278–88.

34. Erekosima N, Suarez-Cuervo C, Ramanathan M, Kim JM, Chelladurai Y, Segal JB, et al. Effectiveness of subcutaneous immunotherapy for allergic rhinoconjunctivitis and asthma: a systematic review. Laryngoscope. 2014;124:616–27.

35. Kim JM, Lin SY, Suarez-Cuervo C, Chelladurai Y, Ramanathan M, Segal JB, et al. Allergen-specific immunotherapy for pediatric asthma and rhinoconjunctivitis: a systematic review. Pediatrics. 2013;131:1155–67.

36. Cardona V, Luengo O, Labrador-Horrillo M. Immunotherapy in allergic rhinitis and lower airway outcomes. Allergy. 2017;72:35–42.

37. Morjaria JB, Caruso M, Rosalia E, Russo C, Polosa R. Preventing progression of allergic rhinitis to asthma. Curr Allergy Asthma Rep. 2014;14:412.

38. Eng PA, Borer-Reinhold M, Heijnen IA, Gnehm HP. Twelve-year follow-up after discontinuation of preseasonal grass pollen immunotherapy in childhood. Allergy. 2006;61:198–201.

39. Burks AW, Calderon MA, Casale T, Cox L, Demoly P, Jutel M, et al. Update on allergy immunotherapy: American Academy of Allergy, Asthma & Immunology/European Academy of Allergy and Clinical Immunology/PRACTALL consensus report. J Allergy Clin Immunol. 2013;131:1288–96.

40. Bahceciler NN, Galip N, Cobanoglu N. Multiallergen-specific immunotherapy in polysensitized patients: where are we? Immunotherapy. 2013;5:183–90.

41. Migueres M, Dávila I, Frati F, Azpeitia A, Jeanpetit Y, Lhéritier-Barrand M, Incorvaia C, Ciprandi G, PlurAL study group. Types of sensitization to aeroallergens: definitions, prevalences and impact on the diagnosis and treatment of allergic respiratory disease. Clin Transl Allergy. 2014;4:16.

42. Sastre J, Landivar ME, Ruiz-García M, Andregnette-Rosigno MV, Mahillo I. How molecular diagnosis can change allergen-specific immunotherapy prescription in a complex pollen area. Allergy. 2012;67:709–11.

43. Cruz AA. The 'united airways' require an holistic approach to management. Allergy. 2005;60:871–4.

44. Fonseca JA, Nogueira-Silva L, Morais-Almeida M, Sa-Sousa A, Azevedo LF, Ferreira J, et al. Control of Allergic Rhinitis and Asthma Test (CARAT) can be used to assess individual patients over time. Clin Transl Allergy. 2012;2:16.

45. Braido F, Baiardini I, Stagi E, Scichilone N, Rossi O, Lombardi C, et al. RhinAsthma patient perspective: a short daily asthma and rhinitis QoL assessment. Allergy. 2012;67:1443–50.

14

Prediction and prevention of allergy and asthma

Jean Bousquet[1,2,3,4,13*], Clive Grattan[5], Thomas Bieber[6], Paolo Matricardi[7], Hans Uwe Simon[8], Ulrich Wahn[9], Antonella Muraro[10], Peter W. Hellings[4,11] and Ioana Agache[12]

Abstract

The European Academy of Allergy and Clinical Immunology (EAACI) owns three journals: Allergy, Pediatric Allergy and Immunology and Clinical and Translational Allergy. One of the major goals of EAACI is to support health promotion in which prevention of allergy and asthma plays a critical role and to disseminate the knowledge of allergy to all stakeholders including the EAACI junior members.

Keywords: Allergy, Asthma, EAACI, Prediction, Prevention

The European Academy of Allergy and Clinical Immunology (EAACI) has three official journals: Allergy, Pediatric Allergy and Immunology and Clinical and Translational Allergy. One of the major goals of EAACI is to support health promotion in which prevention of allergy plays a critical role and to disseminate the knowledge of allergy to all stakeholders including the EAACI junior members [1].

The EAACI journals have reported on the prediction and primary and secondary prevention of allergic diseases and asthma in 2016. This paper summarises these achievements.

Risk and protective factors

IgE-mediated allergy is much more common in Finnish compared with Russian Karelia, although these areas are geographically and genetically close. Many studies are trying to find the reasons explaining these differences. Higher concentrations of common environmental chemicals were measured in Russian compared with Finnish Karelian children and their mothers [2]. The chemicals did not explain the higher prevalence of atopy on the Finnish side.

Atopic dermatitis (AD) is a chronic inflammatory skin condition with a multifactorial pathogenesis. Several perinatal factors may influence the risk of AD. In a Danish nationwide register-based study [3], the risk of developing AD in the first 5 years of life was examined. Low birth weight and preterm birth were inversely associated with a lower risk of AD, while neonatal jaundice and birth during autumn or winter were associated with an increased risk of AD.

The prevalence of childhood AD varies considerably between ethnic groups. The Generation R Study assessed the role of environmental exposures and filaggrin (FLG) mutations on associations between ethnic origin and risk of childhood AD in 5082 children [4]. Compared with Dutch children, Cape Verdean, Dutch Antillean, Surinamese-Creole and Surinamese-Hindustani children had increased risks of AD in the first 4 years of life. Environmental and genetic risk factors partly weakened these associations.

Early gut colonization by *Bifidobacterium breve* and *B. catenulatum* differentially modulates AD risk in children at high risk of developing allergic disease [5]. Faecal samples were collected at age 1 week, 1 month and 3 months from 117 infants at high risk of allergic disease. Temporal variations in *Bifidobacterium* colonization patterns early in life are associated with later development of eczema and/or atopic sensitization in infants at high risk of allergic disease.

Evidence linking maternal psychosocial stress during pregnancy to subsequent child AD is growing, but the

*Correspondence: jean.bousquet@orange.fr
[13] CHU Montpellier, 371 Avenue du Doyen Gaston Giraud, 34295 Montpellier Cedex 5, France
Full list of author information is available at the end of the article

definition of AD is diverse and results are inconsistent. The first systematic review to date addressed prenatal maternal stress and the subsequent risk of atopy-related outcomes in the child [6]. Results suggest a relationship between maternal stress during pregnancy and atopic disorders in the child. However, the existing studies are of diverse quality and the wide definitions of often self-reported stress exposures imply a substantial risk for information bias and false-positive results.

Routine vaccinations can have non-targeted effects on susceptibility to infections and allergic disease. Such effects may depend on age at vaccination, and a delay in pertussis vaccination has been linked to reduced risk of allergic disease. In a population-based cohort of Melbourne, HealthNuts, 4433 12-month-old infants had skin tests and oral challenges to determine food allergy [7]. There was no overall association between delayed Diphtheria, Tetanus, Pertusis (DTaP) vaccination and food allergy; however, children with delayed DTaP had less AD and less use of AD medication. Timing of routine infant immunizations may affect susceptibility to allergic disease.

Body mass index (BMI) and physical activity in early childhood are inconsistently associated with atopic sensitization, AD and asthma in later childhood. Higher BMI and over or under physical activities in early childhood were associated with atopic sensitization, AD and asthma in later childhood [8]. Larger cohorts with repeated measurements of both predictors and outcomes are required to confirm the data.

Greater infant weight gain is associated with lower lung function and increased risk of childhood asthma. The role of early childhood peak growth patterns is unclear. A population-based prospective cohort study among 5364 children assessed repeated growth measurements between 0 and 3 years of age as well as BMI and age at adiposity peak [9]. Respiratory resistance and fractional exhaled nitric oxide were measured at 6 years of age. Greater peak height and weight velocities (PHV) were associated with lower respiratory resistance. Greater peak weight velocity (PWV) and BMI at adiposity peak were associated with increased risks of early and persistent wheezing. Childhood weight status partly explained these associations. No other associations were observed. Follow-up studies at older ages are needed to elucidate whether these effects persist at later ages.

The increased prevalence of atopic diseases has been largely studied in children and adolescents, but fewer data exist in adults. Results from the cross-sectional West Sweden Asthma Study in 30,000 randomly-selected individuals showed that there are different risk factor patterns for asthma, rhinitis and eczema in adults with some risk factors overlapping between these conditions.

Allergic sensitization was a strong risk factor for current asthma and current rhinitis but not for current eczema. Obesity was a risk factor for current asthma and current rhinitis, while farm childhood decreased the risk for current asthma and rhinitis. Occupational exposure to gas dust or fumes and female sex was associated with an increased risk of current asthma and eczema [10].

Allergen exposure is associated with the development of allergic sensitization in childhood as reflected by global variations in sensitization patterns. However, there is little evidence to support a direct association. The Copenhagen Prospective Study on Asthma in Childhood 2000 birth cohort showed in children of 7 and 13 years that perinatal indoor aeroallergen exposure does not seem to affect development of allergic sensitization or rhinitis during childhood [11].

Finally, a hypothesis was proposed: may e-cigarette vaping boost the allergic epidemic by affecting human host defences, *Staphylococcus aureus* virulence and IgE sensitization? [12].

Allergic March

Infants hospitalized for severe bronchiolitis are at increased risk of childhood asthma. A nested cohort study within the Massachusetts General Hospital Obstetric Maternal Study (MOMS) carried out a prospective cohort of pregnant women enrolled during 1998–2006 (n = 5407) [13]. AD was significantly associated with severe bronchiolitis in infancy. The mechanism of the AD-bronchiolitis association is unclear.

Mechanisms

Finnish and Russian Karelian children have a highly contrasting occurrence of asthma and allergy: The methylation levels in the promoter region of the CD14 gene were higher in the Finnish compared to Russian Karelian children. However, the methylation variation of this candidate gene did not explain the asthma and allergy contrast between these two areas and the answer is not simple [14].

The role of FLG mutations during pregnancy and postpartum is unknown. FLG-genotyping was performed in a population-based sample of 1837 women interviewed in the 12th and 30th weeks of pregnancy and 6 months postpartum as part of the Danish National Birth Cohort study 1996–2002. Women with FLG mutations had an increased risk of AD flares during pregnancy and of enduring postpartum physical problems linked to perineal trauma during delivery [15].

First-born children are at higher risk of developing a range of immune-mediated diseases and may have a divergent activated T-cells profile suggesting in utero programming of the child's immune system. In a subgroup of 28 children enrolled in the COPSAC2010 birth cohort, it was found that first-born infants display a reduced anti-inflammatory profile in Tv-cells at birth. This possible in utero 'birth-order' T-cells programming may contribute to a later development of immune-mediated diseases by increasing overall immune reactivity in first-born children as compared to younger siblings [16].

Although total IgE levels have been proposed as a biomarker for disease severity in AD and are increased in the majority of AD patients, they do not correlate with disease severity. During the synthesis of immunoglobulins, free light chains (Ig-FLCs) are produced in excess over heavy chains. In comparison with IgE molecules, Ig-FLCs have a very short serum half-life. Therefore, Ig-FLCs might be more suitable as a biomarker for disease severity during follow-up. However, immunoglobulin free light chains in adult AD patients do not correlate with disease severity [17].

Epigenetics

DNA methylation in adulthood is associated with season of birth, supporting the hypothesis that DNA methylation could mechanistically underlie the effect of season of birth on allergy, although other mechanisms are also likely to be involved [18]. There may be an association between season of birth and blood DNA methylation in adulthood but a recent study was unable to replicate previous findings and the question is still open [19].

Early environmental factors are likely to contribute to CMA. In a small sample size from the Dutch Euro-Prevall birth cohort study (N = 20 CMA, N = 23 controls, N = 10 tolerant boys), general hypermethylation was found in the CMA group compared to control children, while this effect was absent in the tolerant group [20]. Methylation differences were, among others, found in regions of DHX58, ZNF281, EIF42A and HTRA2 genes. Several of these genes are associated with allergic diseases.

Consumption of unboiled farm milk in early life prevents the development of atopic diseases. Milk is a complex signalling and epigenetic imprinting network that promotes stable FoxP3 expression and long-lasting Treg differentiation, crucial postnatal events preventing atopic and autoimmune diseases [21].

Prediction

Profiles of allergic sensitization are poorly documented in infancy. Early polysensitization is associated with allergic multimorbidity in the Pollution and Asthma Risk: an Infant Study (PARIS) birth cohort of infants [22] as early as 18 months of age. Three profiles were found, differing in terms of allergic morbidity at 6 years. Early sensitization can predict allergic multimorbidity in childhood,

and in the case of early polysensitization, multimorbidity is more frequent as early as infancy [23].

The longitudinal pattern of allergen-specific IgE levels from the prenatal stage to early life has remained largely unexplored. 103 mother-infant pairs, part of an ongoing population-based prospective birth cohort study in Taiwan, found that an influence of maternal allergen-specific IgE levels on infant immune response might occur at birth and then wane in infants at 12 months of age [24].

A longitudinal study of maternal body mass index, gestational weight gain, and offspring asthma was carried out in the Growing Up Today Study [25]. Physician-diagnosed asthma during childhood or adolescence was reported by 2694 children (21%). Maternal prepregnancy overweightness and obesity were associated with offspring asthma. The relation of several prenatal factors to risk of childhood asthma supports the early origins hypothesis for asthma.

Prevention

Breastfeeding is associated with a lower risk of asthma symptoms in early childhood, but its effect at older ages remains unclear. The Food Allergy and Intolerance Research (FAIR) cohort (n = 988) [26] showed inconsistent protective effects of nonexclusive and exclusive breastfeeding against long-term allergic outcomes. The Generation R Study [27] examined the associations of duration and exclusiveness of breastfeeding with asthma outcomes in children aged 6 years, and whether these associations were explained by atopic or infectious mechanisms. Breastfeeding patterns may influence wheezing and asthma in childhood, which seem to be partly explained by infectious mechanisms.

Prevention guidelines for infants at high risk of allergic disease recommend hydrolysed formula if formula is introduced before 6 months, but evidence is mixed. Adding specific oligosaccharides may improve outcomes. A partially hydrolysed whey formula containing oligosaccharides does not prevent AD in the first year in high-risk infants [28]. The immunological changes (increased regulatory T-cell and plasmacytoid dendritic cell percentages) that were found require confirmation in a separate cohort.

Data on the long-term impact of hydrolyzed formulas on allergies are scarce. The GINI (German Infant Study on the influence of Nutrition Intervention) trial participants (n = 2252) received one of four formulas in the first four months of life as breast milk substitute if necessary: partial or extensive whey hydrolyzate (pHF-W, eHF-W), extensive casein hydrolyzate (eHF-C) or standard cow's milk formula (CMF) as Ref. [29]. Between 11 and 15 years, the prevalence of asthma and the cumulative incidence of AR were reduced in the eHF-C. The cumulative incidence of AD was reduced in pHF-W and eHF-C, AD prevalence was reduced in eHF-C. No significant effects were found in the eHF-W group on any manifestation, nor was there an effect on sensitization with any formula. In high-risk children, early intervention using different hydrolyzed formulas has variable preventative effects on asthma, allergic rhinitis and AD up to adolescence.

Nutritional adequacy of a cow's milk exclusion diet in infancy is essential since infants with suspected cow's milk allergy are required to follow a strict milk exclusion diet [30]. In a group of UK infants (subgroup of the Prevalence of Infant Food Allergy study), the diets of 39 infants (13 milk-free and 26 controls) were assessed. Although infants consuming a milk-free diet have a nutritional intake that is significantly different to matched controls who are eating an unrestricted diet, this difference is not constant and it is not seen for all nutrients.

The impact of the elimination diet on growth and nutrient intake in children with food protein induced gastrointestinal allergies was examined in children with delayed type allergies [31]. A prospective, observational study was performed at a tertiary gastroenterology department in children ranging in age from 4 weeks to 16 years. With appropriate dietary advice, including optimal energy and protein intake, hypoallergenic formulas and vitamins and mineral supplementation, growth parameters increased from before to after dietary elimination. These factors were positively associated with growth, irrespective of the type of elimination diet and the numbers of foods eliminated.

The prevalence of food hypersensitivity in the UK is still largely open to debate [32]. In a population based birth cohort study conducted in Hampshire, UK as part of the European Initiative on Food Allergy, EuroPrevall, birth cohort study, 1140 infants were recruited with 823 being followed up until 2 years of age. The diagnosis of food allergy was ascertained by positive double-blind, placebo-controlled food challenge (DBPCFC). Cumulative incidence of food hypersensitivity by 2 years of age was 5.0%. The cumulative incidence for individual food allergens were hens' egg 2.7% (1.6–3.8); cows' milk 2.4% (1.4–3.5); peanut 0.7% (0.1–1.3); soy 0.4% (0.0–0.8); wheat 0.2% (0.0–0.5) and 0.1% (0.0–0.32) for fish. Just under half the infants with confirmed food hypersensitivity had no demonstrable IgE.

In the Probiotics in Prevention of Allergy among Children in Trondheim (ProPACT, n = 259) study, AD prevention in children following maternal probiotic supplementation does not appear to be mediated by breast milk TSLP or TGF-beta [33].

The political agenda

Preventive strategies for allergic diseases need to be anchored on a strong political agenda to implement the results of the research into practice. The European Symposium on Precision Medicine in Allergy and Airways Diseases at the European Union Parliament (October 14, 2015) stressed that the socioeconomic impact of allergies and chronic airways diseases cannot be underestimated [34]. Participants underscored the need for optimal patient care in Europe, supporting joint action plans for disease prevention, patient empowerment, and cost-effective treatment strategies. AIRWAYS-ICPs (Integrated care pathways for airway diseases, Action Plan B3 of the European Innovation Partnership on Active and Healthy Ageing, DG Santé and DG Connect) focuses on the prevention and integrated care of chronic diseases. It has proposed a scale-up strategy for the management and prevention of allergic diseases using the recommendations of the European Innovation Partnership on Active and Healthy Ageing [35]. ARIA, the Allergic Rhinitis and its Impact on Asthma (ARIA) initiative commenced during a World Health Organization workshop in 1999, is also targeting preventive strategies to prevent asthma and rhinitis by implementing emerging technologies using the ARIA Allergy Diary app and the ARIA allergy companion app [36]. In close collaboration with the European Forum for Research and Education in Allergy and Airways diseases (EUFOREA) [37], an action plan for increasing awareness on prevention, patient empowerment and cost-effective treatments is being elaborated.

Abbreviations

AD: atopic dermatitis; AR: allergic rhinitis; BMI: body mass index; CMA: cow's milk allergy; CMF: standard cow's milk formula; DTaP: diphtheria, tetanus, pertusis; EAACI: European Academy of Allergy and Clinical Immunology; eHF-C: extensive casein hydrolyzate; eHF-W: extensive whey hydrolyzate; FLG: fillagrin; FoxP3: forkhead box P3; Ig-FLCs: immunoglobulin, free light chains; LC-PUFAs: long chain polyunsaturated fatty acids; pHF-W: partial whey hydrolyzate; PHV: peak height and weight velocities; PWV: peak weight velocity; SNIP: single nucleotide polymorphisms; TGF-β: transforming growth factor-β; Treg: T regulatory cell; TSLP: thymic stromal lymphopoietin.

Authors' contributions

Each author reviewed the referenced papers and the text. The paper was written by JB. All authors read and approved the final manuscript.

Author details
[1] MACVIA-France, Contre les MAladies Chroniques pour un VIeillissement Actif en France European Innovation Partnership on Active and Healthy Ageing Reference Site, Montpellier, France. [2] INSERM U 1168, VIMA: Ageing and Chronic Diseases Epidemiological and Public Health Approaches, Villejuif, France. [3] UMR-S 1168, Université Versailles St-Quentin-en-Yvelines, Montigny le Bretonneux, France. [4] Euforea, Brussels, Belgium. [5] Dermatology Centre, Norfolk and Norwich University Hospital, Norwich, UK. [6] Department of Dermatology and Allergy, Rheinische Friedrich-Wilhelms-University Bonn, Bonn, Germany. [7] AG Molecular Allergology and Immunomodulation, Department of Pediatric Pneumology and Immunology, Charité Medical University, Berlin, Germany. [8] Institute of Pharmacology, University of Bern, Bern, Switzerland. [9] Pediatric Department, Charité, Berlin, Germany. [10] Food Allergy Referral Centre Veneto Region, Department of Women and Child Health, Padua General University Hospital, Padua, Italy. [11] Laboratory of Clinical Immunology, Department of Microbiology and Immunology, KU Leuven, Leuven, Belgium. [12] Faculty of Medicine, Transylvania University, Brasov, Romania. [13] CHU Montpellier, 371 Avenue du Doyen Gaston Giraud, 34295 Montpellier Cedex 5, France.

Acknowledgements
None.

Competing interests
The authors declare that they have no competing interests..

References
1. Tomazic PV, Graessel A, Silva D, Eguiluz-Gracia I, Guibas GV, Grattan C, et al. A mutually beneficial collaboration between the European Academy of Allergy and Clinical Immunology Junior Members and Clinical and Translational Allergy. Clin Transl Allergy. 2016;6:43.
2. Koskinen JP, Kiviranta H, Vartiainen E, Jousilahti P, Vlasoff T, von Hertzen L, et al. Common environmental chemicals do not explain atopy contrast in the Finnish and Russian Karelia. Clin Transl Allergy. 2016;6:14.
3. Egeberg A, Andersen YM, Gislason G, Skov L, Thyssen JP. Neonatal risk factors of atopic dermatitis in Denmark—results from a nationwide register-based study. Pediatr Allergy Immunol. 2016;27(4):368–74.
4. Elbert NJ, Duijts L, den Dekker HT, Jaddoe VW, Sonnenschein-van der Voort AM, de Jongste JC, et al. Role of environmental exposures and filaggrin mutations on associations of ethnic origin with risk of childhood eczema. The Generation R Study. Pediatr Allergy Immunol. 2016;27(6):627–35.
5. Ismail IH, Boyle RJ, Licciardi PV, Oppedisano F, Lahtinen S, Robins-Browne RM, et al. Early gut colonization by *Bifidobacterium breve* and *B. catenulatum* differentially modulates eczema risk in children at high risk of developing allergic disease. Pediatr Allergy Immunol. 2016;27(8):838–46.
6. Andersson NW, Hansen MV, Larsen AD, Hougaard KS, Kolstad HA, Schlunssen V. Prenatal maternal stress and atopic diseases in the child: a systematic review of observational human studies. Allergy. 2016;71(1):15–26.
7. Kiraly N, Koplin JJ, Crawford NW, Bannister S, Flanagan KL, Holt PG, et al. Timing of routine infant vaccinations and risk of food allergy and eczema at one year of age. Allergy. 2016;71(4):541–9.
8. Byberg KK, Eide GE, Forman MR, Juliusson PB, Oymar K. Body mass index and physical activity in early childhood are associated with atopic sensitization, atopic dermatitis and asthma in later childhood. Clin Transl Allergy. 2016;6(1):33.
9. Casas M, den Dekker HT, Kruithof CJ, Reiss IK, Vrijheid M, de Jongste JC, et al. Early childhood growth patterns and school-age respiratory resistance, fractional exhaled nitric oxide and asthma. Pediatr Allergy Immunol. 2016;27(8):854–60.
10. Ronmark EP, Ekerljung L, Mincheva R, Sjolander S, Hagstad S, Wennergren G, et al. Different risk factor patterns for adult asthma, rhinitis and eczema: results from West Sweden Asthma Study. Clin Transl Allergy. 2016;6:28.
11. Schoos AM, Chawes BL, Jelding-Dannemand E, Elfman LB, Bisgaard H. Early indoor aeroallergen exposure is not associated with development of sensitization or allergic rhinitis in high-risk children. Allergy. 2016;71(5):684–91.
12. Bousquet J, Bachert C, Alexander LC, Leone FT. Hypothesis: may e-cigarette smoking boost the allergic epidemic? Clin Transl Allergy. 2016;6:40.
13. Balekian DS, Linnemann RW, Castro VM, Perlis R, Thadhani R, Camargo CA Jr. Pre-birth cohort study of atopic dermatitis and severe bronchiolitis during infancy. Pediatr Allergy Immunol. 2016;27(4):413–8.
14. Khoo SK, Makela M, Chandler D, Schultz EN, Jamieson SE, Goldblatt J, et al. No simple answers for the Finnish and Russian Karelia allergy contrast: methylation of CD14 gene. Pediatr Allergy Immunol. 2016;27(7):721–7.
15. Bager P, Wohlfahrt J, Boyd H, Thyssen JP, Melbye M. The role of filaggrin mutations during pregnancy and postpartum: atopic dermatitis and genital skin diseases. Allergy. 2016;71(5):724–7.
16. Kragh M, Larsen JM, Thysen AH, Rasmussen MA, Wolsk HM, Bisgaard H, et al. Divergent response profile in activated cord blood T cells from first-born child implies birth-order-associated in utero immune programming. Allergy. 2016;71(3):323–32.
17. Thijs JL, Knipping K, Bruijnzeel-Koomen CA, Garssen J, de Bruin-Weller MS, Hijnen DJ. Immunoglobulin free light chains in adult atopic dermatitis patients do not correlate with disease severity. Clin Transl Allergy. 2016;6:44.
18. Lockett GA, Soto-Ramirez N, Ray MA, Everson TM, Xu CJ, Patil VK, et al. Association of season of birth with DNA methylation and allergic disease. Allergy. 2016;71(9):1314–24.
19. Dugue PA, Geurts YM, Milne RL, Lockett GA, Zhang H, Karmaus W, et al. Is there an association between season of birth and blood DNA methylation in adulthood? Allergy. 2016;71(10):1501–4.
20. Petrus NCM, Henneman P, Venema A, Mul A, van Sinderen F, Haagmans M, et al. Cow's milk allergy in Dutch children: an epigenetic pilot survey. Clin Transl Allergy. 2016;6:16.
21. Melnik BC, John SM, Carrera-Bastos P, Schmitz G. Milk: a postnatal imprinting system stabilizing FoxP3 expression and regulatory T cell differentiation. Clin Transl Allergy. 2016;6:18.
22. Gabet S, Just J, Couderc R, Bousquet J, Seta N, Momas I. Early polysensitization is associated with allergic multimorbidity in PARIS birth cohort infants. Pediatr Allergy Immunol. 2016;27(8):831–7.
23. Bousquet J, Anto JM, Akdis M, Auffray C, Keil T, Momas I, et al. Paving the way of systems biology and precision medicine in allergic diseases: the MeDALL success story: mechanisms of the development of ALLergy; EU FP7-CP-IP; Project No: 261357; 2010-2015. Allergy. 2016;71(11):1513–25.
24. Wang JY, Chen CA, Hou YI, Hsiao WL, Huang YW, Tsai YT, et al. Longitudinal pattern of multiplexed immunoglobulin E sensitization from prenatal stage to the first year of life. Pediatr Allergy Immunol. 2016;27(6):620–6.
25. Dumas O, Varraso R, Gillman MW, Field AE, Camargo CA Jr. Longitudinal study of maternal body mass index, gestational weight gain, and offspring asthma. Allergy. 2016;71(9):1295–304.
26. Bion V, Lockett GA, Soto-Ramirez N, Zhang H, Venter C, Karmaus W, et al. Evaluating the efficacy of breastfeeding guidelines on long-term outcomes for allergic disease. Allergy. 2016;71(5):661–70.
27. den Dekker HT, Sonnenschein-van der Voort AM, Jaddoe VW, Reiss IK, de Jongste JC, Duijts L. Breastfeeding and asthma outcomes at the age of 6 years: The Generation R Study. Pediatr Allergy Immunol. 2016;27(5):486–92.
28. Boyle RJ, Tang ML, Chiang WC, Chua MC, Ismail I, Nauta A, et al. Prebiotic-supplemented partially hydrolysed cow's milk formula for the prevention of eczema in high-risk infants: a randomized controlled trial. Allergy. 2016;71(5):701–10.
29. von Berg A, Filipiak-Pittroff B, Schulz H, Hoffmann U, Link E, Sussmann M, et al. Allergic manifestation 15 years after early intervention with hydrolyzed formulas—the GINI Study. Allergy. 2016;71(2):210–9.
30. Maslin K, Oliver EM, Scally KS, Atkinson J, Foote K, Venter C, et al. Nutritional adequacy of a cows' milk exclusion diet in infancy. Clin Transl Allergy. 2016;6:20.
31. Meyer R, De Koker C, Dziubak R, Godwin H, Dominguez-Ortega G, Chebar Lozinsky A, et al. The impact of the elimination diet on growth and nutrient intake in children with food protein induced gastrointestinal allergies. Clin Transl Allergy. 2016;6:25.

32. Garcia-Larsen V, Del Giacco SR, Moreira A, Bonini M, Haahtela T, Bonini S, et al. Dietary intake and risk of asthma in children and adults: protocol for a systematic review and meta-analysis. Clin Transl Allergy. 2016;6:17.

33. Simpson MR, Ro AD, Grimstad O, Johnsen R, Storro O, Oien T. Atopic dermatitis prevention in children following maternal probiotic supplementation does not appear to be mediated by breast milk TSLP or TGF-beta. Clin Transl Allergy. 2016;6:27.

34. Muraro A, Fokkens WJ, Pietikainen S, Borrelli D, Agache I, Bousquet J, et al. European symposium on precision medicine in allergy and airways diseases: Report of the European Union Parliament Symposium (October 14, 2015). Allergy. 2016;71(5):583–7.

35. Bousquet J, Farrell J, Crooks G, Hellings P, Bel EH, Bewick M, et al. Scaling up strategies of the chronic respiratory disease programme of the European Innovation Partnership on Active and Healthy Ageing (Action Plan B3: Area 5). Clin Transl Allergy. 2016;6:29.

36. Bousquet J, Hellings PW, Agache I, Bedbrook A, Bachert C, Bergmann KC, et al. ARIA 2016: care pathways implementing emerging technologies for predictive medicine in rhinitis and asthma across the life cycle. Clin Transl Allergy. 2016;6:47.

37. Hellings PW, Fokkens WJ, Bachert C, Akdis CA, Bieber T, Agache I, et al. Positioning the principles of precision medicine in care pathways for allergic rhinitis and chronic rhinosinusitis—a EUFOREA-ARIA-EPOS-AIRWAYS ICP statement. Allergy. 2017;72(9):1297–305.

Different risk factor patterns for adult asthma, rhinitis and eczema: results from West Sweden Asthma Study

Erik P. Rönmark[1*], Linda Ekerljung[1], Roxana Mincheva[1], Sigrid Sjölander[2], Stig Hagstad[1], Göran Wennergren[3], Eva Rönmark[4], Jan Lötvall[1] and Bo Lundbäck[1]

Abstract

Background: Atopic diseases including asthma, rhinitis and eczema have increased in the second half of the past century. This has been well studied among children and adolescents but with the exception of asthma to a much lesser extent in adults. The adult risk factor pattern of atopic diseases, in particular of eczema, and their relation to allergic sensitization are yet to be fully elucidated. Studies among adults that have compared the risk factor pattern for these conditions in the same material are very few. The objective of this study was to compare the risk factor patterns for asthma, rhinitis and eczema in a randomly selected adult population.

Methods: A questionnaire survey on atopic diseases was dispatched by mail to 30,000 randomly selected individuals in West Sweden aged 16–75 years and 62 % participated. A subgroup of 2000 individuals was selected for clinical examinations including blood sampling for specific serum Immunoglobulin E to common airborne allergens and 1172 attended.

Results: The prevalence of current asthma was 11.8 %, current rhinitis 42.8 %, current eczema 13.5 and 2.3 % had all three conditions while 13.9 % had at least two conditions. No mutual risk factor was identified for all three conditions. Allergic sensitization was a strong risk factor for current asthma (OR 4.1 CI 2.7–6.3) and current rhinitis (OR 5.1 CI 3.8–6.9) but not so for current eczema. Obesity was a risk factor for current asthma and current rhinitis, while farm childhood decreased the risk for current asthma and current rhinitis. Occupational exposure to gas dust or fumes and female sex was associated with an increased risk of current asthma and current eczema.

Conclusions: There are different risk factor patterns for asthma, rhinitis and eczema in adults but some risk factors are overlapping between some of the conditions. The effect of mutable risk factors should be assessed further in longitudinal studies.

Keywords: Asthma, Eczema, Rhinitis, Epidemiology, Prevalence, Population study, Risk factors

Background

The atopic march constitutes the sequential development of atopic diseases [1, 2]. Most often, it starts in early childhood with eczema and progresses with asthma and rhinitis [3–6]. While the exact cause of this temporal pattern remains largely unknown, in recent years the role of the epithelium has gained attention in the pathogenesis of atopic diseases [7, 8]. Filaggrin is an epithelial protein in the epidermis that is responsible for the hydration of stratum corneum [9]. Studies have shown that a mutation in the filaggrin gene predisposes subjects to the development of eczema [10] and mutations in the filaggrin gene are common among subjects with eczema [11]. This impaired skin barrier may lead to allergic sensitization and subsequent development of other atopic diseases such as asthma and rhinitis [12].

*Correspondence: erik.ronmark@gu.se
[1] Department of Internal Medicine, Krefting Research Centre, Institute of Medicine, Sahlgrenska Academy, University of Gothenburg, Box 424, 405 30 Gothenburg, Sweden
Full list of author information is available at the end of the article

Other identified risk factors for atopic diseases in children include exposure to cigarette smoke [13] and family history of atopy [14]. However, the atopic march is mainly related to the incidence of atopic diseases and there is considerate remission of eczema with increasing age [5]. Nevertheless, studies have shown eczema to be common not only among children but also among adults [15–17].

In general, allergic sensitization is associated with asthma, rhinitis and eczema, while the associations with lifestyle and environmental factors show diverging results. Common risk factors for asthma, eczema and rhinitis are infrequently studied simultaneously in adult populations. The aim of this study was to assess individual and common risk factors for asthma, eczema and rhinitis in a randomly selected adult population sample.

Methods
Study area and population
The West Gothia region of Sweden (Fig. 1) has a population of 1.6 million, approximately one-sixth of the total Swedish population. In 2008, a large population based questionnaire survey was dispatched by mail to 30,000 randomly selected subjects in this area. From the metropolitan area of Gothenburg 15,000 subjects were selected and 15,000 subjects from the rest of the county. Response rate was 62 % (18,087 participants). The population study

and a study on effects of late and non-response has previously been described in detail [18, 19]. Among the responders, 2000 randomly selected participants were invited to clinical examinations and 1172 (59 %) individuals participated. Figure 2 shows the study set-up and participation.

Questionnaire and clinical examinations
The questionnaire consisted of three parts administered at the same time. The first part was the Swedish OLIN study questionnaire [20, 21] covering asthma, rhinitis, COPD, respiratory symptoms and possible risk factors of disease such as smoking and family history of airway diseases. The second part included questions regarding occupational exposures, environmental exposures and health status. The third part consisted of the Swedish Global Allergy and Asthma (GA[2]LEN) questionnaire [22] which further assessed respiratory symptoms and diseases and added questions about eczema. The clinical examinations included objective measures of height and weight, a structured interview and a drawn blood sample. Sixty-nine subjects did not participate in the blood sampling either due to unwillingness or technical difficulties but completed the other parts of the examination. The presence of serum Immunoglobulin E (IgE) was assessed using a mixture of 11 common airborne allergens and included timothy, birch, mugwort, olive, parietaria, cat,

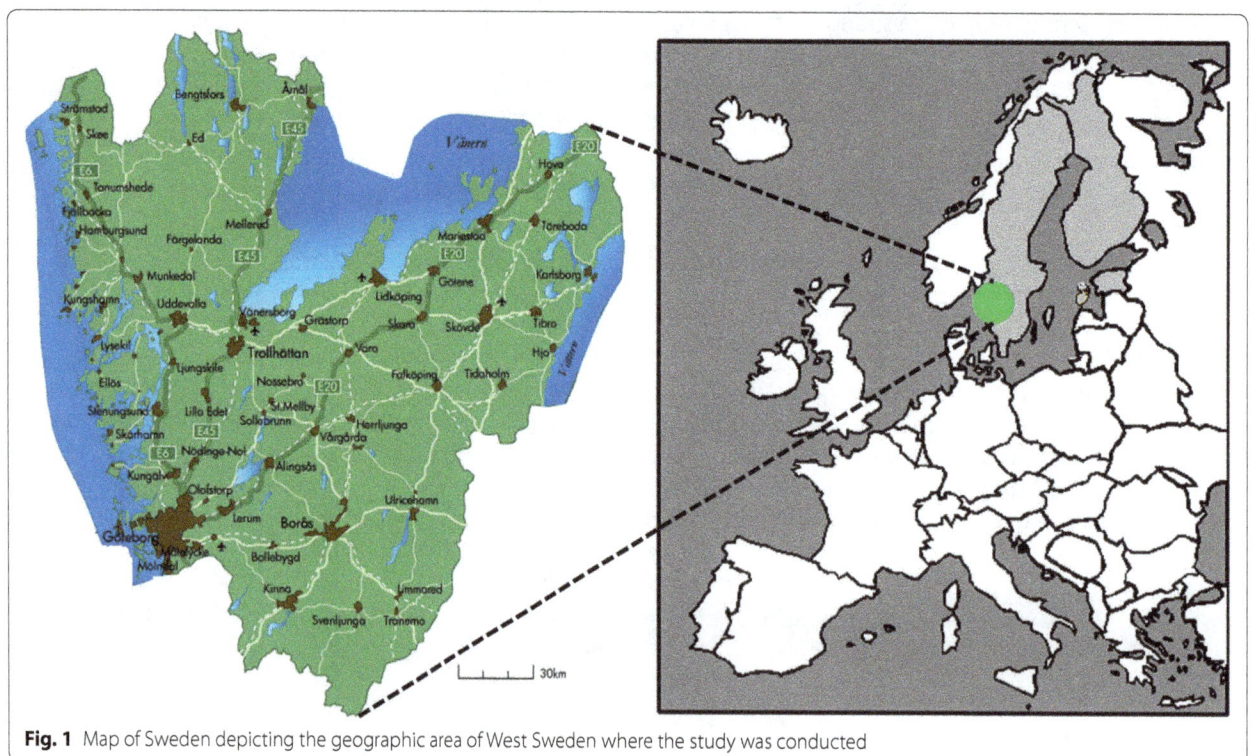

Fig. 1 Map of Sweden depicting the geographic area of West Sweden where the study was conducted

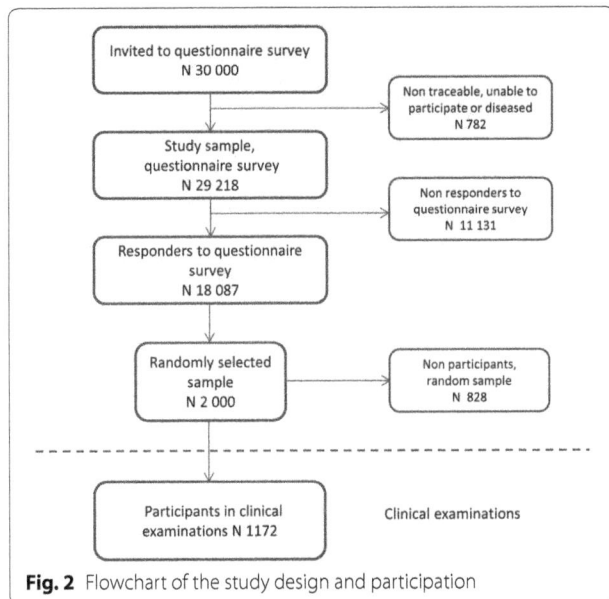

Fig. 2 Flowchart of the study design and participation

dog, horse, *D. pteronyssinus*, *D. farinae* and *C. herbarum* (ImmunoCAP® Phadiatop, Thermo Scientific). A value of ≥ 0.35 kU_A/l was considered a positive test. Body Mass Index (BMI) was calculated by $weight_{(kg)}/(height_{(m)})^2$. BMI was defined as normal if 20–25 kg/m^2, underweight <20 kg/m^2, overweight 25–30 kg/m^2 and more than 30 kg/m^2 considered as obesity.

Definitions

Asthma ever: Either "Have you ever had asthma?" or "Have you ever been diagnosed as having asthma by a physician?"

Current asthma: Asthma ever and a report of either use of asthma medication or recurrent wheeze or attacks of shortness of breath in the last 12 months.

Eczema ever: "Have you ever had eczema or any kind of skin allergy?"

Current eczema: Yes to "Have you ever had an itchy rash which was coming and going for at least 6 months?" and "Have you had this itchy rash in the last 12 months?"

Rhinitis ever: Either "Have you ever had nasal allergies or hay fever?", or *nasal blockage*: "Do you have nasal blockage more or less constantly?", or *runny nose*: "Do you have a runny nose more or less constantly?"

Current rhinitis: Either *nasal blockage* or *runny nose*, or both of the following: "Have you had sneezing, runny nose or nasal blockage apart from colds during the last 12 months?" and "Have these nasal symptoms occurred simultaneously with itching and running eyes?"

Smoking: Smokers reported smoking the year preceding the study and ex-smokers reported having quit smoking

at least 1 year before the study. Non-smokers reported neither smoking nor ex-smoking.

Allergic sensitization: Serum IgE to ImmunoCAP® Phadiatop ≥ 0.35 kU_A/l

Occupational exposure to gas, dust or fumes (GDF): "Have you been substantially exposed to dust, gases or fumes at work?"

Raised on a farm: "Did your family live on a farm during your first 5 years of life?"

Childhood airway infection: "Have you had any severe airway infection or pneumonia before school age, such as whooping cough or croup?"

Childhood daycare: "Did you attend preschool, day care or an orphanage with other children for at least 1 year before school age?"

Analyses

Statistical analyses were performed using IBM SPSS version 20.0.0. The significance level was set to 0.05. Tests for in group differences in proportions were calculated with Fisher's exact test. Tests for trend were computed with a Mantel–Haenszel test where appropriate. Pearson Chi^2 was performed for in group differences in contingency tables larger than two by two. Crude Odds ratios (OR) and 95 % confidence intervals (CI) were calculated for the variables current asthma, current rhinitis and current eczema. Models of multiple logistic regressions were calculated with adjusted ORs and 95 % CIs. Independent covariates were: age divided in three categories, sex, family history of asthma and rhinitis, exposure to gas, dust and fumes at work, raised on a farm, BMI, allergic sensitization, number of siblings and childhood daycare.

Results

Prevalence of asthma, rhinitis, eczema and risk factors

Mean age ± SD of the participants was 50.4 ± 15.4 years with 54 % women. The prevalence of current asthma was 11.8 %, current rhinitis 42.8 % and current eczema 13.5 % (Table 1). Prevalence of asthma ever, eczema ever, rhinitis ever and current rhinitis were all inversely associated with increasing age, as was family history of asthma and rhinitis. Eczema was more common among women and women were also more likely to report a family history of asthma or rhinitis. Usage of rhinitis medications in the last 12 months was more common among younger subjects (P < 0.001). BMI increased by age. Men tended to have a higher BMI and were more exposed to gas, dust or fumes at work compared to women. The prevalence of allergic sensitization was 29.7 %, decreased by age and was more common among men (Table 1).

Figure 3 show the relationship between current asthma, current rhinitis and current eczema. Of all subjects, a

Table 1 Baseline characteristics of the studied population

	Age (years)				Sex			
	18–39	40–59	60–77	P value[1]	Men	Women	P value[2]	Total (95 % CI)
Current asthma	12.3	13.4	9.4	0.216	10.1	13.2	0.122	11.8 (9.9–13.6)
Asthma ever	17.8	16.2	11.8	0.024	14.0	16.2	0.328	15.2 (13.1–17.3)
Current rhinitis	48.8	43.8	36.6	0.001	44.5	41.4	0.314	42.8 (40.0–45.7)
Rhinitis ever	53.7	48.5	39.5	<0.001	50.0	44.4	0.060	47.0 (44.2–50.0)
Current eczema	12.9	17.0	9.7	0.167	11.3	15.4	0.040	13.5 (11.5–15.4)
Eczema ever	49.1	46.8	38.2	0.003	36.5	51.6	<0.001	44.6 (41.8–47.5)
Asthma medication 12 m	11.0	12.5	10.7	0.864	9.8	13.0	0.098	11.5 (9.7–13.4)
Rhinitis medication 12 m	33.7	30.8	19.9	<0.001	27.1	28.9	0.515	28.1 (25.5–30.6)
Allergic sensitization	40.9	31.0	18.6	<0.001	36.0	24.2	<0.001	29.7 (27.0–32.4)
Smoking								
Never smoker	70.6	52.1	49.5	<0.001[3]	58.5	54.5	0.015[3]	56.4 (53.5–59.2)
Ex-smoker	11.0	29.7	37.6		28.3	26.0		27.1 (24.5–29.6)
Current smoker	18.4	18.2	12.9		13.1	19.5		16.5 (14.4–18.7)
Family history								
Asthma	23.8	20.2	15.0	0.004	15.8	22.6	0.004	19.5 (17.2–21.8)
Rhinitis	42.9	35.2	14.0	<0.001	25.3	35.3	<0.001	30.6 (27.9–33.4)
Asthma and rhinitis	16.7	12.6	4.7	<0.001	7.9	14.1	0.002	11.2 (9.4–13.1)
Asthma or rhinitis	49.8	42.1	24.0	<0.001	32.9	43.1	<0.001	38.4 (35.6–41.2)
Body mass index								
Underweight (<20)	10.4	3.0	1.0	<0.001[3]	1.5	7.0	<0.001[3]	4.4 (3.3–5.6)
Normal (20–25)	54.9	34.7	28.0		33.2	42.4		38.1 (35.4–40.9)
Overweight (25–30)	26.1	45.0	52.4		50.7	34.8		42.2 (39.3–45.0)
Obese (>30)	8.6	17.2	18.6		14.6	15.9		15.3 (13.2–17.3)
Occupational GDF	24.3	24.6	25.3	0.750	36.2	14.9	<0.001	24.7 (22.3–27.2)
Metropolitan domicile	70.6	50.9	52.4	<0.001	54.8	58.6	0.214	57.0 (54.0–60.0)
Raised on a farm	7.7	11.8	19.9	<0.001	13.9	12.8	0.604	13.3 (11.4–15.3)

Prevalence (%) and difference (*p* value) by sex and age group. Total prevalence with 95 % confidence intervals (95 % CI)

[1] Test for trend

[2] Fishers exact two sided test

[3] Pearson chi[2] test for in group difference

similar proportion had both current asthma and current rhinitis as current eczema and current rhinitis, 8.5 % and 7.3 % respectively, while 2.6 % had current asthma and current eczema. Only 2.3 % had all three conditions and current rhinitis was the most common single condition (Fig. 3). The relationship between asthma ever, rhinitis ever and eczema ever showed a similar pattern and is available in the appendix (Additional file 1: Figure S1).

Unadjusted risk factors for asthma, rhinitis and eczema

Table 2 shows unadjusted associations for the conditions expressed as odds ratios. Younger age was a significant risk factor for current rhinitis but not for current asthma. For current eczema, only the 40–59 years of age category had an increased risk compared to the oldest. Female sex only increased the risk of current eczema. Family history

of both asthma and rhinitis had the strongest positive association with current asthma (OR 5.4 CI 3.4–8.6) but also significantly increased the risk for current rhinitis and current eczema. Allergic sensitization was a strong risk factor for both current asthma (OR 4.0 CI 2.8–5.4) and current rhinitis (OR 5.8 CI 4.3–7.7) but not significantly so for current eczema (OR 1.4 CI 0.9–1.9). Exposure to gas, dust or fumes at work was a significant risk factor for both current eczema and current asthma (both OR 1.7). Obesity was associated with an increased risk of current rhinitis and current asthma but not of current eczema, while degree of urbanization and metropolitan domicile was not associated with any of the three conditions.

Subjects that grew up on a farm had a lower risk of both current eczema and current rhinitis (OR 0.5

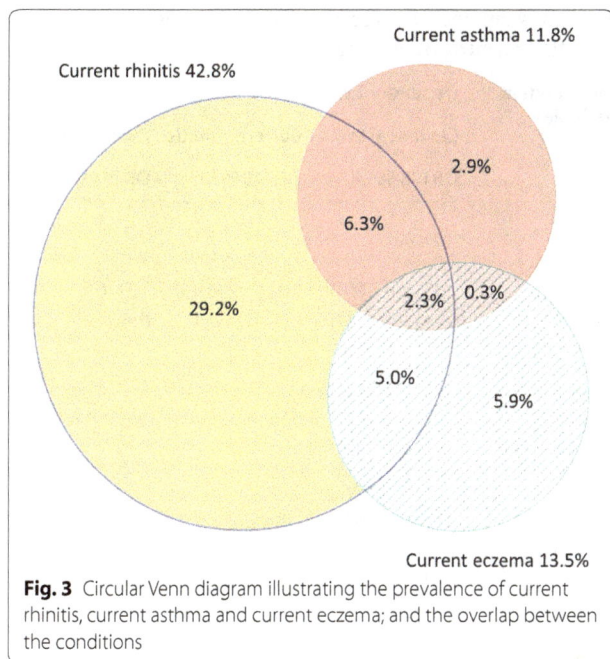

Fig. 3 Circular Venn diagram illustrating the prevalence of current rhinitis, current asthma and current eczema; and the overlap between the conditions

Table 2 Crude odds ratios (OR) and 95 % confidence intervals (CI) for current asthma, current rhinitis and current eczema

Independent variables	Dependent variables		
	Current asthma	Current rhinitis	Current eczema
	OR (95 % CI)	OR (95 % CI)	OR (95 % CI)
Age (years)			
60–77	1	1	1
40–59	1.48 (0.96–2.29)	1.34 (1.02–1.77)	1.91 (1.26–2.90)
18–39	1.34 (0.83–2.17)	1.65 (1.22–2.22)	1.38 (0.86–2.20)
Sex			
Men	1	1	1
Women	1.34 (0.94–1.93)	0.88 (0.70–1.11)	1.45 (1.05–2.00)
Smoking			
Never smoker	1	1	1
Ex-smoker	0.86 (0.56–1.31)	0.96 (0.73–1.26)	1.28 (0.87–1.89)
Current smoker	1.04 (0.64–1.70)	1.15 (0.83–1.59)	1.46 (0.93–2.28)
Family history			
None	1	1	1
Asthma	1.33 (0.58–3.05)	0.72 (0.42–1.25)	1.44 (0.72–2.85)
Rhinitis	1.49 (0.88–2.51)	3.05 (2.20–4.24)	1.32 (0.83–2.08)
Both	5.41 (3.38–8.64)	3.32 (2.23–4.95)	1.82 (1.10–3.00)
Degree of urbanization			
Rural area (<500 inh.)	1	1	1
Village (500–2000 inh.)	0.88 (0.29–2.65)	1.23 (0.65–2.37)	0.97 (0.35–2.74)
Small town (2000–10,000 inh.)	1.28 (0.55–3.00)	1.01 (0.58–1.75)	1.16 (0.51–2.68)
Larger town (>10,000 inh.)	1.29 (0.67–2.48)	1.41 (0.94–2.11)	1.39 (0.74–2.61)
Occupational exposure to GDF			
No	1	1	1
Yes	1.70 (1.16–2.49)	1.10 (0.84–1.44)	1.73 (1.21–2.48)
Metropolitan domicile			
No	1	1	1
Yes	0.86 (0.60–1.23)	1.03 (0.81–1.30)	1.21 (0.86–1.70)
Body mass index			
Normal	1	1	1
Underweight	1.17 (0.47–2.88)	1.34 (0.75–2.38)	1.24 (0.56–2.78)
Overweight	1.07 (0.71–1.63)	0.94 (0.73–1.22)	0.98 (0.67–1.44)
Obese	2.10 (1.29–3.40)	1.79 (1.26–2.53)	1.43 (0.89–2.31)
Allergic sensitization			
No	1	1	1
Yes	4.02 (2.76–5.84)	5.77 (4.34–7.67)	1.35 (0.94–1.93)

CI 0.2–0.9 and 0.5 CI 0.4–0.8) respectively (Table 3). Childhood smoke exposure and maternal smoking in pregnancy was associated with an increased risk of current eczema, while current smoking status was not significantly associated with any of the three conditions. Childhood airway infection increased the risk of asthma. Having one or more sibling increased the risk of current asthma whereas childhood daycare increased the risk of current eczema. Birth weight and educational level were not associated with any of the three conditions (Table 3). Risk factors for eczema ever, asthma ever and rhinitis ever were similar with a few exceptions; most notably allergic sensitization was also positively associated with eczema ever (Additional file 2: Table S1).

Adjusted risk factors for asthma, rhinitis and eczema

Age was not a risk factor for any of the conditions when adjusted odds ratios were calculated in multiple regression models (Table 4). Female sex was a risk factor for both current asthma (OR 1.8 CI 1.2–2.7) and current eczema (OR 1.7 CI 1.2–2.5). Family history of asthma and rhinitis significantly increased the risk of current rhinitis, and the risk of current asthma was of an even greater magnitude, while it was not significantly associated with current eczema. Allergic sensitization was the strongest risk factor for current rhinitis (OR 5.1 CI 3.8–6.9) and the second strongest for current asthma (OR 4.1 2.7–6.3) but was not associated with current eczema.

Exposure to gas dust or fumes as work remained a stable risk factor for current eczema and current asthma after adjustment. Growing up on a farm remained similarly associated with a protective effect on current eczema (OR 0.5 CI 0.3–0.99) and current rhinitis (OR 0.6 CI 0.4–0.96). Obesity was a risk factor for current

Table 3 Crude odds ratios (OR) and 95 % confidence intervals (CI) for current asthma, current rhinitis and current eczema

Independent variables	Dependent variables		
	Current asthma	Current rhinitis	Current eczema
	OR (95 % CI)	OR (95 % CI)	OR (95 % CI)
Raised on a farm			
No	1	1	1
Yes	0.84 (0.48–1.45)	0.54 (0.38–0.78)	0.45 (0.24–0.85)
Number of siblings			
0	1	1	1
1	3.06 (1.29–7.25)	1.37 (0.92–2.06)	0.76 (0.45–1.29)
2 or more	2.76 (1.17–6.49)	1.32 (0.89–1.97)	0.59 (0.35–0.99)
Childhood daycare			
No	1	1	1
Yes	1.14 (0.80–1.63)	1.40 (1.11–1.77)	1.48 (1.06–2.07)
Childhood smoke exposure			
No	1	1	1
Yes	1.05 (0.73–1.50)	0.91 (0.72–1.15)	1.52 (1.06–2.16)
Maternal smoking in pregnancy			
No	1	1	1
Yes	0.70 (0.35–1.37)	1.04 (0.70–1.54)	1.89 (1.13–3.14)
Furry animals in childhood			
Yes	1	1	1
No	1.19 (0.83–1.70)	1.05 (0.75–1.49)	1.24 (0.98–1.57)
Childhood airway infection			
No	1	1	1
Yes	2.35 (1.57–3.51)	0.94 (0.73–1.23)	1.34 (0.92–1.94)
Shared bedroom in childhood			
No	1	1	1
Yes	1.22 (0.85–1.76)	0.91 (0.72–1.16)	0.99 (0.70–1.39)
Birth weight			
3000–4000 g	1	1	1
Less than 2500 g	2.00 (0.89–4.50)	1.22 (0.65–2.31)	0.96 (0.39–2.35)
2500–3000 g	1.41 (0.81–2.45)	1.04 (0.71–1.52)	1.21 (0.73–1.99)
More than 4000 g	0.72 (0.36–1.44)	0.89 (0.60–1.31)	0.54 (0.28–1.04)
Level of education			
Secondary school or less	1	1	1
High school	1.00 (0.59–1.67)	1.10 (0.79–1.54)	1.49 (0.91–2.43)
University	1.09 (0.67–1.78)	1.15 (0.84–1.58)	1.13 (0.69–1.84)

Table 4 Adjusted risk factors for current asthma, current rhinitis and current eczema

Independent variables	Dependent variables		
	Current asthma	Current rhinitis	Current eczema
	OR (95 % CI)	OR (95 % CI)	OR (95 % CI)
Age (years)			
60–77	1	1	1
40–59	1.00 (0.61–1.63)	0.88 (0.64–1.23)	1.51 (0.95–2.38)
18–39	0.73 (0.39–1.37)	0.92 (0.61–1.41)	0.88 (0.49–1.57)
Sex			
Men	1	1	1
Women	1.77 (1.15–2.70)	0.91 (0.69–1.21)	1.71 (1.17–2.51)
Family history			
None	1	1	1
Asthma	1.29 (0.55–3.04)	0.61 (0.34–1.10)	1.45 (0.72–2.94)
Rhinitis	1.16 (0.66–2.03)	2.58 (1.79–3.72)	1.25 (0.77–2.04)
Both	4.33 (2.57–7.30)	2.76 (1.77–4.31)	1.61 (0.94–2.76)
Occupational exposure to GDF			
No	1	1	1
Yes	1.85 (1.20–2.87)	1.03 (0.76–1.41)	2.08 (1.40–3.08)
Raised on a farm			
No	1	1	1
Yes	0.96 (0.52–1.77)	0.64 (0.42–0.96)	0.51 (0.27–0.99)
Body mass index			
Normal	1	1	1
Underweight	0.95 (0.36–2.55)	1.42 (0.74–2.71)	1.00 (0.44–2.30)
Overweight	1.04 (0.65–1.67)	1.04 (0.77–1.41)	1.02 (0.68–1.54)
Obese	1.95 (1.13–3.36)	2.30 (1.53–3.46)	1.34 (0.80–2.24)
Allergic sensitization			
No	1	1	1
Yes	4.11 (2.71–6.25)	5.11 (3.77–6.93)	1.26 (0.85–1.85)
Number of siblings			
0	1	1	1
1	3.09 (1.25–7.63)	1.16 (0.74–1.81)	0.72 (0.42–1.24)
2 or more	2.51 (1.02–6.15)	1.15 (0.74–1.79)	0.55 (0.32–0.94)
Childhood daycare			
No	1	1	1
Yes	0.92 (0.59–1.44)	1.11 (0.81–1.52)	1.40 (0.94–2.10)

Risk is expressed in odds ratios (OR) with 95 % confidence intervals (CI)

asthma and current rhinitis but not for current eczema. Having siblings was a risk factor for current asthma but childhood daycare showed no effect in the multivariate models. Maternal smoking in pregnancy, childhood smoke exposure and smoking status were added separately to the model but were not significantly associated with any of the conditions and did not alter the other risk estimates (not shown). Childhood airway infection was a risk factor for current asthma, OR 2.6 (95 % CI 1.7–4.1) when added separately to the models but did not alter the magnitude of the other risk factors. An additional multivariate analysis was performed to assess the risk factor pattern of subjects with the combination of current asthma and current rhinitis. The results showed that the risk factor pattern in this group was close to identical to subjects with current asthma (data not shown).

Adjusted odds ratios for eczema ever, rhinitis ever and asthma ever showed similar results for most risk factors with some exceptions. Most notably, exposure to gas dust or fumes was not a risk factor for any of the conditions and growing up on a farm had no significant protective on rhinitis ever and eczema ever. However, allergic sensitization was a risk factor for all of eczema ever, rhinitis ever and asthma ever (Additional file 3: Table S2).

Discussion

Main findings

In this population based study of 1172 adults we found that family history of both asthma and allergy was the strongest risk factor for current asthma and it also increased the risk of current rhinitis but not for current eczema after adjustment. Allergic sensitization was an important risk factor for current asthma and current rhinitis, but for not current eczema, and obesity showed the same pattern. Occupational exposure to gas, dust and fumes was positively associated with both current asthma and current eczema but not with current rhinitis. Growing up on a farm had a protective effect on both current eczema and current rhinitis but not on current asthma. Female sex was associated with an increased risk for current asthma and current eczema but not for current rhinitis.

Comparisons to other studies

Comparisons with other studies should be interpreted with caution due to varying definitions of disease. The prevalence of current eczema in our study was 13.5 %. Earlier studies addressing eczema in adults have found similar magnitudes of prevalence with 11.6 % in Sweden [23], 8.1 % in Italy [24], 14.3 % in Denmark [25], 11.5 % in Colombia [26] and 10.2–10.7 % in the United States [16, 17]. Earlier studies of rhinitis have mainly focused on either allergic rhinitis or symptoms of chronic rhinosinusitis. Our definition of current rhinitis included subjects with either allergic rhinitis or other chronic nasal symptoms. The observed prevalence of current rhinitis in our study was 42.8 %. This high prevalence of rhinitis may seem remarkable; however, another recent study in Sweden found that the prevalence of rhinitis symptoms was 51 % [27]. Further, 28.1 % in our study reported use of medication against rhinitis in the last year. Allergic rhinitis has also seen a significant increase in prevalence during the last thirty years [28–30]. The prevalence in Italy has been estimated at 26 % [31] and in southern Finland it has exceeded 40 % [32].

The prevalence of current asthma was 11.8 %. This is of a similar magnitude to Australia where current asthma was present in 8.3–13.1 % depending on age and sex [33], and to Finland where 10.0 % reported asthma and an absolute majority also had symptoms [34]. Other studies have found lower prevalence with 6.6 % in Italy [31] and from 7 to 11 % in Denmark [35, 36]. Noteworthy, all of those studies did not involve older adults and had a more narrow definition of asthma with the Italian study excluding subjects not using medication against asthma.

In agreement with earlier studies [37] we found allergic sensitization to be a strong risk factor for current asthma and current rhinitis. Studies have established that allergic sensitization is a risk factor for childhood eczema [38] but published results among adults are scarce. One pooled study from Europe and the United States [39] found a weak positive association between allergic sensitization and eczema while a stronger association was found in a Danish study [40]. That our study did not show a significant association between eczema and allergic sensitization may reflect a weaker association in adults compared to children, yet also be attributed to the definition of eczema where studies presenting a stronger association often employ traditional definitions of eczema that are affected by asthma and rhinitis [41].

The finding that current asthma and current rhinitis are associated to family histories of those conditions is well known [42, 43], yet the impact of family history of other atopic diseases on adult eczema has not been fully established. One of very few studies on this subject did show an association [44], while in our study no association to either family history of asthma, family history of rhinitis or both was noted. The finding that more women than men suffer from current asthma is in agreement with earlier results [45, 46]. We could also replicate the positive association between female sex and current eczema that previously has been demonstrated in the few studies on this topic [15, 44]. The cause for this gender related difference is largely unknown but different expression of sex hormones may play a role at least for asthma [47].

Occupational exposure to gas, dust or fumes increased the risk for both current asthma and current eczema. In the case of asthma, this has previously been reported [48, 49] and it has been estimated that 14 % of adult onset asthma may be attributed to occupational exposure to GDF [50]. The effect of occupational exposure to GDF on eczema is relatively unknown because most studies on eczema to this date have focused on children. Earlier occupational studies regarding eczema have been limited to contact dermatitis. There are reports highlighting the importance of airborne particles for eczema. A Turkish study [51] found that using wood for house heating was associated with eczema, and in Germany [52] there was an increase in eczema after a large accidental airborne emission of chemicals.

Occupational agents can cause asthma by acting as antigens resulting in an IgE mediated allergic reaction and can also exert a direct effect on the respiratory epithelium with subsequent cell-mediated inflammation that is independent of IgE [53]. The mechanism by how airborne particles from an occupational setting may cause eczema is yet to be elucidated. Recent work with the skin the barrier disruption in focus has gained attention [54] which may explain a plausible mechanism for the role between eczema and occupational exposure.

We found that having lived on a farm during the first 5 years of life was associated with a protective effect on both current rhinitis and current eczema but not current asthma. This contrasts results from studies among children where a protective association with asthma has been shown [55]. The protective effect of farm childhood on rhinitis has been observed in young adults in Finland [56] Germany [57] and Sweden [43]. However, the association between farm living and eczema has not been found in populations of children [58]. In older subjects, a protective effect has been shown in Swedish military conscripts [59]. This is, to our knowledge, the first population based epidemiologic study showing a significant protective association between farm childhood and current eczema in adults.

Our observed positive association between obesity and current asthma has already been established in both cross-sectional [60, 61], case-referent [62] and longitudinal studies [63, 64]. We also found that current rhinitis, but not current eczema was positively associated with obesity. The effect of obesity on rhinitis and eczema is so far infrequently studied with conflicting results. In Japan, a study found that allergic rhinitis was associated with obesity only in conjunction with asthma or wheeze [65]. Another study in Poland found that asthma but not eczema or rhinitis was associated with obesity [66]. However, obese subjects in the United States were more likely to report eczema [15, 67].

Strengths and limitations

There are several methodological strengths and weaknesses with cross-sectional studies of this type. The strength of the randomized population based approach of our study is that it decreases the risk of selection bias. Further, a non-response study comparing the responders to the non-responders of the postal survey has been carried out that did not show any significant differences in terms of diseases or symptoms [19]. While a participation rate of 59 % in the clinical examinations is satisfying and comparable to other international studies, there is a risk of bias with enrichment of subjects with the condition studied. An analysis was performed that compared participants and the non-participants in the clinical examination. No differences were seen in gender, smoking or

reported use of asthma medication. However, prevalence was slightly higher for asthma and rhinitis but we do not believe that this had any major influence on the studied associations. The questions used in the survey were from internationally validated questionnaires and anthropometric parameters were objectively measured. The cross-sectional design of the study has a weakness in its inability to infer causality between the dependent and the independent variables. Associations must thus be regarded with uncertain causality. Recall bias is a concern where for an example individuals with asthma may be better informed of childhood infections compared to healthy subjects. Another weakness is that the questions on eczema may include other non-eczematous types of dermatitis. Validation studies on questions about eczema similar to ours in children have shown good sensitivity but lower specificity [68].

Conclusions

We conclude that there are different risk factor patterns for asthma, rhinitis and eczema among adults. No common risk factor was identified for all three entities. However, some exposures and covariates, such as obesity, farm childhood and allergic sensitization are risk factors for two of the conditions but not all three. Future epidemiological research on the combined determinants of the diseases is needed and especially for rhinitis and eczema.

Abbreviations

BMI: body mass index; CI: confidence interval; GA^{2}LEN: Swedish Global Allergy and Asthma; GDF: occupational exposure to gas, dust or fumes; OR: odds ratio.

Authors' contributions

All authors were involved in the discussions and contributed to writing the manuscript. All authors read and approved the final manuscript.

Author details

[1] Department of Internal Medicine, Krefting Research Centre, Institute of Medicine, Sahlgrenska Academy, University of Gothenburg, Box 424, 405 30 Gothenburg, Sweden. [2] ThermoFisher Scientific, Uppsala, Sweden. [3] Department of Paediatrics, Sahlgrenska Academy, University of Gothenburg, Gothenburg, Sweden. [4] Environmental and Occupational Medicine, The OLIN Unit, Department of Public Health and Clinical Medicine, University of Umeå, Umeå, Sweden.

Competing interests

Dr. Ekerljung reports Grants from AstraZeneca outside the submitted work. Dr. Sjölander is employed by ThermoFisher Scientific, Uppsala, Sweden. Professor Wennergren reports fees for lecturing from Novartis and Meda outside the submitted work. Professor Rönmark reports Grants from AstraZeneca and GSK and personal fees from AstraZeneca outside the submitted work. Professor Lötvall reports Grants from AstraZeneca, GSK, Novartis, Merck and Teva outside the submitted work. Professor Lundbäck reports Grants from AstraZeneca and GSK, personal fees from GSK, AstraZeneca, Novartis and Takeda outside the submitted work. The authors have no other relevant affiliations or financial involvement with any organization or entity with a financial interest in or financial conflict with the subject matter or materials discussed in the manuscript apart from those disclosed.

Funding

The VBG Group Herman Krefting Foundation for Asthma and Allergy Research is gratefully acknowledged for funding of the study. Additional funding was received from the Swedish Heart Lung Foundation, the Swedish Asthma- and Allergy Foundation and the Health Authorities of the Västra Götaland Region.

References

1. Bantz SK, Zhu Z, Zheng T. The atopic march: progression from atopic dermatitis to allergic rhinitis and asthma. J Clin Cell Immunol. 2014;5(2).
2. Spergel JM, Paller AS. Atopic dermatitis and the atopic march. J Allergy Clin Immunol. 2003;112(6 Suppl):S118–27.
3. Gough H, Grabenhenrich L, Reich A, Eckers N, Nitsche O, Schramm D, et al. Allergic multimorbidity of asthma, rhinitis and eczema over 20 years in the German birth cohort MAS. Pediatr Allergy Immunol. 2015;26(5):431–7. doi:10.1111/pai.12410.
4. Illi S, von Mutius E, Lau S, Nickel R, Gruber C, Niggemann B, et al. The natural course of atopic dermatitis from birth to age 7 years and the association with asthma. J Allergy Clin Immunol. 2004;113(5):925–31.
5. Gustafsson D, Sjoberg O, Foucard T. Development of allergies and asthma in infants and young children with atopic dermatitis—a prospective follow-up to 7 years of age. Allergy. 2000;55(3):240–5.
6. Ziyab AH, Raza A, Karmaus W, Tongue N, Zhang H, Matthews S, et al. Trends in eczema in the first 18 years of life: results from the Isle of Wight 1989 birth cohort study. Clin Exp Allergy. 2010;40(12):1776–84. doi:10.1111/j.1365-2222.2010.03633.x.
7. Holgate ST. The epithelium takes centre stage in asthma and atopic dermatitis. Trends Immunol. 2007;28(6):248–51.
8. Bulek K, Swaidani S, Aronica M, Li X. Epithelium: the interplay between innate and Th2 immunity. Immunol Cell Biol. 2010;88(3):257–68.
9. Scott IR, Harding CR. Filaggrin breakdown to water binding compounds during development of the rat stratum corneum is controlled by the water activity of the environment. Dev Biol. 1986;115(1):84–92.
10. Palmer CN, Irvine AD, Terron-Kwiatkowski A, Zhao Y, Liao H, Lee SP, et al. Common loss-of-function variants of the epidermal barrier protein filaggrin are a major predisposing factor for atopic dermatitis. Nat Genet. 2006;38(4):441–6.
11. Rodriguez E, Baurecht H, Herberich E, Wagenpfeil S, Brown SJ, Cordell HJ, et al. Meta-analysis of filaggrin polymorphisms in eczema and asthma: robust risk factors in atopic disease. J Allergy Clin Immunol. 2009;123(6):1361–70 (e7).
12. Weidinger S, O'Sullivan M, Illig T, Baurecht H, Depner M, Rodriguez E, et al. Filaggrin mutations, atopic eczema, hay fever, and asthma in children. J Allergy Clin Immunol. 2008;121(5):1203–9 (e1).
13. Neuman A, Hohmann C, Orsini N, Pershagen G, Eller E, Kjaer HF, et al. Maternal smoking in pregnancy and asthma in preschool children: a pooled analysis of eight birth cohorts. Am J Respir Crit Care Med. 2012;186(10):1037–43. doi:10.1164/rccm.201203-0501OC.
14. Bergmann RL, Edenharter G, Bergmann KE, Lau S, Wahn U. Socioeconomic status is a risk factor for allergy in parents but not in their children. Clin Exp Allergy. 2000;30(12):1740–5.
15. Silverberg JI, Greenland P. Eczema and cardiovascular risk factors in 2 US adult population studies. J Allergy Clin Immunol. 2015;135(3):721–8 (e6).
16. Silverberg JI, Hanifin JM. Adult eczema prevalence and associations with asthma and other health and demographic factors: a US population-based study. J Allergy Clin Immunol. 2013;132(5):1132–8.
17. Hanifin JM, Reed ML. A population-based survey of eczema prevalence in the United States. Dermatitis. 2007;18(2):82–91.
18. Lotvall J, Ekerljung L, Ronmark EP, Wennergren G, Linden A, Ronmark E, et al. West Sweden Asthma Study: prevalence trends over the last 18 years argues no recent increase in asthma. Respir Res. 2009;10:94.
19. Ronmark EP, Ekerljung L, Lotvall J, Toren K, Ronmark E, Lundback B. Large scale questionnaire survey on respiratory health in Sweden: effects of late- and non-response. Respir Med. 2009;103(12):1807–15.
20. Lundback B, Nystrom L, Rosenhall L, Stjernberg N. Obstructive lung disease in northern Sweden: respiratory symptoms assessed in a postal survey. Eur Respir J. 1991;4(3):257–66.
21. Pallasaho P, Lundback B, Laspa SL, Jonsson E, Kotaniemi J, Sovijarvi AR, et al. Increasing prevalence of asthma but not of chronic bronchitis in Finland? Report from the FinEsS-Helsinki Study. Respir Med. 1999;93(11):798–809.
22. Bousquet J, Burney PG, Zuberbier T, Cauwenberge PV, Akdis CA, Bindslev-Jensen C, et al. GA2LEN (Global Allergy and Asthma European Network) addresses the allergy and asthma 'epidemic'. Allergy. 2009;64(7):969–77.
23. Lindberg M, Isacson D, Bingefors K. Self-reported skin diseases, quality of life and medication use: a nationwide pharmaco-epidemiological survey in Sweden. Acta Derm Venereol. 2014;94(2):188–91.
24. Pesce G, Marcon A, Carosso A, Antonicelli L, Cazzoletti L, Ferrari M, et al. Adult eczema in Italy: prevalence and associations with environmental factors. J Eur Acad Dermatol Venereol. 2015;29(6):1180–7.
25. Vinding GR, Zarchi K, Ibler KS, Miller IM, Ellervik C, Jemec GB. Is adult atopic eczema more common than we think?—a population-based study in Danish adults. Acta Derm Venereol. 2014;94(4):480–2.
26. Dennis RJ, Caraballo L, Garcia E, Rojas MX, Rondon MA, Perez A, et al. Prevalence of asthma and other allergic conditions in Colombia 2009–2010: a cross-sectional study. BMC Pulm Med. 2012;12:17.
27. Wang J, Engvall K, Smedje G, Norback D. Rhinitis, asthma and respiratory infections among adults in relation to the home environment in multi-family buildings in Sweden. PLoS ONE. 2014;9(8):e105125.
28. Upton MN, McConnachie A, McSharry C, Hart CL, Smith GD, Gillis CR, et al. Intergenerational 20 year trends in the prevalence of asthma and hay fever in adults: the Midspan family study surveys of parents and offspring. BMJ. 2000;321(7253):88–92.
29. Bjerg A, Ekerljung L, Middelveld R, Dahlen SE, Forsberg B, Franklin K, et al. Increased prevalence of symptoms of rhinitis but not of asthma between 1990 and 2008 in Swedish adults: comparisons of the ECRHS and GA(2)LEN surveys. PLoS ONE. 2011;6(2):e16082.
30. Linneberg A, Jorgensen T, Nielsen NH, Madsen F, Frolund L, Dirksen A. The prevalence of skin-test-positive allergic rhinitis in Danish adults: two cross-sectional surveys 8 years apart. The Copenhagen Allergy Study. Allergy. 2000;55(8):767–72.
31. de Marco R, Cappa V, Accordini S, Rava M, Antonicelli L, Bortolami O, et al. Trends in the prevalence of asthma and allergic rhinitis in Italy between 1991 and 2010. Eur Respir J. 2012;39(4):883–92.
32. Pallasaho P, Juusela M, Lindqvist A, Sovijarvi A, Lundback B, Ronmark E. Allergic rhinoconjunctivitis doubles the risk for incident asthma—results from a population study in Helsinki, Finland. Respir Med. 2011;105(10):1449–56.
33. James AL, Knuiman MW, Divitini ML, Hui J, Hunter M, Palmer LJ, et al. Changes in the prevalence of asthma in adults since 1966: the Busselton health study. Eur Respir J. 2010;35(2):273–8.
34. Kainu A, Pallasaho P, Piirila P, Lindqvist A, Sovijarvi A, Pietinalho A. Increase in prevalence of physician-diagnosed asthma in Helsinki during the Finnish Asthma Programme: improved recognition of asthma in primary care? A cross-sectional cohort study. Prim Care Respir J. 2013;22(1):64–71.
35. Browatzki A, Ulrik CS, Lange P. Prevalence and severity of self-reported asthma in young adults, 1976–2004. Eur Respir J. 2009;34(5):1046–51.
36. Thuesen BH, Heede NG, Tang L, Skaaby T, Thyssen JP, Friedrich N, et al. No association between vitamin D and atopy, asthma, lung function or atopic dermatitis: a prospective study in adults. Allergy. 2015;70(11):1501–4.
37. Warm K, Hedman L, Lindberg A, Lotvall J, Lundback B, Ronmark E. Allergic sensitization is age-dependently associated with rhinitis, but less so with asthma. J Allergy Clin Immunol. 2015. doi:10.1016/j.jaci.2015.06.015.
38. Wuthrich B. Clinical aspects, epidemiology, and prognosis of atopic

dermatitis. Ann Allergy Asthma Immunol. 1999;83(5):464–70.

39. Harrop J, Chinn S, Verlato G, Olivieri M, Norback D, Wjst M, et al. Eczema, atopy and allergen exposure in adults: a population-based study. Clin Exp Allergy. 2007;37(4):526–35.

40. Thyssen JP, Tang L, Husemoen LL, Stender S, Szecsi PB, Menne T, et al. Filaggrin gene mutations are not associated with food and aeroallergen sensitization without concomitant atopic dermatitis in adults. J Allergy Clin Immunol. 2015;135(5):1375–8 **(e1)**.

41. Williams HC, Burney PG, Hay RJ, Archer CB, Shipley MJ, Hunter JJ, et al. The U.K. Working Party's Diagnostic Criteria for Atopic Dermatitis. I. Derivation of a minimum set of discriminators for atopic dermatitis. Br J Dermatol. 1994;131(3):383–96.

42. Backman H, Hedman L, Jansson SA, Lindberg A, Lundback B, Ronmark E. Prevalence trends in respiratory symptoms and asthma in relation to smoking—two cross-sectional studies ten years apart among adults in northern Sweden. World Allergy Organ J. 2014;7(1):1.

43. Eriksson J, Ekerljung L, Lotvall J, Pullerits T, Wennergren G, Ronmark E, et al. Growing up on a farm leads to lifelong protection against allergic rhinitis. Allergy. 2010;65(11):1397–403.

44. Sybilski AJ, Raciborski F, Lipiec A, Tomaszewska A, Lusawa A, Samel-Kowalik P, et al. Epidemiology of atopic dermatitis in Poland according to the Epidemiology of Allergic Disorders in Poland (ECAP) study. J Dermatol. 2015;42(2):140–7.

45. Hedlund U, Eriksson K, Ronmark E. Socio-economic status is related to incidence of asthma and respiratory symptoms in adults. Eur Respir J. 2006;28(2):303–10.

46. Schatz M, Camargo CA Jr. The relationship of sex to asthma prevalence, health care utilization, and medications in a large managed care organization. Ann Allergy Asthma Immunol. 2003;91(6):553–8.

47. Melgert BN, Ray A, Hylkema MN, Timens W, Postma DS. Are there reasons why adult asthma is more common in females? Curr Allergy Asthma Rep. 2007;7(2):143–50.

48. Xu X, Christiani DC. Occupational exposures and physician-diagnosed asthma. Chest. 1993;104(5):1364–70.

49. Halldin CN, Doney BC, Hnizdo E. Changes in prevalence of chronic obstructive pulmonary disease and asthma in the US population and associated risk factors. Chron Respir Dis. 2015;12(1):47–60.

50. Eagan TM, Gulsvik A, Eide GE, Bakke PS. Occupational airborne exposure and the incidence of respiratory symptoms and asthma. Am J Respir Crit Care Med. 2002;166(7):933–8.

51. Talay F, Kurt B, Tug T, Kurt OK, Goksugur N, Yasar Z. The prevalence of asthma and allergic diseases among adults 30–49 years of age in Bolu, Western Black Sea Region of Turkey. Clin Ter. 2014;165(1):e59–63.

52. Traupe H, Menge G, Kandt I, Karmaus W. Higher frequency of atopic dermatitis and decrease in viral warts among children exposed to chemicals liberated in a chemical accident in Frankfurt, Germany. Dermatology. 1997;195(2):112–8.

53. Maestrelli P, Boschetto P, Fabbri LM, Mapp CE. Mechanisms of occupational asthma. J Allergy Clin Immunol. 2009;123(3):531–42 **(quiz 43-4)**.

54. De Benedetto A, Kubo A, Beck LA. Skin barrier disruption: a requirement for allergen sensitization? J Invest Dermatol. 2012;132(3 Pt 2):949–63.

55. Riedler J, Eder W, Oberfeld G, Schreuer M. Austrian children living on a farm have less hay fever, asthma and allergic sensitization. Clin Exp Allergy. 2000;30(2):194–200.

56. Kilpelainen M, Terho EO, Helenius H, Koskenvuo M. Farm environment in childhood prevents the development of allergies. Clin Exp Allergy. 2000;30(2):201–8.

57. Radon K, Schulze A, Nowak D. Inverse association between farm animal contact and respiratory allergies in adulthood: protection, underreporting or selection? Allergy. 2006;61(4):443–6.

58. Flohr C, Pascoe D, Williams HC. Atopic dermatitis and the 'hygiene hypothesis': Too clean to be true? Br J Dermatol. 2005;152(2):202–16.

59. Braback L, Hjern A, Rasmussen F. Trends in asthma, allergic rhinitis and eczema among Swedish conscripts from farming and non-farming environments. A nationwide study over three decades. Clin Exp Allergy. 2004;34(1):38–43.

60. Luder E, Ehrlich RI, Lou WY, Melnik TA, Kattan M. Body mass index and the risk of asthma in adults. Respir Med. 2004;98(1):29–37.

61. Schachter LM, Salome CM, Peat JK, Woolcock AJ. Obesity is a risk for asthma and wheeze but not airway hyperresponsiveness. Thorax. 2001;56(1):4–8.

62. Ronmark E, Andersson C, Nystrom L, Forsberg B, Jarvholm B, Lundback B. Obesity increases the risk of incident asthma among adults. Eur Respir J. 2005;25(2):282–8.

63. Guerra S, Sherrill DL, Bobadilla A, Martinez FD, Barbee RA. The relation of body mass index to asthma, chronic bronchitis, and emphysema. Chest. 2002;122(4):1256–63.

64. Huovinen E, Kaprio J, Koskenvuo M. Factors associated to lifestyle and risk of adult onset asthma. Respir Med. 2003;97(3):273–80.

65. Konno S, Hizawa N, Fukutomi Y, Taniguchi M, Kawagishi Y, Okada C, et al. The prevalence of rhinitis and its association with smoking and obesity in a nationwide survey of Japanese adults. Allergy. 2012;67(5):653–60.

66. Sybilski AJ, Raciborski F, Lipiec A, Tomaszewska A, Lusawa A, Furmanczyk K, et al. Obesity—a risk factor for asthma, but not for atopic dermatitis, allergic rhinitis and sensitization. Public Health Nutr. 2015;18(3):530–6.

67. Silverberg JI, Silverberg NB, Lee-Wong M. Association between atopic dermatitis and obesity in adulthood. Br J Dermatol. 2012;166(3):498–504.

68. Flohr C, Weinmayr G, Weiland SK, Addo-Yobo E, Annesi-Maesano I, Bjorksten B, et al. How well do questionnaires perform compared with physical examination in detecting flexural eczema? Findings from the International Study of Asthma and Allergies in Childhood (ISAAC) Phase Two. Br J Dermatol. 2009;161(4):846–53.

MASK 2017: ARIA digitally-enabled, integrated, person-centred care for rhinitis and asthma multimorbidity using real-world-evidence

J. Bousquet[1,2,3]*, S. Arnavielhe[4], A. Bedbrook[1], M. Bewick[5], D. Laune[4], E. Mathieu-Dupas[4], R. Murray[6], G. L. Onorato[1], J. L. Pépin[7,8], R. Picard[9], F. Portejoie[1], E. Costa[10], J. Fonseca[11,12], O. Lourenço[13], M. Morais-Almeida[14], A. Todo-Bom[15], A. A. Cruz[16,17], J. da Silva[18], F. S. Serpa[19], M. Illario[20], E. Menditto[21], L. Cecchi[22], R. Monti[23], L. Napoli[24], M. T. Ventura[25], G. De Feo[26], D. Larenas-Linnemann[27], M. Fuentes Perez[28], Y. R. Huerta Villabolos[28], D. Rivero-Yeverino[29], E. Rodriguez-Zagal[30], F. Amat[31,32], I. Annesi-Maesano[33], I. Bosse[34], P. Demoly[35], P. Devillier[36], J. F. Fontaine[37], J. Just[31,32], T. P. Kuna[38], B. Samolinski[39], A. Valiulis[40,41], R. Emuzyte[42], V. Kvedariene[43], D. Ryan[44,45], A. Sheikh[46], P. Schmidt-Grendelmeier[47], L. Klimek[48,49], O. Pfaar[48,49], K. C. Bergmann[50,51], R. Mösges[52,53], T. Zuberbier[50,51], R. E. Roller-Wirnsberger[54], P. Tomazic[55], W. J. Fokkens[56], N. H. Chavannes[57], S. Reitsma[56], J. M. Anto[58,59,60,61], V. Cardona[62], T. Dedeu[63,64], J. Mullol[65,66], T. Haahtela[67], J. Salimäki[68], S. Toppila-Salmi[67], E. Valovirta[69,70], B. Gemicioğlu[71], A. Yorgancioglu[72,73], N. Papadopoulos[74,75], E. P. Prokopakis[76], S. Bosnic-Anticevich[77], R. O'Hehir[78,79], J. C. Ivancevich[80], H. Neffen[81], E. Zernotti[82], I. Kull[83], E. Melen[84,85], M. Wickman[86], C. Bachert[87], P. Hellings[3,88,89], S. Palkonen[90], C. Bindslev-Jensen[91], E. Eller[91], S. Waserman[92], M. Sova[93], G. De Vries[94], M. van Eerd[94], I. Agache[95], T. Casale[96], M. Dykewickz[97], R. N. Naclerio[98], Y. Okamoto[99], D. V. Wallace[100] and MASK study group

Abstract

mHealth, such as apps running on consumer smart devices is becoming increasingly popular and has the potential to profoundly affect healthcare and health outcomes. However, it may be disruptive and results achieved are not always reaching the goals. Allergic Rhinitis and its Impact on Asthma (ARIA) has evolved from a guideline using the best evidence-based approach to care pathways suited to real-life using mobile technology in allergic rhinitis (AR) and asthma multimorbidity. Patients largely use over-the-counter medications dispensed in pharmacies. Shared decision making centered around the patient and based on self-management should be the norm. Mobile Airways Sentinel networK (MASK), the Phase 3 ARIA initiative, is based on the freely available MASK app (*the Allergy Diary*, Android and iOS platforms). MASK is available in 16 languages and deployed in 23 countries. The present paper provides an overview of the methods used in MASK and the key results obtained to date. These include a novel phenotypic characterization of the patients, confirmation of the impact of allergic rhinitis on work productivity and treatment patterns in real life. Most patients appear to self-medicate, are often non-adherent and do not follow guidelines. Moreover, *the Allergy Diary* is able to distinguish between AR medications. The potential usefulness of MASK will be further explored by POLLAR (Impact of Air Pollution on Asthma and Rhinitis), a new Horizon 2020 project using the *Allergy Diary*.

Keywords: App, ARIA, Asthma, Care pathways, MASK, mHealth, Rhinitis

*Correspondence: jean.bousquet@orange.fr
[1] MACVIA-France, Fondation Partenariale FMC VIA-LR, CHRU Arnaud de Villeneuve, 371 Avenue du Doyen Gaston Giraud, Montpellier, France
Full list of author information is available at the end of the article

Background

Allergic rhinitis (AR) is the most common chronic disease worldwide. Evidence-based guidelines have improved knowledge on rhinitis and made a significant impact on AR management. However, many patients remain inadequately controlled and the costs for society are enormous, in particular due to the major impact of AR on school and work productivity [1, 2]. Unmet needs have identified clearly many gaps. These include (1) sub-optimal rhinitis and asthma control due to medical, cultural and social barriers [3, 4], (2) poor understanding of endotypes [5], better characterization of phenotypes and multimorbidities [6], better understanding of gender differences [7], (3) assessment of sentinel networks in care pathways for allergen and pollutants exposures, using symptom variation [8], (4) lack of stratification of patients for optimized care pathways [9] and (5) lack of multidisciplinary teams within integrated care pathways, endorsing innovation in real life clinical trials [8] and encouraging patient empowerment [10, 11].

Mobile health (mHealth) is the use of information and communication technology (ICT) for health services and information transfer [12]. mHealth, including apps running on consumer smart devices (i.e., smartphones and tablets), is becoming increasingly popular and has the potential to profoundly impact on healthcare [13]. Novel app-based collaborative systems can have an important role in gathering information quickly and improving coverage and accessibility of prevention and treatment [14]. Implementing mHealth innovations may also have disruptive consequences [15], so it is important to test applicability in each individual situation [16]. A rapid growth of the health apps market has been seen with an estimated 325,000 health apps available in 2017 for most fields of medicine [17]. Benefits and drawbacks have been estimated for a number of disease [18]. The application of mHealth solutions can support the provision of high quality care to patients with AR or asthma, to the satisfaction of both patients and health care professionals, with a reduction in both health care utilization and costs [19]. Appropriately identifying and representing stakeholders' interests and viewpoints in evaluations of mHealth is a critical part of ensuring continued progress and innovation [20]. Patient, caregiver and clinician evaluations and recommendations play an important role in the development of asthma mHealth tools to support the provision of asthma management [21]. Smart devices and internet-based applications are already used in rhinitis and asthma and may help to address some unmet needs [22]. However, these new tools need to be tested and evaluated for acceptability, usability and cost-effectiveness.

Allergic Rhinitis and its Impact on Asthma (ARIA) has evolved from an evidence-based guideline using the best evidence based approach [1, 23–25] to care pathways using mobile technology in AR and asthma multimorbidity [26]. ARIA appears to be close to the patient's needs but real-life data suggest that few patients follow guideline recommendations and that they often self-medicate. Moreover, patients frequently using OTC medications dispensed in pharmacies [27]. Shared decision making (SDM) centered around the patient for self-management should be used more often.

Mobile Airways Sentinel networK (MASK), the Phase 3 ARIA initiative, has been initiated to reduce the global burden of rhinitis and asthma multimorbidity, giving the patient and the health care professional simple tools to better prevent and manage respiratory allergic diseases. More specifically, MASK is focusing on (1) understanding the disease mechanisms and the effects of air pollution in allergic diseases and asthma, (2) better appraising the burden incurred by medical needs and indirect costs, (3) the implementation of multi-sectoral care pathways integrating self-care, air pollution and patient's literacy, using emerging technologies with real world data using the AIRWAYS ICPs algorithm [28], (4) proposing individualized and predictive medicine in rhinitis and asthma multimorbidity, (5) proposing the basis for a sentinel network at the global level for pollution and allergy and (6) assessing the societal implications of exposure to air pollution and allergens and its consequences on health inequalities globally.

The freely available MASK app (*the Allergy Diary*, Android and iOS) [26] is combined with an inter-operable tablet for physicians and other health care professionals (HCPs [29]), using the same extremely simple colloquial language to manage AR (Visual Analogue Scale: VAS) [30, 31]. It is being combined with data on allergen and pollution exposure (POLLAR).

MASK will be scaled up using the EU EIP on AHA strategy [32]. Phase 4 is starting in 2018 and will focus on "change management". MASK is supported by several EU grants and is a WHO GARD (Global Alliance against Chronic Respiratory Diseases) research demonstration project (Table 1).

Methods
Users

The *Allergy Diary* is used by people who searched the internet, Apple App store, Google Play or in any other way. The pages of the App are on the Euforea-ARIA website (www.euforea.eu/about-us/aria.html). A few users were clinic patients to whom the app was recommended by their physicians. Users were not requested to complete the diary for a minimum number of days. However, due to anonymization of data, no specific information on the route of access to the app could be gathered [33, 34].

Table 1 European Union and World Health Organization links of ARIA and MASK

	Date		WHO	EU
ARIA	1999	Workshop	WHO HQ	
	2003–2013	CC rhinitis and asthma	Montpellier	
	2012–	GARD demonstration project	WHO HQ	
	2004–2010	GA2LEN		FP6
	2011–2015	MeDALL		FP7
MASK	2014–	MACVIA-LR		DG Santé-CNECT
	2014–	GARD demonstration project	WHO HQ	
	2014–	EIP on AHA B3		DG Santé-CNECT
	2015–2016	SPAL		Structural and development funds
	2015–2017	Sunfrail		
	2017–	Twinning		DG Santé-CNECT
	2018–	POLLAR		EIT Health

The first question of the App is "I have allergic rhinitis": Yes/No. We tested the sensitivity and specificity of this question [33]. 93.4% users with a positive answer had nasal symptoms versus 12.1% of users with a negative answer. In the first two versions of the App, allergy was not considered in the user's questionnaire and AR cannot be differentiated from chronic rhinosinusitis. It is now included in the third version of the App (June 2018) and we will be able to answer more appropriately to this question in the next study. The results of the pilot study were confirmed in over 9000 users.

Settings
MASK is available in 23 countries and 16 languages. To date (01-09-2018) the app has been used by over 24,000 people.

Ethics and privacy of data
The Allergy Diary is CE1 registered. The terms of use were translated into all languages and customized by lawyers according to the legislation of each country, allowing the use of the results for research and commercial purposes. The example of the UK terms of use have been provided in a previous paper [33].

Geolocation
EU data protection rules have changed since the implementation of the General Data Protection Regulation (Art. 4 para. 1 no. 1 GDPR) [35]. Data anonymization is a method of sanitization for privacy. Anonymization renders personal data "in such a manner that the data subject is not or no longer identifiable" [36]. The European Commission's Article 29 Working Party (WP29) stated already in 2014 with regards to the Directive 95/46/EC [37] that geolocation information is not only personal data but also to be considered as an identifier itself [38, 39]. Processing personal data by means of an app, like e.g. App Diary, besides Directive 95/46/EC [37] also Directive 2002/58/EC [40] as amended by Directive 2009/136/EC [41] applies.

Geolocation was studied for all people who used the Allergy Diary App from December 2015 to November 2017 and who reported medical outcomes. In contradistinction to noise addition (randomization), k-anonymity [42, 43] is an acceptable method for the anonymization of MASK data (generalization) [44] and results can be used for other databases.

Privacy assessment impact
Privacy impact assessments (PIAs), also known as data protection impact assessments (DPIAs) in EU law, is required by GDPR (Article 35 Working Party (WP35). PIA is a systematic process to assess privacy risks to individuals in the collection, use, and disclosure of their personal data. The GDPR introduced PIAs to identify high risks to the privacy rights of individuals when processing their personal data. The assessment shall contain at least:

1. a systematic description of the envisaged processing operations and the purposes of the processing, including, where applicable, the legitimate interest pursued by the controller;
2. an assessment of the necessity and proportionality of the processing operations in relation to the purposes;
3. an assessment of the risks to the rights and freedoms of data subjects and
4. the measures envisaged to address the risks, including safeguards, security measures and mechanisms to ensure the protection of personal data and to dem-

onstrate compliance with this Regulation taking into account the rights and legitimate interests of data subjects and other persons concerned.

When these risks are identified, the GDPR expects that an organization formulates measures to address these risks. Those measures may take the form of technical controls such as encryption or anonymization of data.

The PIA analysis is a self-declarative analysis. In France, the local GDPR representative (*Commission Informatique et Liberté*, CNIL) has provided a software to guide the reflexion around security of personal data and the exposure risks in case of security fails. This software has been used to assess all the risks to be considered through the app uses. The conclusion was that is "negligeable".

The field is moving very fast. In France, June, 10 2018, the modified law "LIL" (*Loi Informatique et Liberté, 2018-493*, https://www.cnil.fr/fr/loi-78-17-du-6-janvier-1978-modifiee) was enacted with a special focus on health-related personal data. Even if the articulation of GDPR and LIL is still unclear, we can anticipate that the app use will remain risk free.

Allergy Diary

The app collects information on AR and asthma symptoms experienced (nasal and ocular) and on disease type (intermittent/persistent) [33] (Table 3). Anonymized and geolocalized users assess daily how symptoms impact their control and AR treatment using the touchscreen functionality on their smart phone to click on five consecutive VAS (i.e. general, nasal and ocular symptoms, asthma and work) (Table 2; Fig. 1). Users input their daily medications using a scroll list that contains all country-specific OTC and prescribed medications available (Fig. 2). The list populated using IMS data and revised by country experts is continuously revised by country experts.

There is a high degree of correlation between these VAS measurements. The example of VAS global measured and VAS nose is presented in Fig. 2.

Outcomes

Five VAS measurements [VAS-global measured, VAS-nose, VAS-eye, VAS-asthma and VAS-work (Table 4)] and a calculated VAS-global score (VAS-nasal + VAS-ocular divided by 2) were assessed [34]. VAS levels range from zero (not at all bothersome) to 100 (very bothersome). Independency of VAS questions was previously confirmed using the Bland and Altman regression analysis [34, 45].

Table 2 Questions on symptoms and impact of symptoms (from Bousquet et al. [33])

Q1: I have rhinitis: Yes/No	Q4: How they affect me: My symptoms (tick)
Q2: I have asthma: Yes/No	❑ Affect my sleep
	❑ Restrict my daily activities
Q3: My symptoms (tick)	❑ Restrict my participation in school or work
	❑ Are troublesome
❑ Runny nose	
❑ Itchy nose	
❑ Sneezing	
❑ Congestion (blocked nose)	
❑ Itchy eyes	
❑ Red eyes	
❑ Watery eyes	

Transfer of personal data from the App to a print

Patients cannot give access to their electronic data to a HCP due to privacy policies. However, they can easily print the daily control of their disease and the medications that they filled in the *Allergy Diary* as follows (Fig. 3).

Additional questionnaires

MASK also includes EQ-5D (EuroQuol) [46–48], Work Productivity and Activity Impairment Allergic Specific (WPAI-AS) [49] and Control of AR and Asthma Test (CARAT) [50–53]. The Epworth Sleepiness Questionnaire [54, 55] is included (June 2018).

Medications

A scroll list is available for all OTC and prescribed medications of the 23 countries. The International Non-proprietary Names classification was used for drug nomenclature [56]. 85 INNs and 505 medications were identified (Fig. 1).

Adherence to treatment

Globally, non-adherence to medications is a major obstacle to the effective delivery of health care. Many mobile phone apps are available to support people to take their medications and to improve medication adherence [57, 58]. However, a recent meta-analysis found that the majority did not have many of the desirable features and were of low quality [57]. However, it is unknown how people use apps, what is considered adherent or non-adherent in terms of app usage, or whether adherence with an app in anyway reflects adherence with medication or control.

In MASK, we did not use adherence questionnaires but first attempted to assess short-term adherence and then to address the long-term issues. [59].

Digitalized ARIA symptom-medication score

Symptom-medication scores are needed to assess the control of allergic diseases. They are currently being

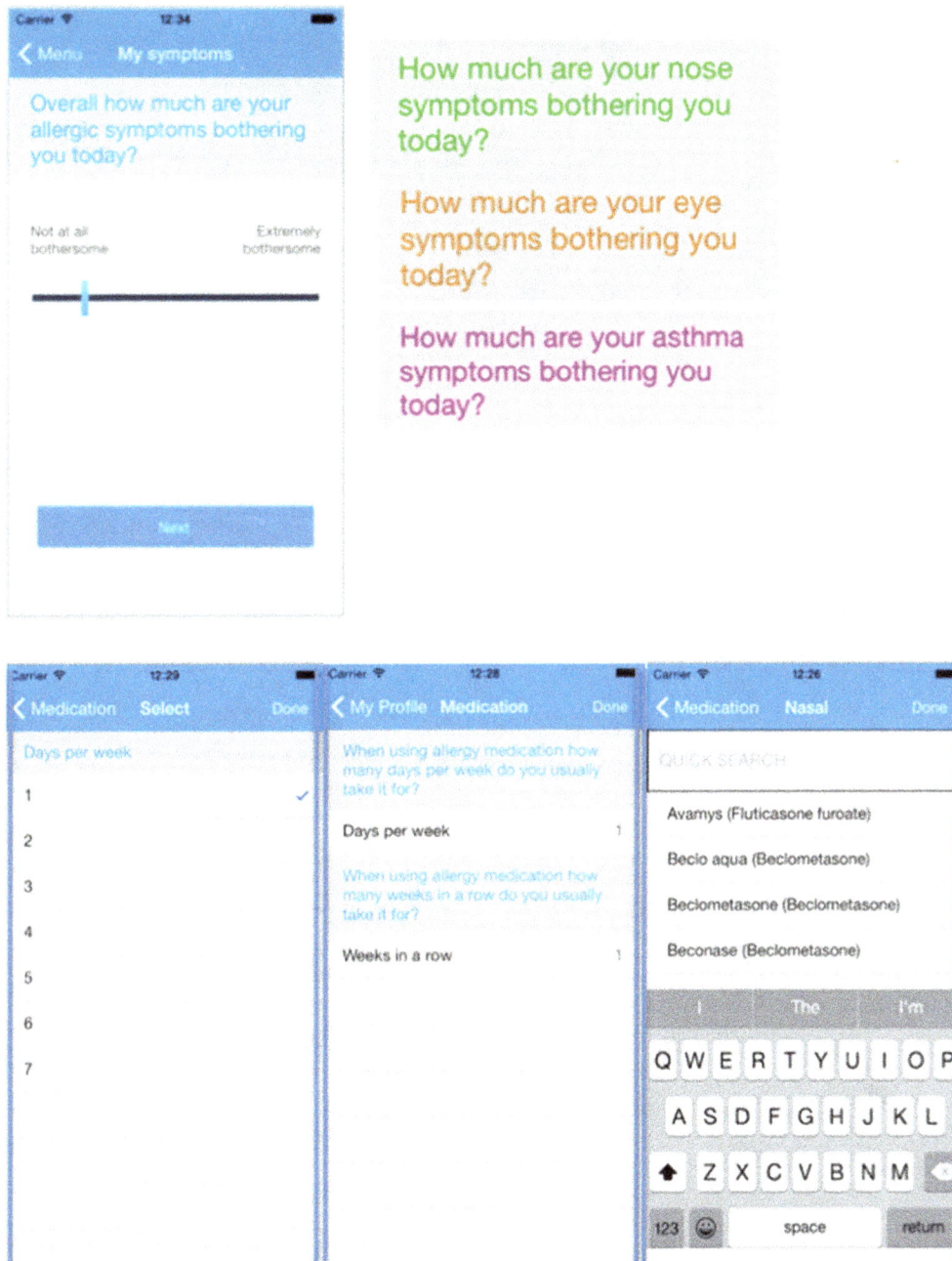

Fig. 1 *Allergy Diary* screens relating to Visual Analogue Scale and medications (from Bousquet et al. [26])

developed for MASK and are being compared with existing ones [60].

MASK algorithm and clinical decision support system

Clinical decision support systems (CDSS) are software algorithms that advise health care providers on the diagnosis and management of patients based on the interaction of patient data and medical information, such as prescribed drugs. CDSS should be based on the best evidence and algorithms to aid patients and health care professionals to jointly determine the treatment and its step-up or step-down strategy for an optimal disease control.

The selection of pharmacotherapy for AR patients depends on several factors, including age, prominent symptoms, symptom severity, AR control, patient preferences and cost. Allergen exposure, pollution and resulting symptoms vary, needing treatment

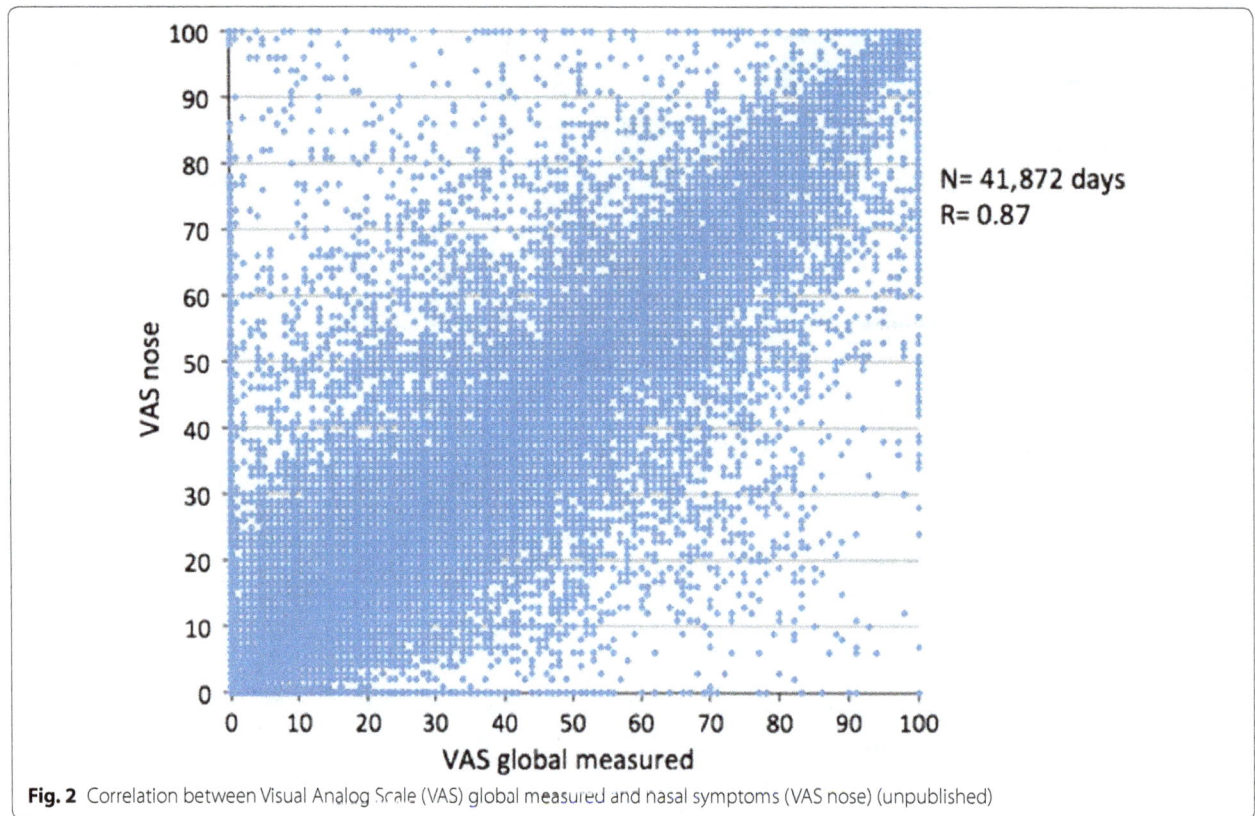

Fig. 2 Correlation between Visual Analog Scale (VAS) global measured and nasal symptoms (VAS nose) (unpublished)

adjustment. In AR, The MASK CDSS is incorporated into an interoperable tablet [29] for HCPs (*ARIA Allergy Diary Companion*) [10, 26]. This is based on an algorithm to aid clinicians to select pharmacotherapy for AR patients and to stratify their disease severity [26] (Fig. 4). It uses a simple step-up/step-down individualized approach to AR pharmacotherapy and may hold the potential for optimal control of symptoms, while minimizing side-effects and costs. However, its use varies depending on the availability of medications in the different countries and on resources. The algorithm is now digitalized and available in English (Fig. 5).

MASK follows the CHRODIS criteria of "Good Practice"

The European Commission is co-funding a large collaborative project named JA-CHRODIS in the context of the 2nd EU Health Programme 2008–2013 [61]. JA-CHRODIS has developed a check-list of 27 items for the evaluation of Good Practices (GP) (http://chrodis.eu/our-work/04-knowledge-platform/). According to the JA-CHRODIS, a Good Practice has been proven to work well and produce good results, and is therefore recommended as a model to be scaled up. The JA-CHRODIS criteria are grouped into nine categories:

- Equity.
- Practice.
- Ethical considerations.
- Evaluation.
- Empowerment and participation.
- Target population.
- Sustainability.
- Governance.
- Scalability

As part of SUNFRAIL, MASK tested the 27 item criteria of CHRODIS and was found to be an example of Good Practice [62].

Pilot study of mobile phone technology in AR

A pilot study in 3260 users found that *Allergy Diary* users were able to properly provide baseline simple phenotypic characteristics. Troublesome symptoms were found mainly in the users with the largest number of symptoms. Around 50% of users with troublesome rhinitis and/or ocular symptoms suffered work impairment. Sleep was impaired by troublesome symptoms and nasal obstruction (Fig. 6). results suggest novel concepts and research questions in AR that may not be identified using classical methods [33].

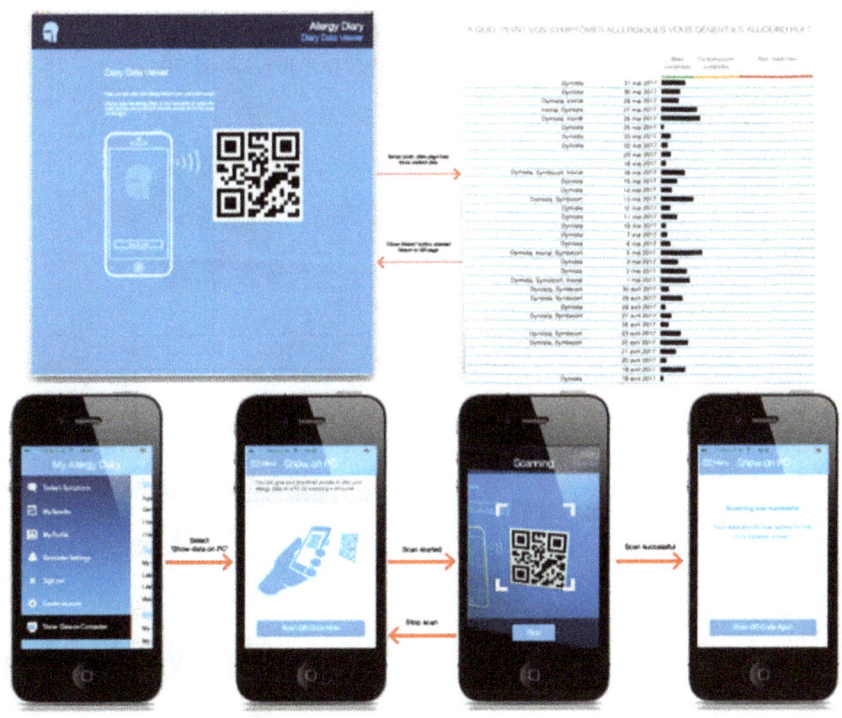

1- Open the Allergy Diary app and choose "Show Data on Computer" in the main menu

2- Go to www.macvia-aria-allergy-diary.com/data on your PC/Laptop (enter this URL in the address bar of the browser from your PC/Laptop)

3- Scan the QR code with the Allergy Diary app

4- The screen with your personal data can be seen

5- And you can also print these data (see figure below)

Fig. 3 Transfer of patient information on a computer and printed information (from Bousquet et al. [46])

Validation of the MASK Visual Analogue Scale on cell phones

VAS included in the *Allergy Diary* was found to be a validated tool to assess control in AR patients following COSMIN guidelines [63] in 1225 users and 14,612 days: internal consistency (Cronbach's α-coefficient > 0.84 and test–retest > 0.7), reliability (intra-class correlation coefficients), sensitivity and acceptability [64]. In addition, e-VAS had a good reproducibility when users (n = 521) answered the e-VAS twice in less than 3 h.

Transfer of innovation of AR and asthma multimorbidity in the elderly: Reference Site Twinning (EIP on AHA)

The EIP on AHA includes 74 Reference Sites. The aim of this TWINNING was to transfer innovation from the MASK App to other reference sites. The phenotypic characteristics of rhinitis and asthma multimorbidity in adults and the elderly are compared using validated mHealth tools (i.e. the Allergy Diary and CARAT) in 23 Reference Sites or regions across Europe and Argentina, Australia, Brazil and Mexico [46]. This will improve understanding, assessment of burden, diagnosis and management of rhinitis in the elderly by comparison with an adult population. The pilot study has been completed in Germany and the project is fully operative using two protocols (Table 3).

Results
Work productivity

AR impairs social life, work and school productivity. Indirect costs associated with lost work productivity are the principal contributor to the total AR costs and result mainly from impaired work performance by presenteeism [2]. The severity of AR symptoms was the most consistent disease-related factor associated with impact of AR on work productivity, although ocular symptoms and sleep disturbances may independently affect work

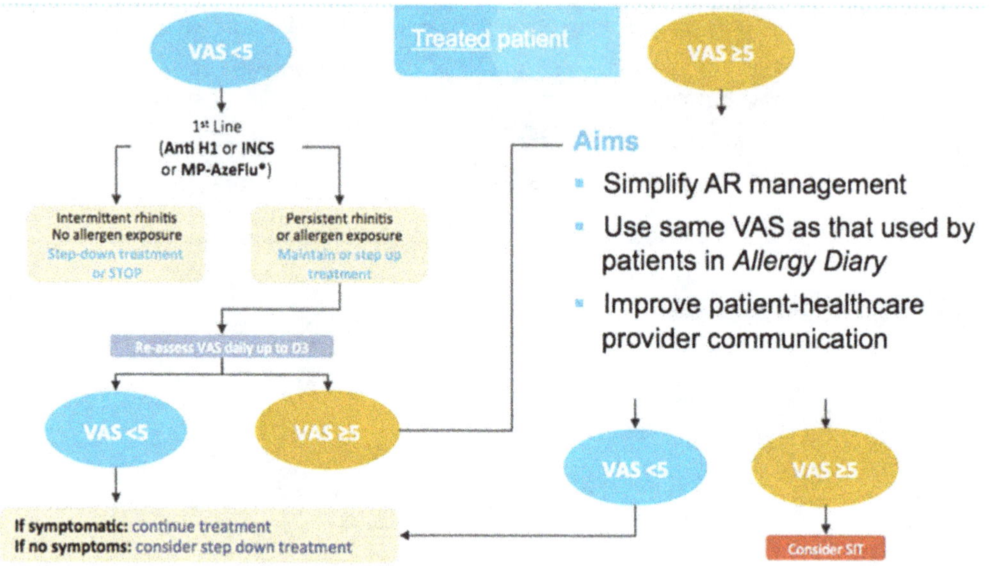

Fig. 4 Clinical decision support systems consensus for allergic rhinitis (from Bousquet et al. [28])

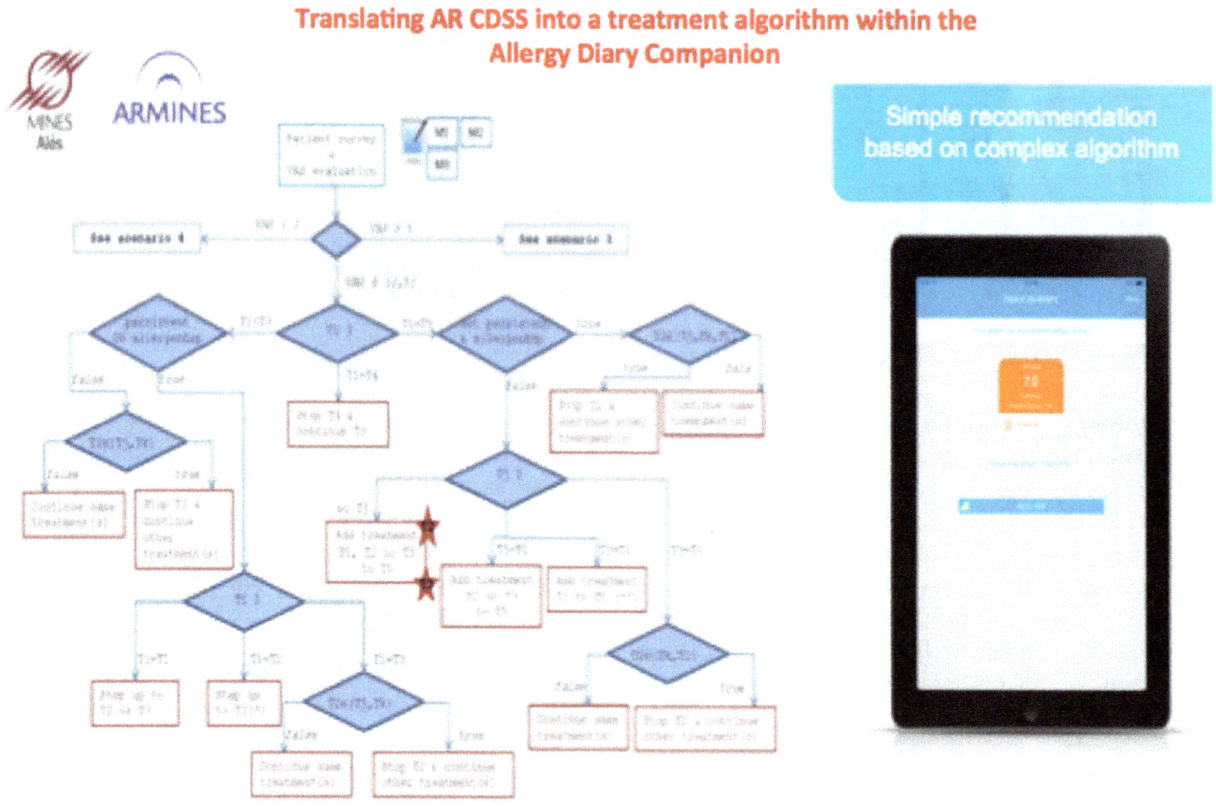

Fig. 5 CDSS digitalization (submitted)

productivity. Overall, the pharmacologic treatment of AR showed a beneficial effect on work productivity.

A cross-sectional study using *Allergy diary* in 1136 users (5659 days) assessed the impact on work productivity of uncontrolled AR assessed by VAS [34]. In users with uncontrolled rhinitis (VAS global measured ≥ 50), approximately 90% had some work impairment and over 50% had severe work impairment

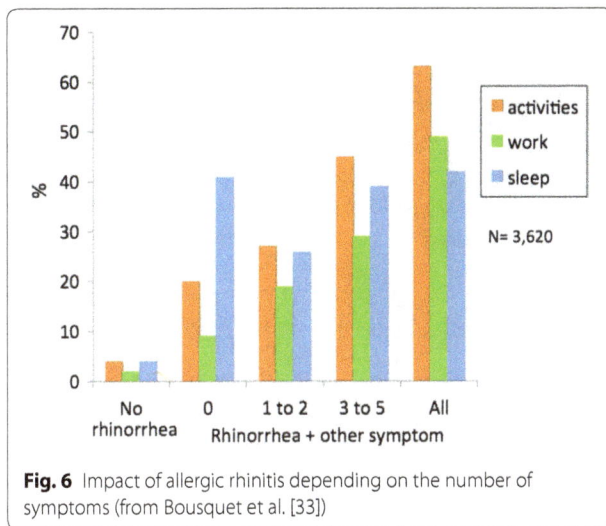

Fig. 6 Impact of allergic rhinitis depending on the number of symptoms (from Bousquet et al. [33])

(VAS-work ≥ 50). There was a significant correlation between VAS-global calculated and VAS-work (Rho = 0.83, p < 0.00001, Spearman rank test). The study has been extended to almost 17,000 days and similar results were observed (Fig. 7).

The baseline study found that bothersome symptoms, nasal obstruction and ocular symptoms were involved in work productivity impact [33] (Fig. 8).

The *Allergy Diary* includes the WPAI:AS in six EU countries. All consecutive users who completed the VAS-work from June 1 to July 31, 2016 were included in the study [66]. A highly significant correlation was found between Questions 4 (impairment of work) and 9 (impairment of activities) in 698 users (Rho = 0.85).

All these studies combine to confirm the impact of uncontrolled AR on work productivity.

Novel phenotypes of allergic diseases

Multimorbidity in allergic airway diseases is well known [6], but no data exist regarding the daily dynamics of symptoms. The *Allergy Diary* assessed the presence and control of daily allergic multimorbidity (asthma, conjunctivitis, rhinitis) and its impact on work productivity in 4025 users and 32,585 days monitored in 19 countries from May 25, 2015 to May 26, 2016. VAS levels < 20/100 were categorized as "Low" burden and VAS levels ≥ 50/100 as "High" burden. VAS global measured levels assessing the global control of the allergic disease were significantly associated with daily allergic multimorbidity. Eight hypothesis-driven patterns were defined based on "Low" and "High" VAS levels. There were < 0.2% days of Rhinitis Low and Asthma High or Conjunctivitis High patterns. There were 5.9% days with a Rhinitis High—Asthma Low pattern. There were 1.7% days with a Rhinitis High—Asthma High—Conjunctivitis Low pattern. A novel Rhinitis High—Asthma High—Conjunctivitis High pattern was identified in 2.9% days and had the greatest impact on uncontrolled VAS global measured and impaired work productivity (Fig. 9). The mobile technology enabled investigation in a novel approach of the intra-individual variability of allergic multimorbidity using days. It identified an unrecognized extreme pattern of uncontrolled multimorbidity [59].

Treatment of allergic rhinitis using mobile technology with real world data

Large observational implementation studies are needed to triangulate the findings from randomized control trials (RCTs) as they reflect "real world" everyday practice. We attempted to provide additional and complementary insights into the real-life AR treatment using mobile technology. The *Allergy Diary* was filled in by 2871 users

Table 3 Twinning protocols (from Bousquet et al., [65])

	Protocol 1	Protocol 2
	Short version	Long version
Allergy Diary	+	+
Equation 5D	Optional	+
Physician's questionnaire		+
Ethics committee	Not needed	Needed (obtained in some Reference Sites)
Inform consent	Terms of Reference on App	From with patient's signature
Recruitment	Any user Persons attending clinic visits can be included	Persons attending clinic visits included with a physician's diagnosis of allergic disease and allergen sensitization (IgE and/or skin tests)
Physician's questionnaire		+

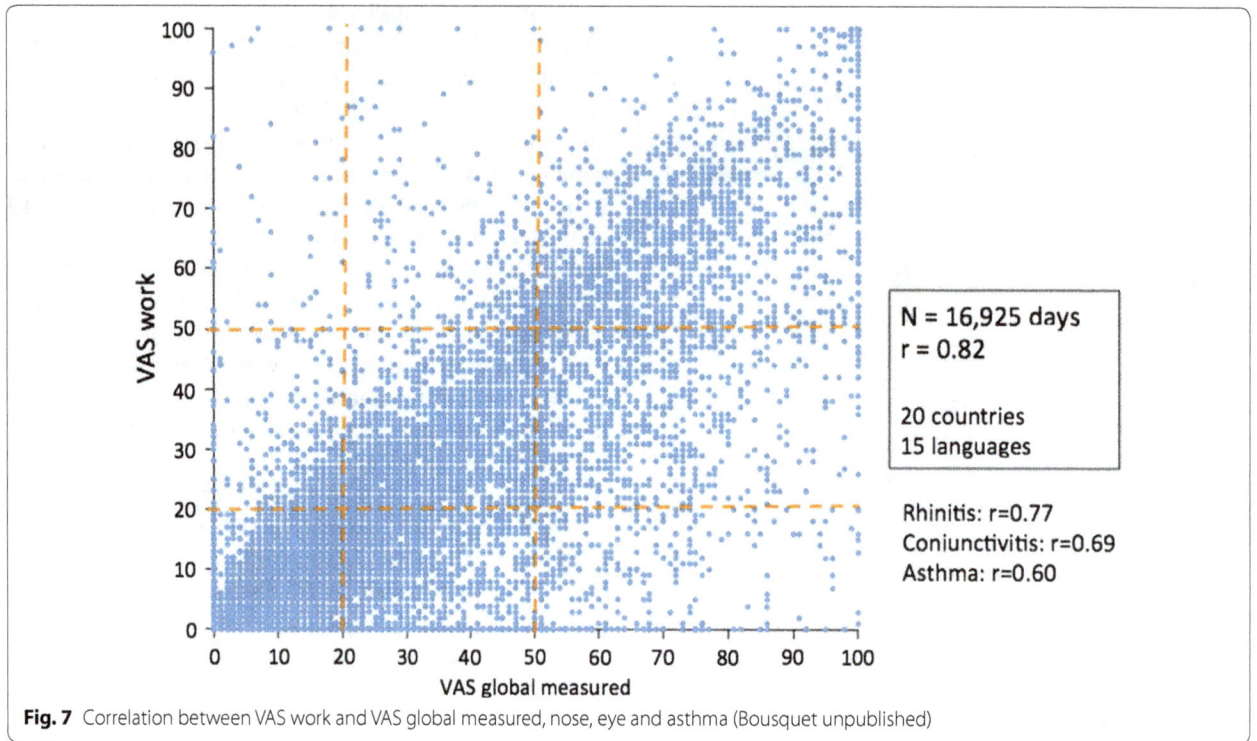

Fig. 7 Correlation between VAS work and VAS global measured, nose, eye and asthma (Bousquet unpublished)

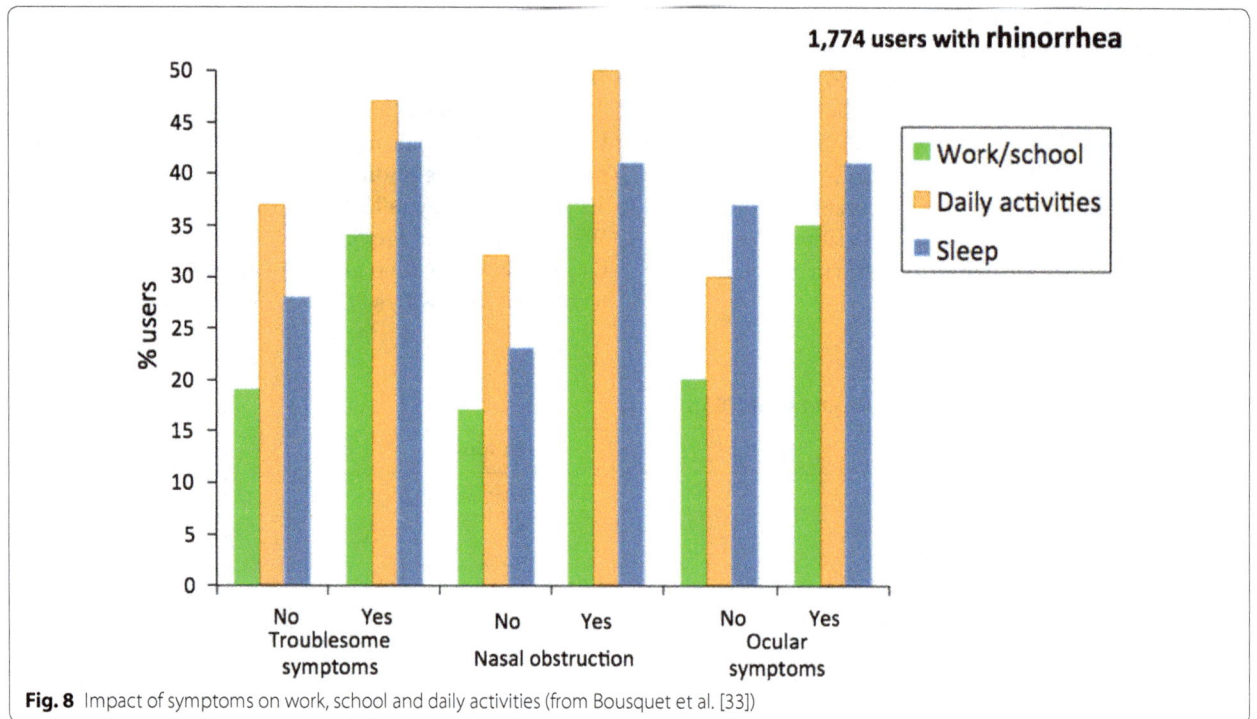

Fig. 8 Impact of symptoms on work, school and daily activities (from Bousquet et al. [33])

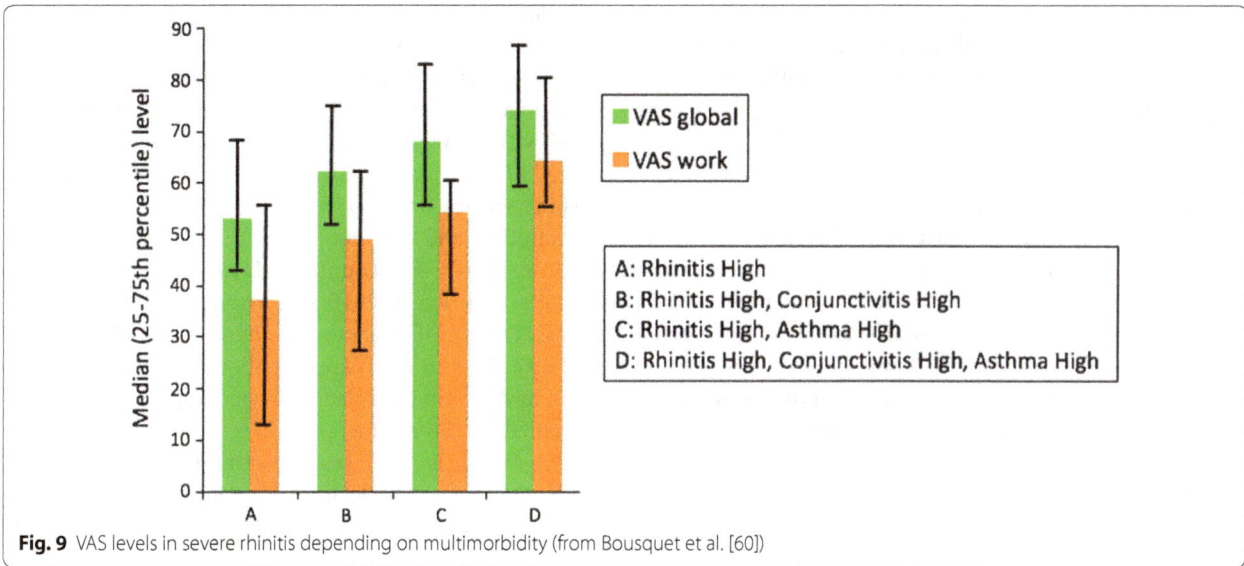

Fig. 9 VAS levels in severe rhinitis depending on multimorbidity (from Bousquet et al. [60])

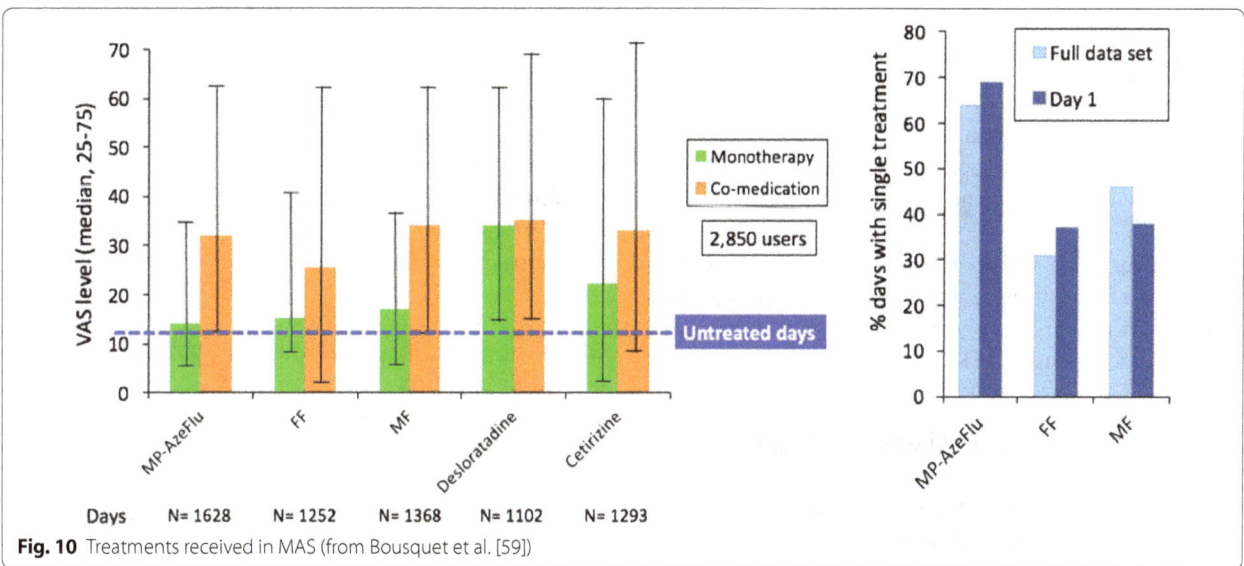

Fig. 10 Treatments received in MAS (from Bousquet et al. [59])

who reported 17,091 days of VAS in 2015 and 2016. Medications were reported for 9634 days. The assessment of days appeared to be more informative than the course of the treatment as, in real life, patients rarely use treatment on a daily basis; rather, they appear to increase treatment use with the loss of symptom control and to stop it when symptoms disappear. The *Allergy Diary* allowed the differentiation between treatments within or

between classes (intranasal corticosteroid use containing medications and oral H1-antihistamines). The control of days differed between no (best control), single or multiple treatments (worst control) (Fig. 10). The study confirms the usefulness of the *Allergy Diary* in accessing and assessing everyday use and practice in AR [59].

Adherence to medications was studied in almost 7000 users reporting medications. 1770 users reported over

7 days of VAS between January 1, 2016 and August 31, 2016 and a major lack of adherence to treatment was observed for all medications (Menditto et al., in preparation).

MASK in the pharmacy

Multidisciplinary integrated care is necessary to reduce the burden of chronic diseases. A significant proportion of patients with AR self-manage their condition and often the pharmacist is the first HCP that a person with nasal symptoms contacts [66, 67]. Pharmacists are trusted in the community and are easily accessible. As such, pharmacists are an important part of the multidisciplinary healthcare team, acting at different steps of rhinitis care pathways.

Pharmacists are important in many areas of intervention in AR:

- Recognizing (identification).
- Risk assessment/stratification.
- OTC treatment.
- Manage refils.
- Patient education.
- Referral to a physician.
- Administration of topical treatment technique and adherence to treatment.

Simple algorithms and tools are essential in the routine implementation of these steps. A first approach was made by ARIA in the pharmacy [68] and is currently being updated using MASK.

POLLAR (Impact of air POLLution on Asthma and Rhinitis)

AR and asthma are impacted by allergens and air pollution. However, interactions between air pollution, sleep [55, 69] and allergic diseases are insufficiently understood. POLLAR aims at combining emerging technologies [search engine TLR2 (technology readiness level); pollution sampler TLR6, App TLR9] with machine learning to (1) understand effects of air pollution in AR and its impact on sleep, work, asthma, (2) propose novel care pathways integrating pollution and patient's literacy, (3) study sleep, (4) improve work productivity, (5) propose the basis for a sentinel network at the EU level for pollution and allergy and (6) assess the societal implications of the interaction.

POLLAR will use the freely existing application for AR monitoring (*Allergy Diary*, 14,000 users, TLR8) combined with a new tool allowing queries on allergen and pollen (TLR2) and existing pollution data. Machine learning will be used to assess the relationship between air pollution and AR comparing polluted and non-polluted areas in 6 EU countries. Data generated in 2018 will be confirmed in 2019 and extended by the individual assessment of pollution (Canarin®, portable sensor, TLR6) in AR and sleep apnea patients used as a control group having impaired sleep. The geographic information system GIS will map the results.

Google Trends (GT) searches trends of specific queries in Google and reflects the real-life epidemiology of AR. We compared GT terms related to allergy and rhinitis in all European Union countries, Norway and Switzerland from January 1, 2011 to December, 20 2016. An annual and clear seasonality of queries was found in most countries but the terms 'hay fever', 'allergy' and 'pollen'—show cultural differences [70]. Using longitudinal data in different countries and multiple terms, we identified an awareness-related spike of searches (December 2016) [70]. In asthma, GTs can identify spikes of mortality as was found in Australia and Kuwait in 2016. However, the usual peaks of asthma during allergen exposure or virus infections cannot be easily monitored [71].

Global applicability of MASK and POLLAR, and their benefits

Although MASK has been devised to optimize care pathways in rhinitis and asthma multimorbidity, its applicability is far more extensive (Table 4).

For MASK, several steps have been achieved.

Conclusion

MASK is a novel approach to obtain real-life data concerning rhinitis and asthma multimorbidity and to help patients and physicians for a better SDM. It can be used for multiple purposes in a friendly manner in order to improve the control of allergic diseases in a cost-effective approach.

MASK 2017: ARIA digitally-enabled, integrated, person-centred care for rhinitis and asthma...

165

Table 4 Global applicability of MASK

Applicability	MASK
Clinical practice	Physicians will be able to read the files of the patients in order to
	Optimize treatment for the patient and, in particular, the current or the next pollen season
	Assess and increase the adherence to treatment
	Help for shared decision making
	Prescribe allergen immunotherapy (AIT) more rapidly when the patient is not controlled despite optimal pharmacologic treatment
	Determine the efficacy of AIT in patients
	The Allergy Diary is an essential tool to provide personalized medicine in AR and asthma
Change management	The first results of MASK indicate that many patients are uncontrolled and non-adherent to treatment
	Moreover, they appear to use their medications as needed and not as a regular basis as prescribed
	Change management is needed
Patient empowerment	Better understanding of the symptoms
	Sentinel network linking aerobiology data and control
	Improved adherence
	Self-management
	Patient empowerment
	Messages sent by the App
Clinical trials	For RCTs, it is essential to have clarity on definitions, and relevant tools. The Allergy Diary allows
	To better stratify the patients needing AIT
	To assess the efficacy of AIT during the trial
	To assess the efficacy when AIT is stopped
	Observational studies are of key importance to confirm RCTs and bring new hypotheses for the treatment of AR and asthma
Registration and reimbursement of medicines	Controlled trials designed with a uniform approach will be more easily evaluated by the Health Technology Assessment agencies (such as NICE) for reimbursement. The Allergy Diary uses EQ-5D, a validated measure of utility
	Better understanding of direct and indirect costs
	Controlled trials designed with a uniform approach will help to synchronize data from real-life world regarding clinical effects and safety/tolerability of new drugs (post-marketing pharmacovigilance
Research on mechanisms and genetics	A uniform definition and a collaborative approach to epidemiological, genetic and mechanistic research are important and will be enhanced by the stratification of patients using the *Allergy Diary*
	Different levels of phenotype characterization (granularity) can be applied to assess phenotypic characterization in old age subjects
Epidemiology	In epidemiologic population studies, standardized definitions and tools are fundamental. The Allergy Diary allows novel approaches combining classical cross-sectional and longitudinal studies with real life studies in large populations
Employers	AR and asthma represent a major burden for the employers, and the estimated annual costs in the EU range from 30 to 60 B€. Better control of the disease was shown to reduce costs. The *Allergy Diary* has the potential to improve the control of allergic diseases and to significantly improve work productivity at the EU level
Public health planning	For public health purposes, a perfect patient characterization in real life is needed to identify the prevalence, burden and costs incurred by patients in order to improve quality of care and optimize health care planning and policies
Reduction of inequities	Inequities still exist in the EU for allergic diseases prevalence and burden (not only sex/gender inequities). POLLAR will attempt to understand them and to propose policies and health promotion strategies

Abbreviations

AHA: active and healthy ageing; AIRWAYS ICPs: integrated care pathways for airway diseases; AR: allergic rhinitis; ARIA: Allergic Rhinitis and Its Impact on Asthma; CARAT: Control of Allergic Rhinitis and Asthma Test; CDSS: clinical decision support system; CNIL: Commission Informatique et Liberté; CRD: Chronic Respiratory Disease; DG CONNECT: Directorate General for Communications Networks, Content & Technology; DG Santé: Directorate General for Health and Food Safety; DG: Directorate General; EFA: European Federation of Allergy and Airways Diseases Patients' Associations; EIP on AHA: European Innovation Partnership on AHA; EIP: European Innovation Partnership; EQ-5D: Euroquol; GARD: WHO Global Alliance against Chronic Respiratory Diseases; GDPR: General Data Protection Regulation; GIS: geographic information system; GP: Good Practice; GT: Google Trends; HCP: health care professional; ICP: integrated care pathway; IMS: Institute of Medical Science; JA-CHRODIS: Joint Action on Chronic Diseases and Promoting Healthy Ageing across the Life Cycle; MACVIA-LR: contre les MAladies Chroniques pour un VIeillissement Actif

(Fighting chronic diseases for AHA); MASK: Mobile Airways Sentinel networK; MeDALL: Mechanisms of the Development of ALLergy (FP7); mHealth: mobile health; NCD: non-communicable disease; OTC: over the counter; PIA: privacy Impact Assessment; POLLAR: Impact of air POLLution on Asthma and Rhinitis; QOL: quality of life; SCUAD: severe chronic upper airway disease; TRL: technology readiness level; TWINNING: transfer of innovation of mobile technology; VAS: Visual Analogue Scale; WHO: World Health Organization; WPAI-AS: Work Productivity and Activity Questionnaire.

Authors' contributions
All authors are MAKS members and have contributed to the design of the project. Many authors also included users and disseminated the project in their own country. All authors read and approved the final manuscript.

Author details
[1] MACVIA-France, Fondation Partenariale FMC VIA-LR, CHRU Arnaud de Villeneuve, 371 Avenue du Doyen Gaston Giraud, Montpellier, France. [2] INSERM U 1168, VIMA: Ageing and Chronic Diseases Epidemiological and Public Health Approaches, Villejuif, Université Versailles St-Quentin-en-Yvelines, UMR-S 1168, Montigny le Bretonneux, France. [3] Euforea, Brussels, Belgium. [4] KYomed-INNOV, Montpellier, France. [5] iQ4U Consultants Ltd, London, UK. [6] MedScript Ltd, Dundalk, Co Louth, Ireland. [7] Laboratoire HP2, Grenoble, INSERM, U1042, Université Grenoble Alpes, Grenoble, France. [8] CHU de Grenoble, Grenoble, France. [9] Conseil Général de l'Economie Ministère de l'Economie, de l'Industrie et du Numérique, Paris, France. [10] UCIBIO, REQUINTE, Faculty of Pharmacy and Competence Center on Active and Healthy Ageing, University of Porto (Porto4Ageing), Porto, Portugal. [11] Center for Health Technology and Services Research- CINTESIS, Faculdade de Medicina, Universidade do Porto, Porto, Portugal. [12] Medida, Lda, Porto, Portugal. [13] Faculty of Health Sciences and CICS – UBI, Health Sciences Research Centre, University of Beira Interior, Covilhã, Portugal. [14] Allergy Center, CUF Descobertas Hospital, Lisbon, Portugal. [15] Imunoalergologia, Centro Hospitalar Universitário de Coimbra and Faculty of Medicine, University of Coimbra, Coimbra, Portugal. [16] ProAR – Nucleo de Excelencia em Asma, Federal University of Bahia, Vitória da Conquista, Brazil. [17] WHO GARD Planning Group, Salvador, Brazil. [18] Allergy Service, University Hospital of Federal University of Santa Catarina (HU-UFSC), Florianópolis, Brazil. [19] Asthma Reference Center, Escola Superior de Ciencias da Santa Casa de Misericordia de Vitoria, Vitória, Esperito Santo, Brazil. [20] Division for Health Innovation, Campania Region and Federico II University Hospital Naples (R&D and DISMET), Naples, Italy. [21] CIRFF, Federico II University, Naples, Italy. [22] SOS Allergology and Clinical Immunology, USL Toscana Centro, Prato, Italy. [23] Department of Medical Sciences, Allergy and Clinical Immunology Unit, University of Torino & Mauriziano Hospital, Torino, Italy. [24] Consortium of Pharmacies and Services COSAFER, Salerno, Italy. [25] Unit of Geriatric Immunoallergology, University of Bari Medical School, Bari, Italy. [26] Department of Medicine, Surgery and Dentistry "Scuola Medica Salernitana", University of Salerno, Salerno, Italy. [27] Center of Excellence in Asthma and Allergy, Hospital Médica Sur, México City, Mexico. [28] Mexico City, Mexico. [29] Puebla, Puebla, Mexico. [30] Ciutad Mexico, Mexico. [31] Allergology Department, Centre de l'Asthme et des Allergies Hôpital d'Enfants Armand-Trousseau (APHP), Paris, France. [32] UPMC Univ Paris 06, UMR_S 1136, Institut Pierre Louis d'Epidémiologie et de Santé Publique, Sorbonne Universités, Equipe EPAR, 75013 Paris, France. [33] Epidemiology of Allergic and Respiratory Diseases, Department Institute Pierre Louis of Epidemiology and Public Health, INSERM, UPMC Sorbonne Université, Medical School Saint Antoine, Paris, France. [34] La Rochelle, France. [35] Department of Respiratory Diseases, Montpellier University Hospital, Montpellier, France. [36] UPRES EA220, Pôle des Maladies des Voies Respiratoires, Hôpital Foch, Université Paris-Saclay, Suresnes, France. [37] Reims, France. [38] Division of Internal Medicine, Asthma and Allergy, Barlicki University Hospital, Medical University of Lodz, Lodz, Poland. [39] Department of Prevention of Environmental Hazards and Allergology, Medical University of Warsaw, Warsaw, Poland. [40] Clinic of Children's Diseases, and Institute of Health Sciences Department of Public Health, Vilnius University Institute of Clinical Medicine, Vilnius, Lithuania. [41] European Academy of Paediatrics (EAP/UEMS-SP), Brussels, Belgium. [42] Clinic of Children's Diseases, Faculty of Medicine, Vilnius University, Vilnius, Lithuania. [43] Faculty of Medicine, Vilnius University, Vilnius, Lithuania. [44] Woodbrook Medical Centre, Loughborough, UK. [45] Allergy and Respiratory Research Group, Usher Institute of Population Health Sciences and Informatics, University of Edinburgh, Medical School, Edinburgh, UK. [46] Centre of Medical Informatics, Usher Institute of Population Health Sciences and Informatics, The University of Edinburgh, Edinburgh, UK. [47] Allergy Unit, Department of Dermatology, University Hospital of Zurich, Zürich, Switzerland. [48] Center for Rhinology and Allergology, Wiesbaden, Germany. [49] Department of Otorhinolaryngology, Head and Neck Surgery, Universitätsmedizin Mannheim, Medical Faculty Mannheim, Heidelberg University, Mannheim, Germany. [50] Comprehensive Allergy-Centre-Charité, Department of Dermatology and Allergy, Charité - Universitätsmedizin Berlin, Berlin, Germany. [51] Global Allergy and Asthma European Network (GA2LEN), Berlin, Germany. [52] Institute of Medical Statistics, and Computational Biology, Medical Faculty, University of Cologne, Cologne, Germany. [53] CRI-Clinical Research International-Ltd, Hamburg, Germany. [54] Department of Internal Medicine, Medical University of Graz, Graz, Austria. [55] Department of ENT, Medical University of Graz, Graz, Austria. [56] Department of Otorhinolaryngology, Academic Medical Centre, Amsterdam, The Netherlands. [57] Department of Public Health and Primary Care, Leiden University Medical Center, Leiden, The Netherlands. [58] ISGlobAL, Centre for Research in Environmental Epidemiology (CREAL), Barcelona, Spain. [59] IMIM (Hospital del Mar Research Institute), Barcelona, Spain. [60] CIBER Epidemiología y Salud Pública (CIBERESP), Barcelona, Spain. [61] Universitat Pompeu Fabra (UPF), Barcelona, Spain. [62] Allergy Section, Department of Internal Medicine, Hospital Vall d'Hebron & ARADyAL Research Network, Barcelona, Spain. [63] AQuAS, Barcelona, Spain. [64] EUREGHA, European Regional and Local Health Association, Brussels, Belgium. [65] Rhinology Unit and Smell Clinic, ENT Department, Hospital Clínic, University of Barcelona, Barcelona, Spain. [66] Clinical and Experimental Respiratory Immunoallergy, IDIBAPS, CIBERES, University of Barcelona, Barcelona, Spain. [67] Skin and Allergy Hospital, Helsinki University Hospital, Helsinki, Finland. [68] Association of Finnish Pharmacists, Helsinki, Finland. [69] Department of Lung Diseases and Clinical Immunology, University of Turku, Turku, Finland. [70] Terveystalo Allergy Clinic, Turku, Finland. [71] Department of Pulmonary Diseases, Cerrahpasa Faculty of Medicine, Istanbul University, Istanbul, Turkey. [72] Department of Pulmonary Diseases, Faculty of Medicine, Celal Bayar University, Manisa, Turkey. [73] GARD Executive Committee, Manisa, Turkey. [74] Center for Pediatrics and Child Health, Institute of Human Development, Royal Manchester Children's Hospital, University of Manchester, Manchester, UK. [75] Allergy Department, 2nd Pediatric Clinic, Athens General Children's Hospital "P&A Kyriakou", University of Athens, 11527 Athens, Greece. [76] Department of Otorhinolaryngology, University of Crete School of Medicine, Heraklion, Greece. [77] Woolcock Institute of Medical Research, University of Sydney and Sydney Local Health District, Glebe, NSW, Australia. [78] Department of Allergy, Immunology and Respiratory Medicine, Alfred Hospital and Central Clinical School, Monash University, Melbourne, VIC, Australia. [79] Department of Immunology, Monash University, Melbourne, VIC, Australia. [80] Servicio de Alergia e Immunologia, Clinica Santa Isabel, Buenos Aires, Argentina. [81] Director of Center of Allergy, Immunology and Respiratory Diseases, Santa Fe, Argentina Center for Allergy and Immunology, Santa Fe, Argentina. [82] Universidad Católica de Córdoba, Córdoba, Argentina. [83] Department of Clinical Science and Education, Karolinska Institutet, Södersjukhuset, Stockholm, Sweden. [84] Sachs' Children and Youth Hospital, Södersjukhuset, Stockholm, Sweden. [85] Institute of Environmental Medicine, Karolinska Institutet, Stockholm, Sweden. [86] Centre for Clinical Research Sörmland, Uppsala University, Eskilstuna, Sweden. [87] Upper Airways Research Laboratory, ENT Department, Ghent University Hospital, Ghent, Belgium. [88] Department of Otorhinolaryngology, Univ Hospitals Leuven, Louvain, Belgium. [89] Academic Medical Center, University of Amsterdam, Amsterdam, The Netherlands. [90] EFA European Federation of Allergy and Airways Diseases Patients' Associations, Brussels, Belgium. [91] Department of Dermatology and Allergy Centre, Odense University Hospital, Odense Research Center for Anaphylaxis (ORCA), Odense, Denmark. [92] Department of Medicine, Clinical Immunology and Allergy, McMaster University, Hamilton, ON, Canada. [93] University Hospital Olomouc, Olomouc, Czech Republic. [94] Peercode BV, Geldermalsen, The Netherlands. [95] Faculty of Medicine, Transylvania University, Brasov, Romania. [96] Division of Allergy/Immunology, University of South Florida, Tampa, USA. [97] Section of Allergy and Immunology, Saint Louis University School of Medicine, Saint Louis, MO, USA. [98] Johns Hopkins School of Medicine, Baltimore, MD, USA. [99] Department of Otorhinolaryngology, Chiba University Hospital, Chiba, Japan. [100] Nova Southeastern University, Fort Lauderdale, Florida, USA.

Acknowledgements
None.

Mask Study Group

J Bousquet[1-3], PW Hellings[4], W Aberer[5], I Agache[6], CA Akdis[7], M Akdis[7], MR Alberti[8], R Almeida[9], F Amat[10], R Angles[11], I Annesi-Maesano[12], IJ Ansotegui[13], JM Anto[14-17], S Arnavielle[18], E Asayag[19], A Asarnoj[20], H Arshad[21], F Avolio[22], E Bacci[23], C Bachert[24], I Baiardini[25], C Barbara[26], M Barbagallo[27], I Baroni[28], BA Barreto[29], X Basagana[14], ED Bateman[30], M Bedolla-Barajas[31], A Bedbrook[2], M Bewick[32], B Beghé[33], EH Bel[34], KC Bergmann[35], KS Bennoor[36], M Benson[37], L Bertorello[23], AZ Białoszewski[38], T Bieber[39], S Bialek[40], C Bindslev-Jensen[41], L Bjermer[42], H Blain[43,44], F Blasi[45], A Blua[46], M Bochenska Marciniak[47], I Bogus-Buczynska[47], AL Boner[48], M Bonini[49], S Bonini[50], CS Bosnic-Anticevich[51], I Bosse[52], J Bouchard[53], LP Boulet[54], R Bourret[55], PJ Bousquet[12], F Braido[25], V Briedis[56], CE Brightling[57], J Brozek[58], C Bucca[59], R Buhl[60], R Buonaiuto[61], C Panaitescu[62], MT Burguete Cabañas[63], E Burte[3], A Bush[64], F Caballero-Fonseca[65], D Caillot[67], D Caimmi[68], MA Calderon[69], PAM Camargos[70], T Camuzat[71], G Canfora[72], GW Canonica[25], V Cardona[73], KH Carlsen[74], P Carreiro-Martins[75], AM Carriazo[76], W Carr[77], C Cartier[78], T Casale[79], G Castellano[80], L Cecchi[81], AM Cepeda[82], NH Chavannes[83], Y Chen[84], R Chiron[68], T Chivato[85], E Chkhartishvili[86], AG Chuchalin[87], KF Chung[88], MM Ciaravolo[89], A Ciceran[90], C Cingi[91], G Ciprandi[92], AC Carvalho Coelho[93], L Colas[94], E Colgan[95], J Coll[96], D Conforti[97], J Correia de Sousa[98], RM Cortés-Grimaldo[99], F Corti[100], E Costa[101], MC Costa-Dominguez[102], AL Courbis[103], L Cox[104], M Crescenzo[105], AA Cruz[106], A Custovic[107], W Czarlewski[108], SE Dahlen[109], C Dario[110], J da Silva[111], Y Dauvilliers[112], U Darsow[113], F De Blay[114], G De Carlo[115], T Dedeu[116], M de Fátima Emerson[117], G De Feo[118], G De Vries[119], B De Martino[120], N de Paula Motta Rubini[121], D Deleanu[122], P Demoly[12,68], JA Denburg[123], P Devillier[124], S Di Capua Ercolano[125], N Di Carluccio[66], A Didier[126], D Dokic[127], MG Dominguez-Silva[128], H Douagui[129], G Dray[103], R Dubakiene[130], SR Durham[131], G Du Toit[132], MS Dykewicz[133], Y El-Gamal[134], P Eklund[135], E Eller[41], R Emuzyte[136], J Farrell[95], A Farsi[81], J Ferreira de Mello Jr[137], J Ferrero[138], A Fink-Wagner[139], A Fiocchi[140], WJ Fokkens[141], JA Fonseca[142], JF Fontaine[143], S Forti[97], JM Fuentes-Perez[144], JL Gálvez-Romero[145], A Gamkrelidze[146], J Garcia-Aymerich[14], CY García-Cobas[147], MH Garcia-Cruz[148], B Gemicioğlu[149], S Genova[150], C George[151], JE Gereda[152], R Gerth van Wijk[153], RM Gomez[154], J Gómez-Vera[155], S González Diaz[156], M Gotua[157], I Grisle[158], M Guidacci[159], NA Guldemond[160], Z Gutter[161], MA Guzmán[162], T Haahtela[163], J Hajjam[164], L Hernández[165], JO'B Hourihane[166], YR Huerta-Villalobos[167], M Humbert[168], G Iaccarino[169], M Illario[170], JC Ivancevich[171], EJ Jares[172], E Jassem[173], SL Johnston[174], G Joos[175], KS Jung[176], M Jutel[177], I Kaidashev[178], O Kalayci[179], AF Kalyoncu[180], J Karjalainen[181], P Kardas[182], T Keil[183], PK Keith[184], M Khaitov[185], N Khaltaev[186], J Kleine-Tebbe[187], L Klimek[188], ML Kowalski[189], M Kuitunen[190], I Kull[191], P Kuna[47], M Kupczyk[47], V Kvedariene[192], E Krzych-Fałta[193], P Lacwik[47], D Larenas-Linnemann[194], D Laune[18], D Lauri[195], J Lavrut[196], LTT Le[197], M Lessa[198], G Levato[199], J Li[200], P Lieberman[201], A Lipiec[193], B Lipworth[202], KC Lodrup Carlsen[203], R Louis[204], O Lourenço[205], JA Luna-Pech[206], K Maciej[47], A Magnan[94], B Mahboub[207], D Maier[208], A Mair[209], I Majer[210], J Malva[211], E Mandajieva[212], P Manning[213], E De Manuel Keenoy[214], GD Marshall[215], MR Masjedi[216], JF Maspero[217], E Mathieu-Dupas[18], JJ Matta Campos[218], AL Matos[219], M Maurer[220], S Mavale-Manuel[221], O Mayora[97], MA Medina-Avalos[222], E Melén[223], F Melo-Gomes[26], EO Meltzer[224], E Menditto[225], J Mercier[226], N Miculinic[227], F Mihaltan[228], B Milenkovic[229], G Moda[230], MD Mogica-Martinez[231], Y Mohammad[232], I Momas[233,234], S Montefort[235], R Monti[236], D Mora Bogado[237], M Morais-Almeida[238], FF Morato-Castro[239], R Mösges[240], A Mota-Pinto[241], P Moura Santo[242], J Mullol[243], L Münter[244], A Muraro[245], R Murray[246], R Naclerio[247], R Nadif[3], M Nalin[28], L Napoli[248], L Namazova-Baranova[249], H Neffen[250], V Niedeberger[251], K Nekam[252], A Neou[253], A Nieto[254], L Nogueira-Silva[255], M Nogues[2,256], F Novellino[257], TD Nyembue[258], RE O'Hehir[259], C Odzhakova[260], K Ohta[261], Y Okamoto[262], K Okubo[263], GL Onorato[2], M Ortega Cisneros[264], S Ouedraogo[265], I Pali-Schöll[266], S Palkonen[115], P Panzner[267], NG Papadopoulos[268], HS Park[269], A Papi[270], G Passalacqua[271], E Paulino[272], R Pawankar[273], S Pedersen[274], JL Pépin[275], AM Pereira[276], M Persico[277], O Pfaar[278,279], J Phillips[280], R Picard[281], B Pigearias[282], I Pin[283], C Pitsios[284], D Plavec[285], W Pohl[286], TA Popov[287], F Portejoie[2], P Potter[288], AC Pozzi[289], D Price[290], EP Prokopakis[291], R Puy[259], B Pugin[292], RE Pulido Ross[293], M Przemecka[47], KF Rabe[294], F Raciborski[193], R Rajabian-Soderlund[295], S Reitsma[141], I Ribeirinho[296], J Rimmer[297], D Rivero-Yeverino[298], JA Rizzo[299], MC Rizzo[300], C Robalo-Cordeiro[301], F Rodenas[302], X Rodo[14], M Rodriguez Gonzalez[303], L Rodriguez-Mañas[304], C Rolland[305], S Rodrigues Valle[306], M Roman Rodriguez[307], A Romano[308], E Rodriguez-Zagal[309], G Rolla[310], RE Roller-Wirnsberger[311], M Romano[28], J Rosado-Pinto[312], N Rosario[313], M Rottem[314], D Ryan[315], H Sagara[316], J Salimäki[317], B Samolinski[193], M Sanchez-Borges[318], J Sastre-Dominguez[319], GK Scadding[320], HJ Schunemann[58], N Scichilone[321], P Schmid-Grendelmeier[322], FS Serpa[323], S Shamai[240], A Sheikh[324], M Sierra[96], FER Simons[325], V Siroux[326], JC Sisul[327], I Skrindo[378], D Solé[328], D Somekh[329], M Sondermann[330], T Sooronbaev[331], M Sova[332], M Sorensen[333], M Sorlini[334], O Spranger[139], C Stellato[118], R Stelmach[335], R Stukas[336], J Sunyer[14-17], J Strozek[193], A Szylling[193], JN Tebyriçá[337], M Thibaudon[338], T To[339], A Todo-Bom[340], PV Tomazic[341], S Toppila-Salmi[163], U Trama[342], M Triggiani[118], C Suppli Ulrik[343], M Urrutia-Pereira[344], R Valenta[345], A Valero[346], A Valiulis[347], E Valovirta[348], M van Eerd[119], E van Ganse[349], M van Hague[350], O Vandenplas[351], MT Ventura[352], G Vezzani[353], T Vasankari[354], A Vatrella[118], MT Verissimo[211], F Viart[78], G Viegi[355], D Vicheva[356], T Vontetsianos[357], M Wagenmann[358], S Walker[359], D Wallace[360], DY Wang[361], S Waserman[362], T Werfel[363], M Westman[364], M Wickman[191], DM Williams[365], S Williams[366], N Wilson[367], J Wright[367], P Wroczynski[40], P Yakovliev[368], BP Yawn[369], PK Yiallouros[370], A Yorgancioglu[371], OM Yusuf[372], HJ Zar[373], L Zhang[374], N Zhong[200], ME Zernotti[375], M Zidarn[376], T Zuberbier[35], C Zubrinich[259], A Zurkuhlen[377]

[1]University Hospital, Montpellier, France. [2]MACVIA-France, Fondation partenariale FMC VIA-LR, Montpellier, France. [3]VIMA. INSERM U 1168, VIMA : Ageing and chronic diseases Epidemiological and public health approaches, Villejuif, Université Versailles St-Quentin-en-Yvelines, UMR-S 1168, Montigny le Bretonneux, France and Euforea, Brussels, Belgium. [4]Laboratory of Clinical Immunology, Department of Microbiology and Immunology, KU Leuven, Leuven, Belgium. [5]Department of Dermatology, Medical University of Graz, Graz, Austria. [6]Transylvania University Brasov, Brasov, Romania. [7]Swiss Institute of Allergy and Asthma Research (SIAF), University of Zurich, Davos, Switzerland. [8]Project Manager, Chairman of the Council of Municipality of Salerno, Italy. [9]Center for Health Technology and Services Research- CINTESIS, Faculdade de Medicina, Universidade do Porto; and Medida, Lda Porto, Portugal. [10]Allergology department, Centre de l'Asthme et des Allergies Hôpital d'Enfants Armand-Trousseau (APHP); Sorbonne Université, UPMC Univ Paris 06, UMR_S 1136, Institut Pierre Louis d'Epidémiologie et de Santé Publique, Equipe EPAR, Paris, France. [11]Innovación y nuevas tecnologías, Salud Sector sanitario de Barbastro, Barbastro, Spain. [12]Epidemiology of Allergic and Respiratory Diseases, Department Institute Pierre Louis of Epidemiology and Public Health, INSERM and Sorbonne Université, Medical School Saint Antoine, Paris, France [13]Department of Allergy and Immunology, Hospital Quirón Bizkaia, Erandio, Spain. [14]ISGlobAL, Centre for Research in Environmental Epidemiology (CREAL), Barcelona, Spain. [15]IMIM (Hospital del Mar Research Institute), Barcelona, Spain. [16]CIBER Epidemiología y Salud Pública (CIBERESP), Barcelona, Spain. [17]Universitat Pompeu Fabra (UPF),Barcelona, Spain. [18]KYomed INNOV, Montpellier, France. [19]Argentine Society of Allergy and Immunopathology, Buenos Aires, Argentina. [20]Clinical Immunology and Allergy Unit, Department of Medicine Solna, Karolinska Institutet, Stockholm, and Astrid Lindgren Children's Hospital, Department of Pediatric Pulmonology and Allergy, Karolinska University Hospital, Stockholm, Sweden. [21]David Hide Asthma and Allergy Research Centre, Isle of Wight, United Kingdom. [22]Regionie Puglia, Bari, Italy. [23]Regione Liguria, Genoa, Italy. [24]Upper Airways Research Laboratory, ENT Dept, Ghent University Hospital, Ghent, Belgium. [25]Allergy and Respiratory Diseases, Ospedale Policlinico San Martino, University of Genoa, Italy. [26]PNDR, Portuguese National Programme for Respiratory Diseases, Faculdade de Medicina de Lisboa, Lisbon, Portugal. [27]Director of the Geriatric Unit, Department of Internal Medicine (DIBIMIS), University of Palermo, Italy. [28]Telbios SRL, Milan, Italy. [29]Universidade do Estado do Pará, Belem, Brazil. [30]Department of Medicine, University of Cape Town, Cape Town, South Africa. [31]Hospital Civil de Guadalajara Dr Juan I Menchaca, Guadalarara, Mexico. [32]iQ4U Consultants Ltd, London, UK. [33]Section of Respiratory Disease, Department of Oncology, Haematology and Respiratory Diseases, University of Modena and Reggio Emilia, Modena, Italy. [34]Department of Respiratory Medicine, Academic Medical Center (AMC), University of Amsterdam, The Netherlands. [35]Comprehensive Allergy Center Charité, Department of Dermatology and Allergy, Charité - Universitätsmedizin Berlin; Global Allergy and Asthma European Network (GA[2]LEN), Berlin, Germany. [36]Deptt of Respiratory Medicine, National Institute of Diseases of the Chest and Hospital, Dhaka, Bangladesh. [37]Centre for Individualized Medicine, Department of Pediatrics, Faculty of Medicine, Linköping, Sweden. [38]Department of Prevention of Environmental Hazards and Allergology, Medical University of Warsaw, Poland. [39]BIEBER. Department of Dermatology and Allergy, Rheinische Friedrich-Wilhelms-University Bonn, Bonn, Germany [40]Dept of Biochemistry and Clinical Chemistry, Faculty of Pharmacy with the Division of Laboratory Medicine, Warsaw Medical University, Warsaw, Poland. [41]Department of Dermatology and Allergy Centre, Odense University Hospital, Odense Research Center for Anaphylaxis (ORCA), Odense, Denmark. [42]Department of Respiratory Medicine and Allergology, University Hospital,

Lund, Sweden. [43]Department of Geriatrics, Montpellier University Hospital, Montpellier, France. [44]EA 2991, Euromov, University Montpellier, France. [45]Department of Pathophysiology and Transplantation, University of Milan, IRCCS Fondazione Ca'Granda Ospedale Maggiore Policlinico, Milan, Italy. [46]Argentine Association of Respiratory Medicine, Buenos Aires, Argentina. [47]Division of Internal Medicine, Asthma and Allergy, Barlicki University Hospital, Medical University of Lodz, Poland. [48]Pediatric Department, University of Verona Hospital, Verona, Italy. [49]Department of Public Health and Infectious Diseases, Sapienza University of Rome, Italy. [50]Second University of Naples and Institute of Translational Medicine, Italian National Research Council. [51]Woolcock Institute of Medical Research, University of Sydney and Woolcock Emphysema Centre and and Sydney Local Health District, Glebe, NSW, Australia. [52]Allergist, La Rochelle, France. [53]Associate professor of clinical medecine, Laval's University, Quebec city, Head of medecine department, Hôpital de la Malbaie, Quebec, Canada. [54]Quebec Heart and Lung Institute, Laval University, Québec City, Quebec, Canada. [55]Centre Hospitalier Valenciennes, France. [56]Head of Department of Clinical Pharmacy of Lithuanian University of Health Sciences, Kaunas, Lithuania. [57]Institute of Lung Health, Respiratory Biomedical Unit, University Hospitals of Leicester NHS Trust, Leicestershire, UK; Department of Infection, Immunity and Inflammation, University of Leicester, Leicester, UK. [58]Department of Health Research Methods, Evidence and Impact, Division of Immunology and Allergy, Department of Medicine, McMaster University, Hamilton, ON, Canada. [59]Chief of the University Pneumology Unit- AOU Molinette, Hospital City of Health and Science of Torino, Italy. [60]Universitätsmedizin der Johannes Gutenberg-Universität Mainz, Mainz, Germany. [61]Pharmacist, Municipality Pharmacy, Sarno, Italy. [62]University of Medicine and Pharmacy Victor Babes, Timisoara, Romania. [63]Instituto de Pediatria, Hospital Zambrano Hellion Tec de Monterrey, Monterrey, Mexico. [64]Imperial College and Royal Brompton Hospital, London, UK. [65]Centro Medico Docente La Trinidad, CaRacas, Venezuela. [66]Regional Director Assofarm Campania and Vice President of the Board of Directors of Cofaser, Salerno, Italy [67]Service de pneumologie, CHU et université d'Auvergne, Clermont-Ferrand, France. [68]Department of Respiratory Diseases, Montpellier University Hospital, France. [69]Imperial College London - National Heart and Lung Institute, Royal Brompton Hospital NHS, London, UK. [70]Federal University of Minas Gerais, Medical School, Department of Pediatrics, Belo Horizonte, Brazil [71]Assitant Director General, Montpellier, Région Occitanie, France. [72]Mayor of Sarno and President of Salerno Province, Director, Anesthesiology Service, Sarno "Martiri del Villa Malta" Hospital, Italy. [73]Allergy Section, Department of Internal Medicine, Hospital Vall d'Hebron & ARADyAL Spanish Research Network, Barcelona, Spain. [74]Department of Paediatrics, Oslo University Hospital and University of Oslo, Oslo, Norway. [75]CEDOC, Integrated Pathophysiological Mechanisms Research Group, Nova Medical School, Campo dos Martires da Patria, Lisbon, and Serviço de Imunoalergologia, Centro Hospitalar de Lisboa Central, EPE, Lisbon, Portugal. [76]Regional Ministry of Health of Andalusia, Seville, Spain. [77]Allergy and Asthma Associates of Southern California, Mission Viejo, CA, USA. [78]ASA - Advanced Solutions Accelerator, Clapiers, France. [79]Division of Allergy/Immunology, University of South Florida, Tampa, Fla, USA. [80]Celentano pharmacy, Massa Lubrense, Italy. [81]SOS Allergology and Clinical Immunology, USL Toscana Centro, Prato, Italy. [82]Allergy and Immunology Laboratory, Metropolitan University Hospital, Branquilla, Columbia. [83]Department of Public Health and Primary Care, Leiden University Medical Center, Leiden, The Netherlands [84]Capital Institute of Pediatrics, Chaoyang district, Beijing, China. [85]School of Medicine, University CEU San Pablo, Madrid, Spain. [86]David Tvildiani Medical University - AIETI Highest Medical School, David Tatishvili Medical Center Tbilisi, Georgia. [87]Pulmonolory Research Institute FMBA, Moscow, Russia and GARD Executive Committee, Moscow, Russia. [88]National Heart & Lung Institute, Imperial College, London, UK. [89]Specialist social worker, Sorrento, Italy. [90]Argentine Federation of Otorhinolaryngology Societies, Buenos Aires, Argentina. [91]Eskisehir Osmangazi University, Medical Faculty, ENT Department, Eskisehir,Turkey. [92]Medicine Department, IRCCS-Azienda Ospedaliera Universitaria San Martino, Genoa, Italy. [93]Universidade Federal da Bahia, Escola de Enfermagem, Brazil. [94]Plateforme Transversale d'Allergologie, Institut du Thorax, CHU de Nantes, Nantes, France. [95]LANUA International Healthcare Consultancy, Northern Ireland, UK. [96]Innovación y nuevas tecnologías, Salud Sector sanitario de Barbastro, Barbastro, Spain. [97]Innovation and Research Office, Department of Health and Social Solidarity, Autonomous Province of Trento, Italy. [98]Life and Health Sciences Research Institute (ICVS), School of Medicine, University of Minho, Braga, Portugal; ICVS/3B's, PT Government Associate Laboratory, Braga/Guimarães, Portugal. [99]Guadalarara, Mexico.

[100]FIMMG (Federazione Italiana Medici di Medicina Generale), Milan, Italy. [101]UCIBIO, REQUINTE, Faculty of Pharmacy and Competence Center on Active and Healthy Ageing of University of Porto(Porto4Ageing), Porto, Portugal. [102]Mexico City, Mexico. [103]IMT Mines Alès, Unversité Montpellier, Alès, France. [104]Department of Medicine, Nova Southeastern University, Davie, University of Miami Dept of Medicine, Miami, Florida, USA. [105]Regional Director Assofarm Campania and Vice President of the Board of Directors of Cofaser, Salerno, Italy. [106]ProAR – Nucleo de Excelencia em Asma, Federal University of Bahia, Brasil and WHO GARD Planning Group, Brazil. [107]Centre for Respiratory Medicine and Allergy, Institute of Inflammation and Repair, University of Manchester and University Hospital of South Manchester, Manchester, UK. [108]Medical Consulting Czarlewski, Levallois, France. [109]The Centre for Allergy Research, The Institute of Environmental Medicine, Karolinska Institutet, Stockholm, Sweden. [110]Azienda Provinciale per i Servizi Sanitari di Trento (APSS-Trento), Italy. [111]Department of Internal Medicine, Federal University of Santa Catarina, Trindade, Florianópolis, Santa Catarina, Brazil. [112]Sleep Unit, Department of Neurology, Hôpital Gui-de-Chauliac Montpellier, Inserm U1061, France. [113]Department of Dermatology and Allergy, Technische Universität München, Munich, Germany; ZAUM-Center for Allergy and Environment, Helmholtz Center Munich, Technische Universität München, Munich, Germany. [114]Allergy Division, Chest Disease Department, University Hospital of Strasbourg, Strasbourg, France. [115]EFA European Federation of Allergy and Airways Diseases Patients' Associations, Brussels, Belgium [116]AQuAS, Barcelna, Spain & EUREGHA, European Regional and Local Health Association, Brussels, Belgium [117]Policlínica Geral do Rio de Janeiro, Rio de Janeiro – Brasil [118]Department of Medicine, Surgery and Dentistry "Scuola Medica Salernitana", University of Salerno, Salerno, Italy. [119]Peercode BV, Geldermalsen,The Netherlands. [120]Social workers oordinator, Sorrento, Italy. [121]Federal University of the State of Rio de Janeiro, School of Medicine and Surgery, Rio de Janeiro, Brazil [122]Allergology and Immunology Discipline, "Iuliu Hatieganu" University of Medicine and Pharmacy, Cluj-Napoca, Romania. [123]Department of Medicine, Division of Clinical Immunology and Allergy, McMaster University, Hamilton, Ontario, Canada. [124]Laboratoire de Pharmacologie Respiratoire UPRES EA220, Hôpital Foch, Suresnes, Université Versailles Saint-Quentin, Université Paris Saclay, France. [125]Farmacie Dei Golfi Group, Massa Lubrense, Italy. [126]Rangueil-Larrey Hospital, Respiratory Diseases Department, Toulouse, France. [127]University Clinic of Pulmology and Allergy, Medical Faculty Skopje, R Macedonia. [128]Mexico City, Mexico. [129]Service de Pneumo-Allergologie, Centre Hospitalo-Universitaire de Béni-Messous, Algiers, Algeria. [130]Clinic of infectious, chest diseases, dermatology and allergology, Vilnius University, Vilnius, Lithuania. [131]Allergy and Clinical Immunology National Heart and Lung Institute, Imperial College London, UK. [132]Guy's and st Thomas' NHS Trust, Kings College London, UK. [133]Section of Allergy and Immunology, Saint Louis University School of Medicine, Saint Louis, Missouri, USA. [134]Pediatric Allergy and Immunology Unit, Children's Hospital, Ain Shams University, Cairo, Egypt. [135]Department of Computing Science, Umeå University, Sweden and Four Computing Oy, Finland. [136]Clinic of Children's Diseases, Faculty of Medicine, Vilnius University, Vilnius, Lithuania. [137]University of São Paulo Medical School, Sao Paulo, Brazil [138]Andalusian Agency for Healthcare Quality, Seville, Spain. [139]Global Allergy and Asthma Platform GAAPP, Vienna, Austria. [140]Division of Allergy, Department of Pediatric Medicine - The Bambino Gesù Children's Research Hospital Holy see, Rome, Italy. [141]Department of Otorhinolaryngology, Amsterdam, University Medical Centres, AMC, Amsterdam the Netherlands. [142]CINTESIS, Center for Research in Health Technologies and Information Systems, Faculdade de Medicina da Universidade do Porto, Porto, Portugal and MEDIDA, Lda, Porto, Portugal [143]Allergist, Reims, France. [144]Hospital general regional 1 "Dr Carlos Mc Gregor Sanchez Navarro" IMSS, Mexico City, Mexico. [145]Regional hospital of ISSSTE, Puebla, Mexico. [146]National Center for Disease Control and Public Health of Georgia, Tbilisi, Georgia. [147]Guadalarara, Mexico. [148]Allergy Clinic, National Institute of Respiratory Diseases, Mexico City, Mexico. [149]Department of Pulmonary Diseases, Istanbul University-Cerrahpasa, Cerrahpasa Faculty of Medicine, Istambul,Turkey. [150]Allergology unit, UHATEM "NIPirogov", Sofia, Bulgaria. [151]Medical University, Faculty of Public Health, Sofia. [152]Allergy and Immunology Division, Clinica Ricardo Palma, Lima, Peru. [153]Department of Internal Medicine, section of Allergology, Erasmus MC, Rotterdam, The Netherlands. [154]Allergy & Asthma Unit, Hospital San Bernardo Salta, Argentina. [155]Allergy Clinic, Hospital Regional del ISSSTE 'Lic. López Mateos', Mexico City, Mexico. [156]Head and Professor, Centro Regional de Excelencia CONACYT y WAO en Alergia, Asma e Inmunologia, Hospital Universitario , Universidad Autónoma de Nuevo León, Monterrey NL, Mexico. [157]Center of Allergy and Immunology, Georgian

Association of Allergology and Clinical Immunology, Tbilisi, Georgia. [158]Latvian Association of Allergists, Center of Tuberculosis and Lung Diseases, Riga, Latvia. [159]Federal District Base Hospital Institute, Brasília, Brazil. [160]Institute of Health Policy and Management iBMG, Erasmus University, Rotterdam, The Netherlands [161]University Hospital Olomouc – National eHealth Centre, Czech Republic. [162]Immunology and Allergy Division, Clinical Hospital, University of Chile, Santiago, Chile. [163]Skin and Allergy Hospital, Helsinki University Hospital, University of Helsinki, Helsinki, Finland. [164]Centich : centre d'expertise national des technologies de l'information et de la communication pour l'autonomie, Gérontopôle autonomie longévité des Pays de la Loire, Conseil régional des Pays de la Loire, Centre d'expertise Partenariat Européen d'Innovation pour un vieillissement actif et en bonne santé, Nantes, France. [165]Autonomous University of Baja California, Ensenada, Baja California, Mexico. [166]Department of Paediatrics and Child Health, University College Cork, Cork, Ireland. [167]Hospital General Regional 1 "Dr. Carlos MacGregor Sánchez Navarro" IMSS, Mexico City, Mexico. [168]Université Paris-Sud; Service de Pneumologie, Hôpital Bicêtre; Inserm UMR_S999, Le Kremlin Bicêtre, France. [169]Dipartimento di medicina, chirurgia e odontoiatria, università di Salerno, Italy. [170]Division for Health Innovation, Campania Region and Federico II University Hospital Naples (R&D and DISMET) Naples, Italy. [171]Servicio de Alergia e Immunologia, Clinica Santa Isabel, Buenos Aires, Argentina. [172]President, Libra Foundation, Buenos Aires, Argentina. [173]Medical University of Gdańsk, Department of Allergology, Gdansk, Poland. [174]Airway Disease Infection Section, National Heart and Lung Institute, Imperial College; MRC & Asthma UK Centre in Allergic Mechanisms of Asthma, London, UK. [175]Dept of Respiratory Medicine, Ghent University Hospital, Ghent, Belgium. [176]Hallym University College of Medicine, Hallym University Sacred Heart Hospital, Gyeonggi-do, South Korea. [177]Department of Clinical Immunology, Wrocław Medical University, Poland. [178]Ukrainina Medical Stomatological Academy, Poltava, Ukraine. [179]Pediatric Allergy and Asthma Unit, Hacettepe University School of Medicine, Ankara, Turkey. [180]Hacettepe University, School of Medicine, Department of Chest Diseases, Immunology and Allergy Division, Ankara, Turkey. [181]Allergy Centre, Tampere University Hospital, Tampere, Finland. [182]First Department of Family Medicine, Medical University of Lodz, Poland. [183]Institute of Social Medicine, Epidemiology and Health Economics, Charité - Universitätsmedizin Berlin, Berlin, and Institute for Clinical Epidemiology and Biometry, University of Wuerzburg, Germany. [184]Department of Medicine, McMaster University, HealthSciences Centre 3V47, West, Hamilton, Ontario, Canada. [185]National Research Center, Institute of Immunology, Federal Medicobiological Agency, Laboratory of Molecular immunology, Moscow, Russian Federation. [186]GARD Chairman, Geneva, Switzerland. [187]Allergy & Asthma Center Westend, Berlin, Germany. [188]Center for Rhinology and Allergology, Wiesbaden, Germany. [189]Department of Immunology and Allergy, Healthy Ageing Research Center, Medical University of Lodz, Lodz, Poland. [190]Children's Hospital and University of Helsinki, Finland. [191]Centre for Clinical Research Sörmland, Uppsala University, Eskilstuna, Sweden. [192]Faculty of Medicine, Vilnius University, Vilnius, Lithuania. [193]Department of Prevention of Envinronmental Hazards and Allergology, Medical University of Warsaw, Poland. [194]Center of Excellence in Asthma and Allergy, Médica Sur Clinical Foundation and Hospital, México City,, Mexico. [195]Presidente CMMC, Milano, Italy. [196]Head of the Allergy Department of Pedro de Elizalde Children's Hospital, Buenos Aires, Argentina. [197]University of Medicine and Pharmacy, Hochiminh City, Vietnam. [198]Federal University of Bahia, Brazil. [199]Sifmed, Milano, Italy. [200]State Key Laboratory of Respiratory Diseases, Guangzhou Institute of Respiratory Disease, the First Affiliated Hospital of Guangzhou Medical University, Guangzhou, China. [201]Departments of Internal Medicine and Pediatrics (Divisions of Allergy and Immunology), University of Tennessee College of Medicine, Germantown, TN, USA. [202]Scottish Centre for Respiratory Research, Cardiovascular & Diabetes Medicine, Medical Research Institute, Ninewells Hospital, University of Dundee, UK. [203]Oslo University Hospital, Department of Paediatrics, Oslo, and University of Oslo, Faculty of Medicine, Institute of Clinical Medicine, Oslo, Norway. [204]Department of Pulmonary Medicine, CHU Sart-Tilman, and GIGA I3 research group, Liege, Belgium. [205]Faculty of Health Sciences and CICS – UBI, Health Sciences Research Centre, University of Beira Interior, Covilhã, Portugal. [206]Department of Philosophical, Methodological and Instrumental Disciplines, CUCS, University of Guadalajara, Guadalajara, Mexico. [207]Department of Pulmonary Medicine, Rashid Hospital, Dubai, UAE. [208]Biomax Informatics AG, Munich, Germany. [209]Director Gerneral for Health and Social Care, Scottish Government, Edinburgh, UK. [210]Department of Respiratory Medicine, University of Bratislava, Bratislava, Slovakia. [211]Coimbra Institute for Clinical and Biomedical Research (iCBR), Faculty of Medicine, University of Coimbra, Portugal; Ageing@Coimbra EIP-AHA Reference Site, Coimbra, Portugal. [212]Medical center Iskar Ltd Sofia, Bulgaria. [213]Department of Medicine (RCSI), Bon Secours Hospital, Glasnevin, Dublin, Ireland. [214]Kronikgune, International Centre of Excellence in Chronicity Research Barakaldo, Bizkaia, Spain [215]Division of Clinical Immunology and Allergy, Laboratory of Behavioral Immunology Research, The University of Mississippi Medical Center, Jackson, Mississippi, USA. [216]Tobacco Control Research Centre;Iranian Anti Tobacco Association, Tehran, Iran. [217]Argentine Association of Allergy and Clinical Immunology, Buenos Aires, Argentina. [218]Mexico City, Mexico. [219]University of Southeast Bahia, Brazil. [220]Allergie-Centrum-Charité at the Department of Dermatology and Allergy, Charité - Universitätsmedizin Berlin, Germany [221]Maputo Central Hospital--Department of Paediatrics, Mozambique. [222]Veracruz, Mexico. [223]Sachs' Children and Youth Hospital, Södersjukhuset, Stockholm and Institute of Environmental Medicine, Karolinska Institutet, Stockholm, Sweden. [224]Allergy and Asthma Medical Group and Research Center, San Diego, California, USA. [225]CIRFF, Federico II University, Naples, Italy. [226]Department of Physiology, CHRU, University Montpellier, Vice President for Research, PhyMedExp, INSERM U1046, CNRS UMR 9214, France. [227]Croatian Pulmonary Society. [228]National Institute of Pneumology M Nasta, Bucharest, Romania. [229]Clinic for Pulmonary Diseases, Clinical Center of Serbia, Faculty of Medicine, University of Belgrade, Serbian Association for Asthma and COPD, Belgrade, Serbia. [230]Regione Piemonte, Torino, Italy. [231]Col Jardines de Sta Monica, Tlalnepantla, Mexico. [232]National Center for Research in Chronic Respiratory Diseases, Tishreen University School of Medicine, Latakia, Syria. [233]Department of Public health and health products, Paris Descartes University-Sorbonne Paris Cité, EA 4064 and Paris Municipal Department of social action, childhood, and health, Paris, France. [234]Paris municipal Department of social action, childhood, and health, Paris, France. [235]Lead Respiratory Physician Mater Dei Hospital Malta, Academic Head of Dept and Professor of Medicine University of Malta, Deputy Dean Faculty of Medicine and Surgery University of Medicine, La Valette, Malta. [236]Department of Medical Sciences, Allergy and Clinical Immunology Unit, University of Torino & Mauriziano Hospital, Torino, Italy. [237]Instituto de Prevision Social IPS HC, Socia de la SPAAI, Tesorera de la SLAAI, Asuncion, Paraguay. [238]Allergy Center, CUF Descobertas Hospital, Lisbon, Portugal. [239]Universidade de São Paulo, São Paulo, Brazil. [240]Institute of Medical Statistics, and Computational Biology, Medical Faculty, University of Cologne, Germany and CRI-Clinical Research International-Ltd, Hamburg, Germany. [241]General Pathology Institute, Faculty of Medicine, University of Coimbra, Portugal; Ageing@Coimbra EIP-AHA Reference Site, Coimbra, Portugal. [242]Federal University of Bahia, Brazil. [243]Rhinology Unit & Smell Clinic, ENT Department, Hospital Clínic; Clinical & Experimental Respiratory Immunoallergy, IDIBAPS, CIBERES, University of Barcelona, Spain. [244]Danish Commitee for Health Education, Copenhagen East, Denmark. [245]Food Allergy Referral Centre Veneto Region, Department of Women and Child Health, Padua General University Hospital, Padua, Italy. [246]Director, Medical Communications Consultant, MedScript Ltd, Dundalk, Co Louth, Ireland and Honorary Research Fellow, OPC, Cambridge, UK Ireland. [247]Johns Hopkins School of Medicine, Baltimore, Maryland, USA. [248]General Manager of COFASER - Pharmacy Services Consortium, Salerno, Italy. [249]Scientific Centre of Children's Health under the MoH, Moscow, Russian National Research Medical University named Pirogov, Moscow, Russia. [250]Director of Center of Allergy, Immunology and Respiratory Diseases, Santa Fe, Argentina Center for Allergy and Immunology, Santa Fe, Argentina. [251]Dept of Otorhinolaryngology, Medical University of Vienna, AKH, Vienna, Austria. [252]Hospital of the Hospitaller Brothers in Buda, Budapest, Hungary. [253]Die Hautambulanz and Rothhaar study center, Berlin, Germany. [254]Neumología y Alergología Infantil, Hospital La Fe, Valencia, Spain. [255]Center for Health Technology and Services Research - CINTESIS and Department of Internal Medicine, Centro Hospitalar Sao Joao, Porto, Portugal. [256]Caisse d'assurance retraite et de la santé au travail du Languedoc-Roussillon (CARSAT-LR), Montpellier, France. [257]Director of Department of Pharmacy of University of Naples Federico II, Naples, Italy. [258]ENT Department, University Hospital of Kinshasa, Kinshasa, Congo. [259]Department of Allergy, Immunology and Respiratory Medicine, Alfred Hospital and Central Clinical School, Monash University, Melbourne, Victoria, Australia; Department of Immunology, Monash University, Melbourne, Victoria, Australia. [260]Medical center "Research expert", Varna, Bulgaria. [261]National Hospital Organization, Tokyo National Hospital, Tokyo, Japan. [262]Dept of Otorhinolaryngology, Chiba University Hospital, Chiba, Japan. [263]Dept of Otolaryngology, Nippon Medical School, Tokyo, Japan. [264]Jalisco, Guadalarara. [265]Centre Hospitalier Universitaire Pédiatrique Charles de Gaulle, Ouagadougou, Burkina Faso. [266]Dept of Comparative

Medicine; Messerli Research Institute of the University of Veterinary Medicine and Medical University, Vienna, Austria.[267]Department of Immunology and Allergology, Faculty of Medicine and Faculty Hospital in Pilsen, Charles University in Prague, Pilsen, Czech Republic. [268]Division of Infection, Immunity & Respiratory Medicine, Royal Manchester Children's Hospital, University of Manchester, Manchester, UK, and Allergy Department, 2nd Pediatric Clinic, Athens General Children's Hospital "P&A Kyriakou," University of Athens, Athens, Greece. [269]Department of Allergy and Clinical Immunology, Ajou University School of Medicine, Suwon, South Korea. [270]Respiratory Medicine, Department of Medical Sciences, University of Ferrara, Ferrara, Italy. [271]Allergy and Respiratory Diseases, Ospedale Policlino San Martino -University of Genoa, Italy. [272]Farmacias Holon, Lisbon, Portugal. [273]Department of Pediatrics, Nippon Medical School, Tokyo, Japan. [274]University of Southern Denmark, Kolding, Denmark. [275]Université Grenoble Alpes, Laboratoire HP2, Grenoble, INSERM, U1042 and CHU de Grenoble, France. [276]Allergy Unit, CUF-Porto Hospital and Institute; Center for Research in Health Technologies and information systems CINTESIS, Universidade do Porto, Portugal. [277]Sociologist, municipality area n33, Sorrento, Italy. [278]Center for Rhinology and Allergology, Wiesbaden, Germany. [279]Department of Otorhinolaryngology, Head and Neck Surgery, Universitätsmedizin Mannheim, Medical Faculty Mannheim, Heidelberg University, Mannheim, Germany. [280]Centre for empowering people and communites, Dublin, UK. [281]Conseil Général de l'Economie Ministère de l'Economie, de l'Industrie et du Numérique, Paris, France. [282]Société de Pneumologie de Langue Française, Espace francophone de Pneumologie, Paris, France. [283]Département de pédiatrie, CHU de Grenoble, Grenoble France. [284]Medical School, University of Cyprus, Nicosia, Cyprus. [285]Children's Hospital Srebrnjak, Zagreb, School of Medicine, University J.J. Strossmayer, Osijek, Croatia. [286]Karl Landsteiner Institute for Clinical and Experimental Pneumology, Hietzing Hospital, Vienna, Austria. [287]University Hospital 'Sv. Ivan Rilski'", Sofia, Bulgaria. [288]Allergy Diagnostic and Clinical Research Unit, University of Cape Town Lung Institute, Cape Town, South Africa. [289]Vice-Presidente of IML, Milano, Italy. [290]Centre of Academic Primary Care, Division of Applied Health Sciences, University of Aberdeen, Aberdeen, United Kingdom ; Observational and Pragmatic Research Institute, Singapore, Singapore. [291]Department of Otorhinolaryngology University of Crete School of Medicine, Heraklion, Greece. [292]European Forum for Research and Education in Allergy and Airway Diseases (EUFOREA), Brussels, Belgium. [293]Cancun, Quintana Roo, Mexico. [294]LungenClinic Grosshansdorf, Airway Research Center North, Member of the German Center for Lung Research (DZL), Grosshansdorf, Germany Department of Medicine, Christian Albrechts University, Airway Research Center North, Member of the German Center for Lung Research (DZL), Kiel, Germany. [295]Department of Nephrology and Endocrinology, Karolinska University Hospital, Stockholm, Sweden. [296]Farmácia São Paio, Vila Nova de Gaia, Porto, Portugal. [297]St Vincent's Hospital and University of Sydney, Sydney, New South Wales, Australia. [298]Puebla, Mexico. [299]Serviço de Pneumologia-Hosp das Clinicas UFPE-EBSERH, Recife, Brazil. [300]Universidade Federal de São Paulo, São Paulo, Brazil. [301]Centre of Pneumology, Coimbra University Hospital, Portugal. [302]Polibienestar Research Institute, University of Valencia, Valencia, Spain. [303]Pediatric Allergy and Clinical Immunology, Hospital Angeles Pedregal, Mexico City, Mexico. [304]Getafe University Hospital Department of Geriatrics, Madrid, Spain. [305]Association Asthme et Allergie, Paris, France. [306]Universidade Federal do Rio de Janeiro, Rio de Janeiro, Brazil. [307]Primary Care Respiratory Research Unit Institutode Investigación Sanitaria de Palma IdisPa, Palma de Mallorca, Spain. [308]Allergy Unit, Presidio Columbus, Rome, Catholic University of Sacred Heart, Rome and IRCCS Oasi Maria SS, Troina, Italy. [309]Mexico City, Mexico. [310]Regione Piemonte, Torino, Italy. [311]Medical University of Graz, Department of Internal Medicine, Graz, Austria. [312]Serviço de Imunoalergologia Hospital da Luz Lisboa Portugal. [313]Hospital de Clinicas, University of Parana, Brazil. [314]Division of Allergy Asthma and Clinical Immunology, Emek Medical Center, Afula, Israel. [315]Honorary Clinical Research Fellow, Allergy and Respiratory Research Group, The University of Edinburgh, Edinburgh, UK. [316]Showa University School of Medicine, Tokyo, Japan. [317]Association of Finnish Pharmacies. [318]Allergy and Clinical Immunology Department, Centro Médico-Docente la, Trinidad and Clínica El Avila, Caracas, Venezuela. [319]Faculty of Medicine, Autnonous University of Madrid, Spain. [320]The Royal National TNE Hospital, University College London, UK. [321]DIBIMIS, University of Palermo, Italy. [322]Allergy Unit, Department of Dermatology, University Hospital of Zurich, Zürich, Switzerland. [323]Asthma Reference Center, Escola Superior de Ciencias da Santa Casa de Misericordia de Vitoria - Esperito Santo, Brazil. [324]THe Usher Institute of Population Health Sciences and Informatics, The University of Edinburgh, Edinburgh, UK. [325]Department of Pediatrics & Child Health,

Department of Immunology, Faculty of Medicine, University of Manitoba, Winnipeg, Manitoba, Canada. [326]INSERM, Université Grenoble Alpes, IAB, U 1209, Team of Environmental Epidemiology applied to Reproduction and Respiratory Health, Université Joseph Fourier, Grenoble, France. [327]Sociedad Paraguaya de Alergia Asma e Inmunologi´a, Paraguay. [328]Division of Allergy, Clinical Immunology and Rheumatology, Department of Pediatrics, Federal University of São Paulo, São Paulo, Brazil. [329]European Health Futures Forum (EHFF), Dromahair, Ireland. [330]ENT, Aachen, Germany. [331]Kyrgyzstan National Centre of Cardiology and Internal medicine, Euro-Asian respiratory Society, Bishkek, Kyrgyzstan. [332]University Hospital Olomouc, Czech Republic. [333]Department of Paediatric and Adolescent medicine, University Hospital of North Norway, Tromsø, Paediatric Research Group, Deptarment of Clinical Medicine, Faculty of Health Sciences, UiT The Arctic University of Norway, Tromsø, Norway. [334]Presidente, IML (Lombardy Medical Initiative), Bergamo, Italy. [335]Pulmonary Division, Heart Institute (InCor), Hospital da Clinicas da Faculdade de Medicina da Universidade de Sao Paulo, Sao Paulo, Brazil. [336]Public Health Institute of Vilnius University, Vilnius, Lithuania. [337]Universidade Federal do Estado do Rio de Janeiro, Rio de Janeiro - Brazil [338]RNSA (Réseau National de Surveillance Aérobiologique), Brussieu, France. [339]The Hospital for Sick Children, Dalla Lana School of Public Health, University of Toronto, Canada. [340]Imunoalergologia, Centro Hospitalar Universitário de Coimbra and Faculty of Medicine, University of Coimbra, Portugal. [341]Department of ENT, Medical University of Graz, Austria. [342]Campania Region, Division on Pharmacy and devices policy, Naples, Italy. [343]Department of Respiratory Medicine, Hvidovre Hospital & University of Copenhagen, Denmark. [344]Universidade Federal dos Pampas, Uruguaiana, Brazil. [345]Division of Immunopathology, Department of Pathophysiology and Allergy Research, Center for Pathophysiology, Infectiology and Immunology, Medical University of Vienna, Vienna, Austria. [346]Pneumology and Allergy Department CIBERES and Clinical & Experimental Respiratory Immunoallergy, IDIBAPS, University of Barcelona, Spain. [347]Vilnius University Institute of Clinical Medicine, Clinic of Children's Diseases, and Institute of Health Sciences, Department of Public Health, Vilnius, Lithuania; European Academy of Paediatrics (EAP/UEMS-SP), Brussels, Belgium. [348]Department of Lung Diseases and Clinical Immunology Allergology, University of Turku and Terveystalo allergy clinic, Turku, Finland. [349]PELyon; HESPER 7425, Health Services and Performance Resarch - Université Claude Bernard Lyon France.[350]Immunology and Allergy Unit, Department of Medicine Solna, Karolinska Institutet and University Hospital, Stockholm. [351]Department of Chest Medicine, Centre Hospitalier Universitaire UCL Namur, Université Catholique de Louvain, Yvoir, Belgium. [352]University of Bari Medical School, Unit of Geriatric Immunoallergology, Bari, Italy. [353]Pulmonary Unit, Department of Medical Specialties, Arcispedale SMaria Nuova/IRCCS, AUSL di Reggio Emilia, Italy. [354]FILHA, Finnish Lung Association, Helsinki, Finland. [355]Pulmonary Environmental Epidemiology Unit, CNR Institute of Clinical Physiology, Pisa, Italy ; and CNR Institute of Biomedicine and Molecular Immunology "A Monroy", Palermo, Italy. [356]Medical University, Plovdiv, Bulgaria, Department of Otorhinolaryngology, Plovdiv, Bulgaria. [357]Sotiria Hospital, Athens, Greece. [358]Dept of Otorhinolaryngology, Universitätsklinikum Düsseldorf, Germany. [359]Asthma UK, Mansell street, London, UK. [360]Nova Southeastern University, Fort Lauderdale, Florida, USA. [361]Department of Otolaryngology, Yong Loo Lin School of Medicine, National University of Singapore, Singapore, Singapore. [362]Department of Medicine, Clinical Immunology and Allergy, McMaster University, Hamilton, Ontario, Canada. [363]Division of Immunodermatology and Allergy Research, Department of Dermatology and Allergy, Hannover Medical School, Hannover, Germany. [364]Department of Medicine Solna, Immunology and Allergy Unit, Karolinska Institutet and Department of ENT diseases, Karolinska University Hospital, Stockholm, Sweden. [365]Eshelman School of Pharmacy, University of North Carolina, Chapel Hill, NC, USA. [366]International Primary Care Respiratory Group IPCRG, Aberdeen, Scotland. [367]Bradford Institute for Health Research, Bradford Royal Infirmary, Bradford, UK. [368]Allergologist - Medical College of Medical Faculty, Thracian University, Stara Zagora, Bulgaria. [369]Department of Research, Olmsted Medical Center, Rochester, Minnesota, USA. [370]Cyprus International Institute for Environmental & Public Health in Association with Harvard School of Public Health, Cyprus University of Technology, Limassol, Cyprus; Department of Pediatrics, Hospital "Archbishop Makarios III", Nicosia, Cyprus. [371]Celal Bayar University Department of Pulmonology, Manisa, Turkey. [372]The Allergy and Asthma Institute, Pakistan. [373]Department of Paediatrics and Child Health, Red Cross Children's Hospital, and MRC Unit on Child & Adolescent Health, University of Cape Town, Cape Town, South Africa. [374]Department of Otolaryngology Head and Neck Surgery, Beijing TongRen Hospital and Beijing

Institute of Otolaryngology, Beijing, China. [375]Universidad Católica de Córdoba, Córdoba, Argentina. [376]University Clinic of Respiratory and Allergic Diseases, Golnik, Slovenia. [377]Gesundheitsregion KölnBonn - HRCB Projekt GmbH, Kohln, Germany. [378]Akershus University Hospital, Department of Otorhinolaryngology, Akershus, Norway.

Competing interests

SBA reports personal fees from Boehringer Ingelheim, GSK, AstraZeneca, TEVA, grants from TEVA, MEDA outside the submitted work. JB reports personal fees and other from Chiesi, Cipla, Hikma, Menarini, Mundipharma, Mylan, Novartis, Sanofi-Aventis, Takeda, Teva, Uriach, other from Kyomed, outside the submitted work. AAC reports grants and personal fees from GlaxoSmithKline, personal fees from Boehrinher Ingelheim, personal fees from AstraZeneca, personal fees from Novartis, personal fees from Merk, Sharp & Dohma, personal fees from MEDA Pharma, personal fees from EUROFARMA, personal fees from Sanofi Aventis, outside the submitted work. MD reports other from Allergan, outside the submitted work. WF reports grants from Meda, outside the submitted work. TH reports personal fees from Mundipharma, Novartis, and Orion Pharma, outside the submitted work. JJ reports grants and personal fees from novartis, ALK abello, personal fees from thermofischer, astra zeneca outside the submitted work. PK reports personal fees from Adamed, Boehringer Ingelheim, AstraZeneca, Chiesi, FAES, Berlin Chemie, Novartis, Polpharma, Allergopharma, outside the submitted work. VK has received payment for consultancy from GSK and for lectures from Stallergens, Berlin-CHemie outside the submitted work. DLL reports personal fees from GSK, Astrazeneca, MEDA, Boehringer Ingelheim, Novartis, Grunenthal, UCB, Amstrong, Siegfried, DBV Technologies, MSD, Pfizer, grants from Sanofi, Astrazeneca, Novartis, UCB, GSK, TEVA, Chiesi, Boehringer Ingelheim, outside the submitted work. RM reports personal fees from ALK, grants from ASIT biotech, Leti, BitopAG, Hulka, Ursapharm, Optima; personal fees from allergopharma, Nuvo, Meda, Friulchem, Hexal, Servier, Bayer, Johnson&Johnson, Klosterfrau, GSK, MSD, FAES, Stada, UCB, Allergy Therapeutics; grants and personal fees from Bencard, Stallergenes; grants, personal fees and non-financial support from Lofarma; non-financial support from Roxall, Atmos, Bionorica, Otonomy, Ferrero; personal fees and non-financial support from Novartis. NP reports personal fees from Novartis, Faes Farma, BIOMAY, HAL, Nutricia Research, Menarini, Novartis, MEDA, Abbvie, MSD, Omega Pharma, Danone, grants from Menarini, outside the submitted work. JLP reports grants from Air Liquide Foundation, AGIR à dom, Astrazeneca, Fisher & Paykel, Mutualia, Philips, Resmed, Vitalaire, other from AGIR à dom, Astrazeneca, Boehringer Ingelheim, Jazz Pharmaceutical, Night Balance, Philips, Resmed, Sefam, outside the submitted work. OP reports grants and personal fees from ALK-Abelló, Allergopharma, Stallergenes Greer, HAL Allergy Holding B.V./HAL Allergie GmbH, Bencard Allergie GmbH/Allergy Therapeutics, Lofarma, Biotech Tools S.A., Laboratorios LETI/LETI Pharma, Anergis S.A., grants from Biomay, Nuvo, Circassia, Glaxo Smith Kline, personal fees from Novartis Pharma, MEDA Pharma, Mobile Chamber Experts (a GA[2]LEN Partner), Pohl-Boskamp, Indoor Biotechnologies, grants from, outside the submitted work. AMTB reports grants and personal fees from Novartis, Boehringer Ingelheim, Mundipharma, GSK (GlaxoSmithKline), personal fees from Teva Pharma, AstraZeneca, grants from Leti, outside the submitted work. SW reports personnal fees from Merck, GSK, Novartis, Behring, Shire, Sanofi, Barid Aralez, Mylan Meda, Pediapharm outside the submitted work.

Funding

FMC VIA LR.

References

1. Bousquet J, Khaltaev N, Cruz AA, Denburg J, Fokkens WJ, Togias A, et al. Allergic rhinitis and its impact on asthma (ARIA) 2008 update (in collaboration with the World Health Organization, GA(2)LEN and AllerGen). Allergy. 2008;63(Suppl 86):8–160.
2. Vandenplas O, Vinnikov D, Blanc PD, Agache I, Bachert C, Bewick M, et al. Impact of rhinitis on work productivity: a systematic review. J Allergy Clin Immunol Pract. 2018;6(4):1274–86.
3. Bousquet J, Bachert C, Canonica GW, Casale TB, Cruz AA, Lockey RJ, et al. Unmet needs in severe chronic upper airway disease (SCUAD). J Allergy Clin Immunol. 2009;124(3):428–33.
4. Bousquet J, Mantzouranis E, Cruz AA, Ait-Khaled N, Baena-Cagnani CE, Bleecker ER, et al. Uniform definition of asthma severity, control, and exacerbations: document presented for the World Health Organization Consultation on Severe Asthma. J Allergy Clin Immunol. 2010;126(5):926–38.
5. De Greve G, Hellings PW, Fokkens WJ, Pugin B, Steelant B, Seys SF. Endotype-driven treatment in chronic upper airway diseases. Clin Transl Allergy. 2017;7:22.
6. Cingi C, Gevaert P, Mosges R, Rondon C, Hox V, Rudenko M, et al. Multimorbidities of allergic rhinitis in adults: European Academy of Allergy and Clinical Immunology task force report. Clin Transl Allergy. 2017;7:17.
7. Frohlich M, Pinart M, Keller T, Reich A, Cabieses B, Hohmann C, et al. Is there a sex-shift in prevalence of allergic rhinitis and comorbid asthma from childhood to adulthood? A meta-analysis. Clin Transl Allergy. 2017;7:44.
8. Bousquet J, Addis A, Adcock I, Agache I, Agusti A, Alonso A, et al. Integrated care pathways for airway diseases (AIRWAYS-ICPs). Eur Respir J. 2014;44(2):304–23.
9. Hellings PW, Fokkens WJ, Bachert C, Akdis CA, Bieber T, Agache I, et al. Positioning the principles of precision medicine in care pathways for allergic rhinitis and chronic rhinosinusitis—an EUFOREA-ARIA-EPOS-AIRWAYS ICP statement. Allergy. 2017;72(9):1297–305.
10. Bousquet J, Schunemann HJ, Fonseca J, Samolinski B, Bachert C, Canonica GW, et al. MACVIA-ARIA Sentinel NetworK for allergic rhinitis (MASK-rhinitis): the new generation guideline implementation. Allergy. 2015;70(11):1372–92.
11. Hellings PW, Fokkens WJ, Akdis C, Bachert C, Cingi C, Dietz de Loos D, et al. Uncontrolled allergic rhinitis and chronic rhinosinusitis: where do we stand today? Allergy. 2013;68(1):1–7.
12. mHealth. New horizons for health through mobile technologies. Global Observatory for eHealth series—Vol. 3 WHO Library Cataloguing-in-Publication Data. 2011; http://www.who.int/goe/publications/goe_mhealth_web.pdf. Accessed 30 Sept 2018.
13. Ozdalga E, Ozdalga A, Ahuja N. The smartphone in medicine: a review of current and potential use among physicians and students. J Med Internet Res. 2012;14(5):e128.
14. Freifeld CC, Chunara R, Mekaru SR, Chan EH, Kass-Hout T, Ayala Iacucci A, et al. Participatory epidemiology: use of mobile phones for community-based health reporting. PLoS Med. 2010;7(12):e1000376.
15. Keijser W, de-Manuel-Keenoy E, d'Angelantonio M, Stafylas P, Hobson P, Apuzzo G, et al. DG Connect funded projects on information and communication technologies (ICT) for old age people: Beyond Silos, CareWell and SmartCare. J Nutr Health Aging. 2016;20(10):1024–33.
16. Mozaffar H, Cresswell KM, Williams R, Bates DW, Sheikh A. Exploring the roots of unintended safety threats associated with the introduction of hospital ePrescribing systems and candidate avoidance and/or mitigation strategies: a qualitative study. BMJ Qual Saf. 2017;26(9):722–733.
17. Talboom-Kamp EP, Verdijk NA, Harmans LM, Numans ME, Chavannes NH. An eHealth platform to manage chronic disease in primary care: an innovative approach. Interact J Med Res. 2016;5(1):e5.
18. Lee L, Sheikh A. Understanding stakeholder interests and perspectives in evaluations of health IT. Stud Health Technol Inf. 2016;222:53–62.
19. Geryk LL, Roberts CA, Sage AJ, Coyne-Beasley T, Sleath BL, Carpenter DM. Parent and clinician preferences for an asthma app to promote adolescent self-management: a formative study. JMIR Res Protoc. 2016;5(4):e229.
20. Bousquet J, Chavannes NH, Guldemond N, Haahtela T, Hellings PW, Sheikh A. Realising the potential of mHealth to improve asthma and allergy care: how to shape the future. Eur Respir J. 2017;49(5):1700447.

21. Lau AY, Arguel A, Dennis S, Liaw ST, Coiera E. "Why Didn't it Work?" Lessons from a randomized controlled trial of a web-based personally controlled health management system for adults with asthma. J Med Internet Res. 2015;17(12):e283.

22. Simpson AJ, Honkoop PJ, Kennington E, Snoeck-Stroband JB, Smith I, East J, et al. Perspectives of patients and healthcare professionals on mHealth for asthma self-management. Eur Respir J. 2017. https://doi.org/10.1183/13993003.01966-2016.

23. Bousquet J, Van Cauwenberge P, Khaltaev N. Allergic rhinitis and its impact on asthma. J Allergy Clin Immunol. 2001;108(5 Suppl):S147–334.

24. Brozek JL, Bousquet J, Baena-Cagnani CE, Bonini S, Canonica GW, Casale TB, et al. Allergic Rhinitis and its Impact on Asthma (ARIA) guidelines: 2010 revision. J Allergy Clin Immunol. 2010;126(3):466–76.

25. Brozek JL, Bousquet J, Agache I, Agarwal A, Bachert C, Bosnic-Anticevich S, et al. Allergic Rhinitis and its Impact on Asthma (ARIA) guide- lines—2016 revision. J Allergy Clin Immunol. 2017;140(4):950–8.

26. Bousquet J, Hellings PW, Agache I, Bedbrook A, Bachert C, Bergmann KC, et al. ARIA 2016: care pathways implementing emerging technologies for predictive medicine in rhinitis and asthma across the life cycle. Clin Transl Allergy. 2016;6:47.

27. Lombardi C, Musicco E, Rastrelli F, Bettoncelli G, Passalacqua G, Canonica GW. The patient with rhinitis in the pharmacy. A cross-sectional study in real life. Asthma Res Pract. 2015;1:4.

28. Bousquet J, Schunemann HJ, Hellings PW, Arnavielhe S, Bachert C, Bedbrook A, et al. MACVIA clinical decision algorithm in adolescents and adults with allergic rhinitis. J Allergy Clin Immunol. 2016;138(2):367–74 (e2).

29. Bourret R, Bousquet J, Mercier J, Camuzat T, Bedbrook A, Demoly P, et al. MASK rhinitis, a single tool for integrated care pathways in allergic rhinitis. World Hosp Health Serv. 2015;51(3):36–9.

30. Hellings PW, Muraro A, Fokkens W, Mullol J, Bachert C, Canonica GW, et al. A common language to assess allergic rhinitis control: results from a survey conducted during EAACI 2013 Congress. Clin Transl Allergy. 2015;5:36.

31. Klimek L, Bergmann KC, Biedermann T, Bousquet J, Hellings P, Jung K, et al. Visual analogue scales (VAS): measuring instruments for the documentation of symptoms and therapy monitoring in cases of allergic rhinitis in everyday health care: position Paper of the German Society of Allergology (AeDA) and the German Society of Allergy and Clinical Immunology (DGAKI), ENT Section, in collaboration with the working group on Clinical Immunology, Allergology and Environmental Medicine of the German Society of Otorhinolaryngology, Head and Neck Surgery (DGHNOKHC). Allergo J Int. 2017;26(1):16–24.

32. Bousquet J, Farrell J, Crooks G, Hellings P, Bel EH, Bewick M, et al. Scaling up strategies of the chronic respiratory disease programme of the Euro- pean Innovation Partnership on Active and Healthy Ageing (Action Plan B3: Area 5). Clin Transl Allergy. 2016;6:29.

33. Bousquet J, Caimmi DP, Bedbrook A, Bewick M, Hellings PW, Devillier P, et al. Pilot study of mobile phone technology in allergic rhinitis in Euro- pean countries: the MASK-rhinitis study. Allergy. 2017;72(6):857–65.

34. Bousquet J, Bewick M, Arnavielhe S, Mathieu-Dupas E, Murray R, Bed- brook A, et al. Work productivity in rhinitis using cell phones: the MASK pilot study. Allergy. 2017;72(10):1475–84.

35. Aristodimou A, Antoniades A, Pattichis CS. Privacy preserving data pub- lishing of categorical data through k-anonymity and feature selection. Healthc Technol Lett. 2016;3(1):16–21.

36. Aldeen YA, Salleh M, Razzaque MA. A comprehensive review on privacy preserving data mining. Springerplus. 2015;4:694.

37. Protection of personal data. Article 29 data protection working party. Opinion 05/2014 on anonymisation techniques. European Commission Justice Data Protection. 2014;0829/14/EN WP216. http://ec.europa.eu/justice/data-protection/index_en.htm. Accessed 30 Sept 2018.

38. Regulation (EU) 2016/679 of the European Parliamant and of the Council of 27 April 2016 on the protection of natural persons with regard to the processing of personal data and on the free movement of such data, and repealing Directive 95/46/EC (General Data Protection Regulation). Offi- cial Organ of the European Union. 2016. http://eur-lex.europa.eu/legal -content/EN/TXT/PDF/?uri=CELEX:32016R0679&from=EN. Accessed 30 Sept 2018.

39. Article 28 EU General Data Protection Regulation (EU-GDPR). 2018. https ://www.eugdpr.org/. Accessed 30 Sept 2018.

40. Directive 2002/58/EC of the European Parliament and of the Council of 12 July 2002 concerning the processing of personal data and the protec- tion of privacy in the electronic communications sector (Directive on privacy and electronic communications). Off J Eur Commun L 201, 37; 31 July 2002.

41. Directive 2009/136/EC of The European Parliament and of the Council of 25 November 2009 amending Directive 2002/22/EC on universal service and users' rights relating to electronic communications networks and services, Directive 2002/58/EC concerning the processing of personal data and the protection of privacy in the electronic communications sec- tor and Regulation (EC) No 2006/2004 on cooperation between national authorities responsible for the enforcement of consumer protection laws. Off J Eur Union, L 337, 11; 18 December 2009.

42. Sweeney L. k-anonymity: a model for protecting privacy. Int J Uncertain Fuz Knowl Syst. 2002;10:557–70.

43. El Emam K, Dankar FK, Issa R, et al. A globally optimal k-anonymity method for the de-identification of health data. J Am Med Inform Assoc. 2009;16:670–82.

44. Samreth D, Arnavielhe S, Ingenrieth F, Bedbrook A, Onorato GL, Murray R, et al. Geolocation with respect to personal privacy for the Allergy Diary app—a MASK study. World Allergy Organ J. 2018;11(1):15. https://doi.org/10.1186/s40413-018-0194-3.

45. Bland JM, Altman DG. Statistical methods for assessing agree- ment between two methods of clinical measurement. Lancet. 1986;1(8476):307–10.

46. Bousquet J, Agache I, Aliberti MR, Angles R, Annesi-Maesano I, Anto JM, et al. Transfer of innovation on allergic rhinitis and asthma multimorbid- ity in the elderly (MACVIA-ARIA)—EIP on AHA Twinning Reference Site (GARD research demonstration project). Allergy. 2018;73(1):77–92.

47. Konig HH, Bernert S, Angermeyer MC, Matschinger H, Martinez M, Vilagut G, et al. Comparison of population health status in six european coun- tries: results of a representative survey using the EQ-5D questionnaire. Med Care. 2009;47(2):255–61.

48. Smith AF, Pitt AD, Rodruiguez AE, Alio JL, Martl N, Teus M, et al. The economic and quality of life impact of seasonal allergic conjunctivitis in a Spanish setting. Ophthalmic Epidemiol. 2005;12(4):233–42.

49. Bousquet J, VandenPlas O, Bewick M, Arnavielhe S, Bedbrook A, Murray R, et al. The Work Productivity and Activity Impairment Allergic Specific (WPAI-AS) Questionnaire using mobile technology: the MASK study. J Investig Allergol Clin Immunol. 2018;28(1):42–4.

50. Azevedo P, Correia de Sousa J, Bousquet J, Bugalho-Almeida A, Del Giacco SR, Demoly P, et al. Control of Allergic Rhinitis and Asthma Test (CARAT): dissemination and applications in primary care. Prim Care Respir J. 2013;22(1):112–6.

51. Fonseca JA, Nogueira-Silva L, Morais-Almeida M, Azevedo L, Sa-Sousa A, Branco-Ferreira M, et al. Validation of a questionnaire (CARAT10) to assess rhinitis and asthma in patients with asthma. Allergy. 2010;65(8):1042–8.

52. Nogueira-Silva L, Martins SV, Cruz-Correia R, Azevedo LF, Morais-Almeida M, Bugalho-Almeida A, et al. Control of allergic rhinitis and asthma test— a formal approach to the development of a measuring tool. Respir Res. 2009;10:52.

53. van der Leeuw S, van der Molen T, Dekhuijzen PN, Fonseca JA, van Gemert FA, Gerth van Wijk R, et al. The minimal clinically important dif- ference of the control of allergic rhinitis and asthma test (CARAT): cross- cultural validation and relation with pollen counts. NPJ Prim Care Respir Med. 2015;25:14107.

54. Johns MW. Reliability and factor analysis of the Epworth Sleepiness Scale. Sleep. 1992;15(4):376–81.

55. Leger D, Annesi-Maesano I, Carat F, Rugina M, Chanal I, Pribil C, et al. Allergic rhinitis and its consequences on quality of sleep: an unexplored area. Arch Intern Med. 2006;166(16):1744–8.

56. Kopp-Kubel S. International Nonproprietary Names (INN) for pharmaceu- tical substances. Bull World Health Organ. 1995;73(3):275–9.

57. Santo K, Richtering SS, Chalmers J, Thiagalingam A, Chow CK, Redfern J. Mobile phone apps to improve medication adherence: a systematic stepwise process to identify high-quality apps. JMIR Mhealth Uhealth. 2016;4(4):e132.

58. Thakkar J, Kurup R, Laba TL, Santo K, Thiagalingam A, Rodgers A, et al. Mobile telephone text messaging for medication adherence in chronic disease: a meta-analysis. JAMA Intern Med. 2016;176(3):340–9.

59. Bousquet J, Arnavielhe S, Bedbrook A, Alexis-Alexandre G, van Eerd M, Murray R, et al. Treatment of allergic rhinitis using mobile technology with real world data: the MASK observational pilot study. Allergy. 2018;73(9):1763–74.

60. Devillier P, Chassany O, Vicaut E, de Beaumont O, Robin B, Dreyfus JF, et al. The minimally important difference in the Rhinoconjunctivitis Total Symptom Score in grass-pollen-induced allergic rhinoconjunctivitis. Allergy. 2014;69(12):1689–95.

61. Onder G, Palmer K, Navickas R, Jureviciene E, Mammarella F, Strandzheva M, et al. Time to face the challenge of multimorbidity. A European perspective from the joint action on chronic diseases and promoting healthy ageing across the life cycle (JA-CHRODIS). Eur J Intern Med. 2015;26(3):157–9.

62. Bousquet J, Onorato GL, Bachert C, Barbolini M, Bedbrook A, Bjermer L, et al. CHRODIS criteria applied to the MASK (MACVIA-ARIA Sentinel NetworK) Good Practice in allergic rhinitis: a SUNFRAIL report. Clin Transl Allergy. 2017;7:37.

63. Mokkink LB, Terwee CB, Patrick DL, Alonso J, Stratford PW, Knol DL, et al. The COSMIN study reached international consensus on taxonomy, terminology, and definitions of measurement properties for health-related patient-reported outcomes. J Clin Epidemiol. 2010;63(7):737–45.

64. Caimmi D, Baiz N, Tanno LK, Demoly P, Arnavielhe S, Murray R, et al. Validation of the MASK-rhinitis visual analogue scale on smartphone screens to assess allergic rhinitis control. Clin Exp Allergy. 2017;47(12):1526–33.

65. Bousquet J, Devillier P, Anto JM, Bewick M, Haahtela T, Arnavielhe S, et al. Daily allergic multimorbidity in rhinitis using mobile technology: a novel concept of the MASK study. Allergy. 2018;73(8):1622–31.

66. Tan R, Cvetkovski B, Kritikos V, Price D, Yan K, Smith P, et al. Identifying the hidden burden of allergic rhinitis (AR) in community pharmacy: a global phenomenon. Asthma Res Pract. 2017;3:8.

67. Carr WW, Yawn BP. Management of allergic rhinitis in the era of effective over-the-counter treatments. Postgrad Med. 2017;129(6):572–80.

68. Members of the Workshop. ARIA in the pharmacy: management of allergic rhinitis symptoms in the pharmacy. Allergic rhinitis and its impact on asthma. Allergy. 2004;59(4):373–87

69. Bousquet J, Cruz A, Robalo-Cordeiro C. Obstructive sleep apnoea syndrome is an under-recognized cause of uncontrolled asthma across the life cycle. Rev Port Pneumol. 2016;22(1):1–3

70. Bousquet J, Agache I, Anto JM, Bergmann KC, Bachert C, Annesi-Maesano I, et al. Google Trends terms reporting rhinitis and related topics differ in European countries. Allergy 2017;72(8):1261–6.

71. Bousquet J, O'Hehir RE, Anto JM, D'Amato G, Mösges R, Hellings PW, Van Eerd M, Sheikh A. Assessment of thunderstorm-induced asthma using Google Trends. J Allergy Clin Immunol. 2017;140(3):891–3.

Alpha 1 antitrypsin distribution in an allergic asthmatic population sensitized to house dust mites

I. Suárez-Lorenzo[1]* , F. Rodríguez de Castro[2], D. Cruz-Niesvaara[3], E. Herrera-Ramos[4], C. Rodríguez-Gallego[4] and T. Carrillo-Diaz[5]

Abstract

Background and objective: Severe alpha1 antitrypsin deficiency has been clearly associated with pulmonary emphysema, but its relationship with bronchial asthma remains controversial. Some deficient alpha 1 antitrypsin (AAT) genotypes seem to be associated with asthma development. The objective of this study was to analyze the distribution of AAT genotypes in asthmatic patients allergic to house dust mites (HDM), and to asses a possible association between these genotypes and severe asthma.

Methods: A cross-sectional cohort study of 648 patients with HDM allergic asthma was carried out. Demographic, clinical and analytical variables were collected. PI*S and PI*Z AAT deficient alleles of the SERPINA1 gene were assayed by real-time PCR.

Results: Asthma was intermittent in 253 patients and persistent in 395 patients (246 mild, 101 moderate and 48 severe). One hundred and forty-five asthmatic patients (22.4%) with at least one mutated allele (S or Z) were identified. No association between the different genotypes and asthma severity was found. No significant differences in all clinical and functional tests, as well as nasal eosinophils, IgA and IgE serum levels were observed. Peripheral eosinophils were significantly lower in patients with the PI*MS genotype (p = 0.0228). Neither association between deficient AAT genotypes or serum ATT deficiency (AATD) and development of severe asthma, or correlation between ATT levels and FEV1 was observed.

Conclusion: In conclusion, the distribution of AAT genotypes in HDM allergic asthmatic patients did not differ from those found in Spanish population. Neither severe ATTD or deficient AAT genotypes appear to confer different clinical expression of asthma.

Keywords: Alpha 1 antitrypsin, Alpha 1 antitrypsin deficiency, House dust mites, Asthma, Allergy

Background

Alpha-1 antitrypsin (AAT) is a serine proteinase inhibitor (PI) that protects alveoli against the destructive effects of neutrophil elastase, proteinase 3 and cathepsin G, which cause destruction of pulmonary parenchyma [1, 2]. Alpha-1 antitrypsin deficiency (AATD) is an autosomal codominant genetic condition first described by Laurell and Erikson in 1963 [3]. Multiple genetic variants in the gene encoding AAT, *SERPINA1*, are associated with low serum AAT levels. The most common deficient alleles are protease inhibitor PI*S and PI*Z, being PI*M the normal variant. Pi*ZZ individuals have severe AAT deficiency, with only 10% of normal serum levels as compared to Pi*MM subjects. Individuals homozygous for the Pi*S (Pi*SS) alleles have approximately 60% of normal serum ATT levels [4, 5]. Although AATD was initially thought of as a rare disease, it has proven to be underdiagnosed in many countries [5, 6]. The distribution of deficient alleles depends on the location; for example, Z variant is more

---

*Correspondence: isadora.suarez101@alu.ulpgc.es
[1] Postgraduate and Doctoral School, Universidad de Las Palmas de Gran Canaria, Camino Real de San Roque, 1, 35015 Las Palmas de Gran Canaria, Las Palmas, Spain
Full list of author information is available at the end of the article

prevalent in North and Western Europe, while S variant has a higher prevalence in the South of Europe, particularly in Spain [7]. Nowadays, different national registries provide the exact prevalence of AATD. However, it is still not considered sufficiently by physicians in the diagnostic phase [8, 9].

Worldwide, AATD has been frequently related to chronic obstructive pulmonary disease (COPD), premature emphysema and liver failure [10–13], but its relationship with asthma remains controversial [14]. AATD is associated with wheezing and dyspnea, which are also characteristic symptoms of asthma. That is why it is sometimes difficult to differentiate between these conditions [14–16] and, according to the American Thoracic Society (ATS)/European Respiratory Society (ERS) and the World Health organization (WHO), diagnosis of asthma is one of the clinical indications for genetic AATD testing [17, 18].

The aim of this study is to analyze the distribution of the most common ATT genotypes in a cohort of asthmatic patients sensitized to house dust mites (HDM). Furthermore, this study attempts to investigate the influence of ATTD and the presence of certain genotypes on the severity of allergic asthma.

Methods

A cross-sectional cohort study of HDM-sensitive asthmatic patients (skin prick test and specific immunoglobulin E) was carried out. Asthmatic subjects were recruited through the Allergy Clinic of the "Hospital Universitario de Gran Canaria Doctor Negrín" (Canary Islands). All of them were Caucasian, aged over 12. They all had a diagnosis of asthma, with or without rhinitis or other allergic conditions, and complained of typical asthma symptoms such as wheezing, dyspnea and/or other symptoms which they had suffered from over the previous two years. Patients were divided into four groups (intermittent and persistent mild, moderate and severe), according to the severity of their disease and following the Spanish asthma guideline—GEMA4.0 [19]. Written informed consent was obtained from all subjects before participating in the study, which was approved by the Ethics Committee of the hospital.

Asthma was diagnosed on the basis of a history of asthma symptoms and clinical examination (dyspnea, chest tightness, wheezing, cough), and a significant reversibility of their forced expiratory volume in one second (FEV1), as measured with a spirometer (Flowscreen, Viasys, Germany) upon treatment with bronchodilators, at least in one visit during the patient follow-up [19]. Fractional exhaled nitric oxide (FeNO) was also performed (NIOX-MINO® Aerocrine).

Skin-prick tests were performed with several dust mite allergens (*Dermatophagoides pteronyssinus*, *Dermatophagoides farinae*, *Blomia tropicalis*, *Acarus siro*, *Lepidoglyphus destructor* and *Tyrophagus putrescientae*) from ALK Abelló, Spain. A positive skin-prick test was defined as a mean wheal diameter of at least 3 mm or larger than that of the negative control following current guidelines [20].

In all subjects, blood eosinophils and neutrophils, and total serum immunoglobulin A (IgA), immunoglobulin E (IgE) and specific IgE to *D. pteronyssinus*, *D. farinae*, *B. tropicalis*, *A. siro*, *L. destructor* and *T. putrescientae* (ImmunoCap, Phadia, Sweden) were determined. ATT serum levels were measured by nephelometry (BNII, Siemens, Erlangen, Germany).

ATT genotypes were determined by using real-time polymerase chain reaction (PCR) and LigthCycler 2.0 for the detection of the mutation according to the technique previously described [21].

Statistical analysis was performed using the nonparametric Kruskal–Wallis test for quantitative variables and Chi square or Fisher tests for qualitative variables. Binary logistic regression was used to determine the association between genotypes and the presence or absence of severe persistent asthma, adjusting for age, smoking habit, significant comorbidity, previous treatment received and some analytical values. The possible correlation between the serum levels of ATT and bronchial functional test parameters was evaluated by Spearman's rank correlation coefficient. A value of $p < 0.05$ was considered to be statistically significant. All analyses were performed using the R Project (Version 1.0.153) [22].

Results

During a period of 22 months, 648 asthmatic patients over 12 years (median age 29 years) who were allergic to HDM were recruited into the study. Four hundred and twenty-five (66%) were females and 54 (8%) were smokers. Demographic and clinical characteristics of the patients are listed in Table 1.

According to the GEMA4.0, 253 asthmatic patients were classified as intermittent and 395 as persistent (246 mild, 101 moderate, and 48 severe). Patients with severe asthma were significantly older ($p = 1.72^{-12}$) as has been previously reported [23]. In addition, a slightly higher percentage of ex-smokers were seen in the group with severe asthma ($p = 0.0301$), which was considered in the posterior multivariate analysis. Regarding the clinical comorbidity, there was a significantly higher proportion of patients with conjunctivitis in the intermittent asthma group ($p = 0.008201$) and polyposis in the moderate group ($p = 0.00013$), while no significance was observed in terms of rhinitis, chronic sinusitis, atopic dermatitis,

Table 1 Demographic, clinical and analytical features of the studied population

	Global (n = 648)	Intermittent (n = 253)	Mild (n = 246)	Moderate (n = 101)	Severe (n = 48)	P value*
Sex, n (%)						0.316
Male	233 (34)	90 (36)	84 (34)	38 (38)	11 (23)	
Female	425 (66)	163 (64)	162 (66)	62 (62)	37 (77)	
Age, years						$1.72e-12$[‡]
Median (IQ_{25-75})	29 (20–38)	27 (20–36)	27 (19–35)	34 (24–44)	41 (34–53)	
Smoker n (%)	54 (8)	24 (9.5)	21 (8.5)	9 (9)	0	0.369
Obesity n (%)	115 (18)	46 (18.2)	36 (14.9)	19 (19.2)	13 (27)	0.221
Conjunctivitis n (%)	107 (16.5)	54 (21.3)	40 (16.3)	11 (11)	2 (4.2)	0.008201[‡]
Rhinitis n (%)	640 (98.8)	250 (98.8)	244 (99.2)	99 (99)	47 (97.9)	0.885
Polyposis n (%)	17 (2.62)	1 (0.8)	2 (0.8)	9 (9)	4 (8.3)	0.00013[‡]
Chronic sinusitis n (%)	32 (4.94)	11 (4.3)	11 (4.5)	8 (8)	2 (4.2)	0.519
Atopic dermatitis n (%)	23 (3.55)	12 (4.7)	5 (2)	5 (5)	1 (2.1)	0.295
Previous pneumonia n (%)	5 (0.77)	1 (0.4)	2 (0.8)	1 (1)	1 (2.1)	0.332
FEV1 (l)						$3.98e-22$[‡]
Median (IQ_{25-75})	2.9 (2.5–3.4)	3.1 (2.7–3.6)	2.9 (2.6–3.5)	2.6 (2.2–3.1)	2.0 (1.7–2.5)	
FEV1 (%)						$1.14e-24$[‡]
Median (IQ_{25-75})	90 (81–100)	95 (88–104)	90.5 (84–98)	78 (68–90)	74 (60–81)	
Feno (ppb)						0.873
Median (IQ_{25-75})	40 (23–72)	41 (23–73)	41 (26–72)	35.5 (19–69)	38 (21–60)	
Total IgE (IU/ml)[§]						0.0789
Median (IQ_{25-75})	255 (117–563)	225 (111.5–533)	274 (113–615)	305 (124–711)	213 (93–426)	
IgE Dermatophagoides pteronyssinus						0.0637
Median (IQ_{25-75})	42 (15–100)	34 (13–99)	51 (21–101)	44 (16–100)	42 (5.8–98)	
IgE Dermatophagoides farinae						0.119
Median (IQ_{25-75})	27 (11–79)	21 (10–66)	34 (12–81)	26 (11–85)	32 (5.7–78.8)	
IgE Blomia tropicalis						0.931
Median (IQ_{25-75})	7 (2.1–21)	7 (2–19)	6.8 (3–23)	8.8 (2.1–20)	6.9 (3–19)	
IgE Lepidoglyphus destructor						0.448
Median (IQ_{25-75})	2.4 (1–7)	2.6 (0.9–6)	2.1 (1–6)	2.1 (1–11)	4.1 (2–9)	
IgE Tyrophagus putrescientae						0.743
Median (IQ_{25-75})	2 (1–7.5)	3 (1–7)	2 (1–7)	2 (1–8.5)	3.1 (1–1.9)	
IgE Acarus siro						0.389
Median (IQ_{25-75})	2.6 (1–7)	2.7 (0.9–7.5)	2.4 (1–7)	5 (1–9)	1.3 (0.7–1.8)	
IgA (mg/dL)[§]						0.00024[‡]
Median (IQ_{25-75})	217 (162–279)	220.5 (164–292)	205.5 (157–260)	205.5 (161–271.5)	268 (220–334)	
Eosinophils (10^9/L)[§]						0.153
Median (IQ_{25-75})	0.3 (0.2–0.5)	0.3 (0.2–0.5)	0.3 (0.2–0.5)	0.3 (0.2–0.5)	0.3 (0.1–0.5)	
Nasal cytology eosinophils (%)						0.265
Median (IQ_{25-75})	37.5 (10–70)	40 (10–70)	40 (15–70)	30 (5–50)	40 (5–60)	
AAT (mg/dL)[§]						0.945
Median (IQ_{25-75})	134 (118–154)	135 (115–159)	134 (118–154)	133 (116–149)	135 (119–144)	

FEV1 (forced expiratory volume in the 1 s), FENO (fractional exhaled nitric oxide), IgE (immunoglobulin E), IgA (immunoglobulin A), AAT (alpha1 antitrypsin)

* Kruskal–Wallis statistic analysis for continuous non normal variables and Chi square or F-test for nominal ones

[‡] Statistical significance, p value < 0.01

[§] Normal value IgE: 10–179 IU/ml; Normal value of IgA: 80–310 mg/dl; Normal value of blood eosinophils: 0–0.54 × 109/L; Normal value ATT: 100–200 mg/dL (1.0–2.0 g/L)

previous pneumonias or even frequent respiratory infections the year before entering the study. Respiratory function values and analytical determinations are also represented in Table 1.

Median blood eosinophil count was 0.3×10^9/L (0.2–0.5). Median percentage of eosinophils found in the nasal cytology was 37.5% (10–70), with no significant differences among all stages of disease severity. The median serum IgE was high, 255 IU/ml (117–563) as compared to the normal value (< 100 IU/ml), but there was no significant difference among asthma groups. The values of specific IgE were quite similar among all groups. IgA serum levels were significantly higher in patients with severe asthma (268 mg/dl- normal value 80–310 mg/dl) as compared to the other groups (moderate [205.5 mg/dl], mild [205.5 mg/dl] and intermittent [220.5 mg/dl]) (p = 0.00024).

Median AAT value was 134 mg/dl (118-154), within normal range (100–200 mg/dL), and no significant difference was observed according to the severity of the disease. Sixty-six (10.2%) asthmatics had serum AAT levels below the lower limit of normal (< 100 mg/dl) and only three (0.5%) had severe deficiency (< 57 mg/dl) [24].

One hundred and forty-five patients (22.4%) had a deficient AAT genotype. No individual with severe AAT deficiency genotype (PI*ZZ) was identified in our series.

Demographic and clinical characteristics according to PI genotype are shown in Table 2. The distribution of all different severity asthma stages among all AAT genotypes was similar, and no significant difference was observed. However, peripheral eosinophils were significantly lower in the PI*MS group (p = 0.0228). As was expected, the serum levels of ATT were lower in PI*MZ and PI*SZ groups (p = 1.18^{-25}). Analytical and functional respiratory test variables are illustrated in Table 3. Finally, we did not find any significant association between AATD and AAT genotypes and the risk of having severe persistent asthma (Table 4).

Discussion

Many authors have suggested an increased risk of asthma with some AAT genotypes. Eden et al. [16] showed that 44% of patients with AATD (20–25% of them with an allergy) had asthma, which was three times more prevalent in PI*MZ subjects than in PI*ZZ individuals. Other investigators have found an even higher percentage of asthmatics among PI*SS population when compared to subjects without deficient alleles [25]. We have not found any clinical association between AATD and AAT genotypes and severity of asthma among HDM sensitized patients. Indeed, the distribution of deficient genotypes among all asthma severity categories was very similar to that described previously in Spanish asthmatic population (Table 5).

The balance between normal lung inflammation and repair is a complex process that involves pro- and anti-inflammatory cytokines and the accumulation of inflammatory and immune effector cells [26]. In this work,

Table 2 Demographic and clinical characteristics according to alpha 1 antitrypsin genotypes

	PI*MM (n = 503)	PI*MS (n = 110)	PI*MZ (n = 15)	PI*SS (n = 14)	PI*SZ (n = 6)	P value
Sex n (%)						0.525
Male	178 (35)	35 (32)	3 (20)	6 (43)	1 (17)	
Female	325 (65)	75 (68)	12 (80)	8 (57)	5 (83)	
Age, years						0.818
Median (IQ$_{25-75}$)	28 (20–38)	31 (23–38)	30 (24–38)	32 (20–36)	20.5 (19–36)	
Smokers n (%)	37 (7.4)	11 (10)	4 (26.7)	2 (14.3)	0	0.0882
Intermittent asthma n (%)	191 (38)	45 (41)	4 (26.7)	9 (64.3)	4 (66.7)	0.134
Mild persistent asthma (%)	194 (38.6)	39(35.5)	6(40)	5(35.7)	2(33.3)	0.981
Moderate persistent asthma n (%)	78 (15.5)	18 (16.4)	4 (26.7)	0	0	0.303
Severe persistent asthma n (%)	39 (7.8)	8 (7.3)	1 (6.7)	0	0	0.958
Polyposis n (%)	9 (1.8)	6 (5.5)	2 (13.3)	0	0	0.104
Chronic sinusitis n (%)	24 (4.8)	3 (2.7)	2 (13.3)	2 (14.3)	1 (16.7)	0.0516
Atopic dermatitis n (%)	17 (3.4)	4 (3.6)	0	1 (7.1)	1 (16.7)	0.271
Previous pneumonia n (%)	4 (0.8)	1 (0.9)	0	0	0	1
> 3infections/year n (%)	4 (0.8)	0	0	0	0	1
Previous treatment: oral glucocorticosteroids n (%)	10 (2)	2 (1.8)	0	0	0	1
Previous treatment: immunotherapy n (%)	38 (7.6)	10 (9.1)	0	0	0	0.804
Previous treatment: omalizumab n (%)	1 (0.2)	0	0	0	0	1

* Kruskal–Wallis statistic analysis for continuous non normal variables and Chi square or F-test for nominal ones

Table 3 Analytical and functional respiratory tests according to alpha 1 antitrypsin genotype

	PI*MM (n = 503)	PI*MS (n = 110)	PI*MZ (n = 15)	PI*SS (n = 14)	PI*SZ (n = 6)	P value*
FEV1 (l)						0.23
Median (IQ$_{25-75}$)	2.9 (2.5–3.4)	2.9 (2.4–3.4)	2.9 (2.7–3.3)	3.1 (2.8–3.7)	3.3 (3.2–3.3)	
FEV1 (%)						0.0763
Median (IQ$_{25-75}$)	90 (81–100)	91 (76–101)	92 (84–105)	97 (86–99)	101 (99–111)	
Total IgE (IU/dL)§						0.194
Median (IQ$_{25-75}$)	272 (124–576)	207 (74–538)	165 (115–399)	151 (127–646)	169 (90–582)	
IgE Dermatophagoides pteronyssinus						0.372
Median (IQ$_{25-75}$)	45 (17–100)	31 (9–101)	70 (11–101)	34 (20–89)	61 (30–101)	
IgE Dermatophagoides farinae						0.273
Median (IQ$_{25-75}$)	29 (12–80)	17 (6.6–54)	41 (14–79)	24 (8.8–74)	31 (21–84)	
IgE Blomia tropicalis						0.89
Median (IQ$_{25-75}$)	7 (2.1–22)	8 (2.5–19)	6 (5.2–9.6)	9.5 (2–18)	4.5 (1–8.5)	
IgE Lepidoglyphus destructor						0.348
Median (IQ$_{25-75}$)	2 (1–6)	3.1 (1.1–8)	4 (3.6–10)	4 (2–8)	2.2 (2–16)	
IgE Tyrophagus putrescientae						0.409
Median (IQ$_{25-75}$)	2.3 (1–8)	2.3 (1.4–5)	1 (1–1.01)	1.6 (0.7–8)	2.1	
IgE Acarus siro						0.129
Median (IQ$_{25-75}$)	2 (0.9–7)	4 (3–5)	10 (4.3–35)	5.5 (1–11)	23.3	
IgA (mg/dL)§						0.333
Median (IQ$_{25-75}$)	216.5 (164–285)	204 (150.8–261)	261 (181–331)	224 (193–238)	255 (160–267)	
Eosinophils (10^9/L)§						0.0228‡
Median(IQ$_{25-75}$)	0.3 (0.2–0.5)	0.3 (0.2–0.4)	0.4 (0.3–0.6)	0.5 (0.3–0.6)	0.3 (0.2–0.4)	
Nasal cytology eosinophils (%)						0.378
Median (IQ$_{25-75}$)	40 (10–70)	20 (7.5–60)	45 (33–65)	50 (30–65)	50	
AAT (mg/dL)§						1.18e–25‡
Median (IQ$_{25-75}$)	138 (123–159)	116 (104–137)	80 (78–87)	89 (86–96)	64 (61.3–70.5)	

FEV1 (forced expiratory volume in the 1 s), IgE (immunoglobulin E), IgA (immunoglobulin A), AAT (alpha1 antitrypsin)

* Kruskal–Wallis statistic analysis

‡ Statistical significance, p value < 0.05

§ Normal value IgE: 10–179 IU/ml; Normal value of IgA: 80–310 mg/dl; Normal value of blood eosinophils: 0–0.54 × 109/L; Normal value ATT: 100–200 mg/dL (1.0–2.0 g/L)

Table 4 Relationship between AATD or AAT genotypes and severe persistent asthma

	Severe persistent asthma OR (95%CI)	P value*	Multivariable correction**
PI*MM	1.2700 (0.6–2.69)	0.532	0.382
PI*MS	0.9760 (0.44–2.15)	0.953	0.665
PI*SS	0.00000078 (0–Inf)	0.983	0.992
PI*MZ	0.8910 (0.12–6.92)	0.912	0.953
PI*SZ	0.000000791 (0–Inf)	0.989	0.995
SAATD	6.3600 (0.57–71.5)	0.134	0.711
AATD	0.5680 (0.17–1.88)	0.355	0.992

PI: protease inhibitor, SAATD (severe alpha 1 antitrypsin deficiency, < 57 mg/dl), AATD (alpha1 antitrypsin deficit, < 100 mg/dl)

* Binary logistic regression

** Adjusted for age, conjunctivitis, polyposis, ex-smokers, passive smokers

contrary to previous investigations, we studied a specific group of asthmatic patients sensitized to HDM. It has been proved that mites produce a huge inflammatory reaction in the lung, not only through CD4 + Th2 cells that induce an IgE allergic response, but also through the innate immune system [27]. Different researchers have provided ample evidence that some components of *D pteronyssinus*, such as group 1 allergens (Der p 1), can activate different routes that alter the immune system [28]. Other allergens, such as Der p 3 and Der p 6, also seem to contribute to the HDM allergic response [29]. It is even more intriguing how these allergens can also directly damage the respiratory epithelium by activating mast cell independent of IgE [30].

ATT inhibits neutrophil serine proteases and can regulate the chemotaxis of neutrophils in two different ways:

Table 5 Protease inhibitor genotype distribution in different populations

	PI*MM	PI*MS	PI*MZ	PI*SS	PI*SZ	PI*ZZ
Our population (n = 648)	503 (77.62%)	110 (16.98%)	15 (2.31%)	14 (2.16%)	6 (0.93%)	0
Spanish population [7]	–	1/5 (20%)	1/33 (3%)	1/92 (1.1%)	1/278 (0.36%)	1/3344 (0.03%)
Miravitles et al. study [37]	333 (75.7%)	84 (19.1%)	14 (3.2%)	–	0	0

PI (protease inhibitor)

inhibition of IL8-CXCR1 interaction and modulation of ADAM17 activity impeding FcγRIIIb release [31]. The inactivation of ATT by some major components of *D pteronyssinus*, such as Der p 1, has already been proven [32]. The majority of our patients (96.5%) were sensitized to this mite and consequently, the anti-inflammatory action of ATT can be missing in this population. Thus, it is conceivable to think that there could be a possible association between AATD and severity of allergic asthma. However, we have not been able to find a significant association between AATD and severe asthma, as it was reported previously by van Veen et al. in asthmatic patients without a known sensitivity [33]. Neither total IgE nor HDM specific IgE were higher in the most severe asthmatic cases [34]. What we observed is higher serum levels of IgA in patients with severe asthma, as has already been reported [35]. That is why we included serum IgA in the multivariate analysis.

We have also assessed the distribution of different AAT genotypes in our series, which does not differ from the general population in our country [7, 36]. Furthermore, asthmatic carriers of deficient genotypes did not have different clinical expression of asthma, as it was reported before in a non-selected population of asthmatic patients [37] and in a population with severe asthma [33]. AAT serum levels were lower in asthmatic carriers of Z allele [38, 39], but there was no correlation of functional respiratory values neither with serum AAT levels nor AAT genotypes. These results are similar to those reported by others [33, 40]. Nevertheless, another study, conducted with children, suggested that, although low levels of AAT do not enhance the risk of developing asthma, an impaired AAT balance may potentially increase the vulnerability for decrease in lung function and bronchial hyperreactivity in asthmatic children [41].

In contrast to previous reports [37], we have found lower levels of blood eosinophils in PI*MS subjects in comparison to other genotypes. Likewise, the percentage of eosinophils in nasal cytology was also lower in the PI*MS group, though not significantly.

We recognize that our study has some limitations. First of all, we did not predict the required sample size by power calculation, but we strongly believe that this sample of patients truly reflects what happens to the asthmatic population. Moreover, our series is the largest sample studied at the moment. Secondly, we could not find any patient heterozygous for Z allele but this genotype is extremely uncommon and less prevalent in Spain. Finally, we only measured serum ATT levels and we do not know if the local production of ATT by pulmonary epithelial cells and macrophages may balance the low serum ATT levels.

To conclude, we could not find any association between AATD and asthma severity among patients sensitized to HDM. Our findings support what has been reported by others in smaller series of asthmatics. The proportion of asthmatics with deficient AAT genotypes in our series is similar to the proportion in the general population. Although the blood count and nasal eosinophils values seem to be different among the different genotypes, more studies are needed to confirm this due to the scarcity of asthmatic allergic populations with alleles PI*Z.

Abbreviations
ATT: alpha1 antitrypsin; ATTD: alpha 1 antitrypsin deficiency; COPD: chronic obstructive pulmonary disease; FeNO: fractional exhaled nitric oxide; FEV1: forced expiratory volume in 1 s; FVC: forced vital capacity; HDM: house dust mites; ICS: inhalated glucocorticosteroids; IgA: immunoglobulin A; IgE: immunoglobulin E; LABA: long-acting β2-agonists; PI: protease inhibitor; SABA: short-acting β2-agonists; SATTD: severe alpha 1 antitrypsin deficiency.

Authors' contributions
ISL, FRC, DCN, EHR, CRG, TCD: Conceived ideas or/and experiment design. ISL, DCN, TCD: Data collection. ISL: Data analysis. ISL, FRC, CRG, TCD: Interpretation of results. ISL, FRC, DCN, EHR, CRG, TCD: Revision of the content. All authors read and approved the final manuscript.

Author details

[1] Postgraduate and Doctoral School, Universidad de Las Palmas de Gran Canaria, Camino Real de San Roque, 1, 35015 Las Palmas de Gran Canaria, Las Palmas, Spain. [2] Pneumology Unit, Hospital Universitario de Gran Canaria Doctor Negrín, Las Palmas de Gran Canaria, Spain. [3] Allergy Unit, Hospital General de Fuerteventura, Puerto del Rosario, Spain. [4] Immunology Unit, Hospital Universitario de Gran Canaria Doctor Negrín, Las Palmas de Gran Canaria, Spain. [5] Allergy Unit, Hospital Universitario de Gran Canaria Doctor Negrín, Las Palmas de Gran Canaria, Spain.

Acknowledgements

The authors are very grateful to ALK-Abelló for the financial support.

Competing interests

The authors declare that they have no competing interests.

Funding

Instituto de Salud Carlos III. Award number PI12/01565 (Recipient Carlos Rodriguez-Gallego). Instituto de Salud Carlos III. Award number PI10/01718 (Recipient Carlos Rodriguez-Gallego).

References

1. Cosio MG, Bazzan E, Rigobello C, Tinè M, Turato G, Baraldo S, et al. Alpha-1 antitrypsin deficiency: beyond the protease/antiprotease paradigm. Ann Am Thorac Soc. 2016;13(Suppl 4):S305–10.

2. McCarthy C, Reeves EP, McElvaney NG. The role of neutrophils in alpha-1 antitrypsin deficiency. Ann Am Thorac Soc. 2016;13(Suppl 4):S297–304.

3. Laurell C-B, Eriksson S. The electrophoretic α1-globulin pattern of serum in α1-antitrypsin deficiency 1963. COPD. 2013;10(Suppl 1):3–8.

4. Dickens JA, Lomas DA. Why has it been so difficult to prove the efficacy of alpha-1-antitrypsin replacement therapy? Insights from the study of disease pathogenesis. Drug Des Devel Ther. 2011;5:391–405.

5. de Serres FJ, Blanco I. Prevalence of α1-antitrypsin deficiency alleles PI*S and PI*Z worldwide and effective screening for each of the five phenotypic classes PI*MS, PI*MZ, PI*SS, PI*SZ, and PI*ZZ: a comprehensive review. Ther Adv Respir Dis. 2012;6(5):277–95.

6. Stockley RA, Dirksen A, Stolk J. Alpha-1 antitrypsin deficiency: the European experience. COPD. 2013;10(Suppl 1):50–3.

7. Blanco I, de Serres FJ, Fernandez-Bustillo E, Lara B, Miravitlles M. Estimated numbers and prevalence of PI*S and PI*Z alleles of alpha1-antitrypsin deficiency in European countries. Eur Respir J. 2006;27(1):77–84.

8. Lara B, Blanco I, Martínez MT, Rodríguez E, Bustamante A, Casas F, et al. Spanish registry of patients with alpha-1 antitrypsin deficiency: database evaluation and population analysis. Arch Bronconeumol. 2017;53(1):13–8.

9. Lara B, Miravitlles M. Spanish registry of patients with alpha-1 antitrypsin deficiency; comparison of the characteristics of PISZ and PIZZ individuals. COPD. 2015;12(Suppl 1):27–31.

10. Sørheim I-C, Bakke P, Gulsvik A, Pillai SG, Johannessen A, Gaarder PI, et al. α1-Antitrypsin protease inhibitor MZ heterozygosity is associated with airflow obstruction in two large cohorts. Chest. 2010;138(5):1125–32.

11. Dahl M, Hersh CP, Ly NP, Berkey CS, Silverman EK, Nordestgaard BG. The protease inhibitor PI*S allele and COPD: a meta-analysis. Eur Respir J. 2005;26(1):67–76.

12. Hersh CP, Dahl M, Ly NP, Berkey CS, Nordestgaard BG, Silverman EK. Chronic obstructive pulmonary disease in alpha1-antitrypsin PI MZ heterozygotes: a meta-analysis. Thorax. 2004;59(10):843–9.

13. Mehta AJ, Thun GA, Imboden M, Ferrarotti I, Keidel D, Künzli N, et al. Interactions between SERPINA1 PiMZ genotype, occupational exposure and lung function decline. Occup Environ Med. 2014;71(4):234–40.

14. Siri D, Farah H, Hogarth DK. Distinguishing alpha1-antitrypsin deficiency from asthma. Ann Allergy Asthma Immunol. 2013;111(6):458–64.

15. Strange C. Airway disease in alpha-1 antitrypsin deficiency. COPD. 2013;10(Suppl 1):68–73.

16. Eden E, Strange C, Holladay B, Xie L. Asthma and allergy in alpha-1 antitrypsin deficiency. Respir Med. 2006;100(8):1384–91.

17. American Thoracic Society, European Respiratory Society. American Thoracic Society/European Respiratory Society statement: standards for the diagnosis and management of individuals with alpha-1 antitrypsin deficiency. Am J Respir Crit Care Med. 2003;168(7):818–900.

18. Alpha 1-antitrypsin deficiency: memorandum from a WHO meeting. Bull World Health Organ. 1997;75(5):397–415.

19. GEMA 4.0 [Internet]. Gemasma. [cited 2017 Oct 26]. https://www.gemasma.com/.

20. Bousquet J, Heinzerling L, Bachert C, Papadopoulos NG, Bousquet PJ, Burney PG, et al. Practical guide to skin prick tests in allergy to aeroallergens. Allergy. 2012;67(1):18–24.

21. Ahsen N von, Oellerich M, Schütz E. Use of two reporter dyes without interference in a single-tube rapid-cycle PCR: α1-antitrypsin genotyping by multiplex real-time fluorescence PCR with the lightcycler. Clinical Chemistry [Internet]. 2000 Feb 1 [cited 2018 Apr 12];46(2):156–61. http://clinchem.aaccjnls.org/content/46/2/156.

22. R Core Team. R: A language and environment for statistical computing. [Internet]. Vienna, Austria.: R Foundation for Statistical Computing, 2017. https://www.R-project.org/.

23. Mincheva R, Ekerljung L, Bossios A, Lundbäck B, Lötvall J. High prevalence of severe asthma in a large random population study. J Allergy Clin Immunol. 2018;141(6):2256–64.

24. Stoller JK, Lacbawan FL, Aboussouan LS. Alpha-1 Antitrypsin deficiency. In: Adam MP, Ardinger HH, Pagon RA, Wallace SE, Bean LJ, Mefford HC, et al. editors. GeneReviews(®) [Internet]. Seattle (WA): University of Washington, Seattle; 1993 [cited 2017 Oct 24]. http://www.ncbi.nlm.nih.gov/books/NBK1519/.

25. McGee D, Schwarz L, McClure R, Peterka L, Rouhani F, Brantly M, et al. Is PiSS alpha-1 antitrypsin deficiency associated with disease? Pulm Med. 2010;2010:570679.

26. Stockley RA. The multiple facets of alpha-1-antitrypsin. Ann Transl Med. 2015;3(10):130.

27. Calderón MA, Linneberg A, Kleine-Tebbe J, De Blay F, de Rojas DHF, Virchow JC, et al. Respiratory allergy caused by house dust mites: What do we really know? J Allergy Clin Immunol. 2015;136(1):38–48.

28. Bouchecareilh M, Balch WE. Proteostasis, an emerging therapeutic paradigm for managing inflammatory airway stress disease. Curr Mol Med. 2012;12(7):815–26.

29. Jacquet A, Campisi V, Szpakowska M, Dumez M-E, Galleni M, Chevigné A. Profiling the extended cleavage specificity of the house dust mite protease allergens Der p 1, Der p 3 and Der p 6 for the prediction of new cell surface protein substrates. Int J Mol Sci. 2017;18(7):1373.

30. Takai T, Ikeda S. Barrier dysfunction caused by environmental proteases in the pathogenesis of allergic diseases. Allergol Int. 2011;60(1):25–35.

31. Bergin DA, Reeves EP, Meleady P, Henry M, McElvaney OJ, Carroll TP, et al. α-1 Antitrypsin regulates human neutrophil chemotaxis induced by soluble immune complexes and IL-8. J Clin Invest. 2010;120(12):4236–50.

32. Kalsheker NA, Deam S, Chambers L, Sreedharan S, Brocklehurst K, Lomas DA. The house dust mite allergen Der p1 catalytically inactivates alpha 1-antitrypsin by specific reactive centre loop cleavage: a mechanism that promotes airway inflammation and asthma. Biochem Biophys Res Commun. 1996;221(1):59–61.

33. van Veen IH, ten Brinke A, van der Linden AC, Rabe KF, Bel EH. Deficient alpha-1-antitrypsin phenotypes and persistent airflow limitation in severe asthma. Respir Med. 2006;100(9):1534–9.

34. Davila I, Valero A, Entrenas LM, Valveny N, Herráez L, SIGE Study Group. Relationship between serum total IgE and disease severity in patients with allergic asthma in Spain. J Investig Allergol Clin Immunol. 2015;25(2):120–7.

35. Kim W-J, Choi IS, Kim CS, Lee J-H, Kang H-W. Relationship between serum IgA level and allergy/asthma. Korean J Intern Med. 2017;32(1):137–45.

36. Blanco I, Fernández-Bustillo E, de Serres FJ, Alkassam D, Rodríguez Menéndez C. PI*S and PI*Z alpha 1-antitrypsin deficiency: estimated prevalence and number of deficient subjects in Spain. Med Clin (Barc). 2004;123(20):761–5.

37. Miravitlles M, Vilà S, Torrella M, Balcells E, Rodríguez-Frías F, de la Roza C, et al. Influence of deficient alpha1-anti-trypsin phenotypes on clinical characteristics and severity of asthma in adults. Respir Med. 2002;96(3):186–92.

38. Ferrarotti I, Thun GA, Zorzetto M, Ottaviani S, Imboden M, Schindler C, et al. Serum levels and genotype distribution of α1-antitrypsin in the general population. Thorax. 2012;67(8):669–74.

39. Zorzetto M, Russi E, Senn O, Imboden M, Ferrarotti I, Tinelli C, et al. SERPINA1 gene variants in individuals from the general population with reduced alpha1-antitrypsin concentrations. Clin Chem. 2008;54(8):1331–8.

40. Silva GE, Sherrill DL, Guerra S, Barbee RA. A longitudinal study of alpha1-antitrypsin phenotypes and decline in FEV1 in a community population. Chest. 2003;123(5):1435–40.

41. von Ehrenstein OS, Maier EM, Weiland SK, Carr D, Hirsch T, Nicolai T, et al. Alpha1 antitrypsin and the prevalence and severity of asthma. Arch Dis Child. 2004;89(3):230–1.

Permissions

List of Contributors

Mayra Álvarez-Santos, Patricia Ramos-Ramírez, Fernando Gutiérrez-Aguilar, Sandra Sánchez-Hernández and Blanca Bazan-Perkins
Instituto Nacional de Enfermedades Respiratorias Ismael Cosío Villegas, Departamento de Hiperreactividad Bronquial, Calzada de Tlalpan 4502, Mexico

Ricardo Lascurain
Departamento de Bioquímica, Facultad de Medicina, Universidad Nacional Autónoma de México, México, DF, Mexico

Raúl Olmos-Zuñiga and Rogelio Jasso-Victoria
Departamento de Cirugía Experimental, Instituto Nacional de Enfermedades, Respiratorias Ismael Cosío Villegas, Calzada de Tlalpan 4502, Mexico

Norma A Bobadilla
Molecular Physiology Unit, Instituto de Investigaciones Biomédicas, Universidad Nacional Autónoma de México, México, Mexico
Instituto Nacional de Ciencias Médicas y Nutrición Salvador Zubirán, Department of Nephrology, México, Mexico

Wei Tang, Steven G. Smith, Wei Du, Akash Gugilla, John Paul Oliveria, Karen Howie, Brittany M. Salter, Gail M. Gauvreau, Paul M. O'Byrne and Roma Sehmi
Division of Respirology, Department of Medicine, McMaster University, Hamilton, ON L6M 1A6, Canada

Wei Tang, Wei Du and Juan Du
Department of Respirology and Critical Medicine, Ruijin Hospital, Shanghai Jiaotong University School of Medicine, Shanghai, China

Vanessa Garcia-Larsen, James F. Potts and Peter G. J. Burney
Population Health and Occupational Medicine Group, National Heart and Lung Institute, Imperial College London, London, UK

Rhonda Arthur
Department of Nutrition, King's College London, London, UK

Peter H. Howarth
Faculty of Medicine, University of Southampton, London, UK

Matti Ahlström and Tari Haahtela
Skin and Allergy Hospital, Helsinki University Hospital, Southampton, Finland

Carlos Loureiro and Ana Todo Bom
Immuno-allergology Department, Coimbra University Hospital, Helsinki, Portugal

Grzegorz Brożek
Department of Epidemiology, College of Medicine, Medical University of Silesia, Katowice, Poland

Joanna Makowska and Marek L. Kowalski
Department of Immunology, Rheumatology and Allergy, Medical University of Lodz, Coimbra, Poland

Trine Thilsing
Research Unit for Occupational and Environmental Medicine, Institute of Clinical Research, University of Southern Denmark Coimbra, Denmark

Thomas Keil
Institute of Social Medicine, Epidemiology and Health Economics, Charité - Universitätsmedizin Berlin, Lodz, Germany
Institute of Clinical Epidemiology and Biometry, Würzburg University, Würzburg, Germany

Paolo M. Matricardi
Deptartment of Pediatrics, Charité – Universitätsmedizin Berlin, Berlin, Germany

Kjell Torén
Section of Occupational and Environmental Medicine, University of Gothenburg, Odense, Sweden

Thibaut van Zele
Upper Airway Research Laboratory, Ghent University, Ghent, Belgium

Claus Bachert
Division of ENT Diseases, Karolinska Institute, Stockholm, Sweden

Barbara Rymarczyk
Clinical Department of Internal Diseases, Allergology and Clinical Immunology, Medical University of Silesia, Katowice, Poland

Christer Janson
Department of Medical Sciences, Respiratory, Allergy and Sleep Research, Uppsala University, Ghent, Sweden

Bertil Forsberg
Division of Occupational and Environmental Medicine, Department of Public Health and Clinical Medicine, Umeå University, Chorzów, Sweden

Ewa Niżankowska-Mogilnicka
Jagiellonian University School of Medicine, Krakow, Poland

Vanessa Garcia-Larsen
Respiratory Epidemiology, Occupational Medicine and Public Health Group, National Heart and Lung Institute, Imperial College London, Emmanuel Kaye Building, Manresa Road, London SW3 6LR, UK

Felix Asamoah
Centre for Environmental and Preventive Medicine, Wolfson Institute of Preventive Medicine, London, UK
Barts and the London School of Medicine and Dentistry, Queen Mary University of London, London, UK
Neonatal Unit, Homerton University Hospital NHS Foundation Trust, London, UK

Artemisia Kakourou
Department of Hygiene and Epidemiology, University of Ioannina School of Medicine, Ioannina, Greece

Sangeeta Dhami
Evidence-Based Health Care Ltd, Edinburgh, UK

Susanne Lau
Charite Medical University, Berlin, Germany

Ioana Agache
Department of Allergy and Clinical Immunology, Faculty of Medicine, Transylvania University Brasov, Brasov, Romania

Antonella Muraro
Food Allergy Referral Centre Veneto Region, University Hospital of Padua, Padua, Italy

Graham Roberts
The David Hide Asthma and Allergy Research Centre, St Mary's Hospital, Newport, Isle of Wight, UK
NIHR Biomedical Research Centre, University Hospital Southampton NHS Foundation Trust and Faculty of Medicine, University of Southampton, Southampton, UK
Faculty of Medicine, University of Southampton, Southampton, UK

Cezmi Akdis
Swiss Institute for Allergy and Asthma Research, Davos, Switzerland

Matteo Bonini
Sapienza University Rome, Rome, Italy

Ozlem Cavkaytar
Department of Allergy and Clinical Immunology, Sami Ulus Maternity and Children Training and Research Hospital, Ankara Turkey

Breda Flood
European Federation of Allergy and Airways Diseases Patients Association, Brussels, Belgium

Kenji Izuhara
Saga Medical School, Saga, Japan

Marek Jutel
Wroclaw Medical University, Wrocław, Poland

Ömer Kalayci
Department of Otorhinolaryngology, Head and Neck Surgery, Universitätsmedizin Mannheim, Medical Faculty Mannheim, Heidelberg University, Mannheim, Germany
Center for Rhinology and Allergology, Wiesbaden, Germany
Hacettepe University, Ankara, Turkey

Aziz Sheikh
Asthma UK Centre for Applied Research, Usher Institute of Population Health Sciences and Informatics, The University of Edinburgh, Edinburgh, UK

Mônica Versiani Nunes Pinheiro de Queiroz
Department of Pediatrics, School of Medicine, Federal University of Ouro Preto, Ouro Preto, Brazil

Cristina Gonçalves Alvim
Department of Pediatrics, School of Medicine, Federal University of Minas Gerais, Belo Horizonte, Brazil

Álvaro A. Cruz
ProAR – Federal University of Bahia, Salvador, Brazil

Mônica Versiani Nunes Pinheiro de Queiroz
Departamento de Clínicas Pediátrica e do Adulto, Escola de Medicina, Universidade Federal de Ouro Preto, Rua Dois 697, Ouro Preto, MG 35400-000, Brazil

Leyla Pur Ozyigit
Department of Allergy and Immunology, Koç University, School of Medicine, Istanbul, Turkey

Hideaki Morita and Mubeccel Akdis
Swiss Institute of Allergy and Asthma Research, University of Zurich, Zurich, Switzerland
Christine Kühne-Center for Allergy Research and Education, Davos, Switzerland

Paulo Camargos
Pediatric Pulmonology Unit, University Hospital, Federal University of Minas Gerais, Avenida Alfredo Balena 190, Room 267, Belo Horizonte 30130-100, Brazil

Alessandra Affonso, Geralda Calazans, Lidiana Ramalho, Marisa L. Ribeiro, Nulma Jentzsch and Simone Senna
Municipal Public Health Department, Belo Horizonte, Brazil

Renato T. Stein
Laboratory Renato T. Stein3of Pediatric Respirology, Infant Center, Institute of Biomedical Research, Pontifícia Universidade Católica do Rio Grande do Sul, Porto Alegre, Brazil

M. Fröhlich, M. Pinart and S. Roll
Institute of Social Medicine, Epidemiology and Health Economics, Charité -Universitätsmedizin Berlin, Berlin, Germany

M. Fröhlich
Clinic for Neonatology, Charité - Universitätsmedizin Berlin, Berlin, Germany

M. Pinart
Max-Delbrück-Centrum für Molekulare Medizin, Research Team Molecular Epidemiology, Berlin, Germany

M. Pinart and J. M. Antó
ISGlobal, Centre for Research in Environmental Epidemiology (CREAL), Barcelona, Spain
IMIM (Hospital del Mar Research Institute), Barcelona, Spain
Universitat Popmpeu Fabra (UPF), Barcelona, Spain
CIBER Epidemiología y Salud Pública (CIBERESP), Barcelona, Spain

A. Reich
Epidemiology, German Rheumatism Research Centre, Berlin, Germany

B. Cabieses
Facultad de Medicina Clínica Alemana, Universidad del Desarrollo, Santiago, Chile

D. S. Postma
Department of Pulmonology, University Medical Center Groningen, University of Groningen, Groningen, The Netherlands

T. Keil
Institute of Clinical Epidemiology and Biometry, University of Wuerzburg, Würzburg, Germany

Rita Amaral, João A. Fonseca, Tiago Jacinto and Ana M. Pereira
CINTESIS- Center for Health Technology and Services Research, Faculty of Medicine, University of Porto, Edifício Nascente, Piso 2, Rua Dr. Plácido da Costa, s/n, 4200-450 Porto, Portugal

Rita Amaral and Tiago Jacinto
Department of Cardiovascular and Respiratory Sciences, Porto Health School, Porto, Portugal

João A. Fonseca
MEDCIDS- Department of Community Medicine, Information, and Health Sciences, Faculty of Medicine, University of Porto, Porto, Portugal

Tiago Jacinto and Ana M. Pereira
Department of Allergy, Instituto and Hospital CUF, Porto, Portugal

Andrei Malinovschi
Department of Medical Sciences: Clinical Physiology, Uppsala University, Uppsala, Sweden

Christer Janson
Department of Medical Sciences: Respiratory Medicine and Allergology, Uppsala University, Uppsala, Sweden

Kjell Alving
Department of Women's and Children's Health: Paediatric Research, Uppsala University, Uppsala, Sweden

Jon Genuneit and Annina M. Seibold
Institute of Epidemiology and Medical Biometry, Ulm University, Helmholtzstr.22, 89081 Ulm, Germany

Christian J. Apfelbacher
Institute of Epidemiology and Preventive Medicine, University of Regensburg, Regensburg, Germany

George N. Konstantinou
Department of Allergy and Clinical Immunology, 424 General Military Training Hospital, Thessaloniki, Greece

Jennifer J. Koplin
Murdoch Children's Research Institute, University of Melbourne, Melbourne, Australia

Stefania La Grutta
Institute of Biomedicine and Molecular Immunology, National Research Council of Italy, Palermo, Italy

Kirsty Logan
Division of Asthma, Allergy and Lung Biology, Children's Allergies Department, King's College London, London, UK

Carsten Flohr
Unit for Population-Based Dermatology Research, St John's Institute of Dermatology, King's College London and Guy's and St Thomas' NHS Foundation, London, UK

Michael R. Perkin
Population Health Research Institute, St George's, University of London, London, UK

G. Rentzos
Section of Allergology, University Hospital of Sahlgrenska, 413 45 Gothenburg, Sweden

L. Johanson and L. Ekerljung
Krefting Research Centre, Department of Internal Medicine and Clinical Nutrition, University of Gothenburg, Gothenburg, Sweden

E. Telemo
Department for Rheumatology and Inflammation Research, Sahlgrenska Academy, University of Gothenburg, Gothenburg, Sweden

S. Sjölander
R&D, ImmunoDiagnostics, Thermofischer Scientific, Uppsala, Sweden

Jean Bousquet
MACVIA-France, Fondation partenariale FMC VIA-LR, Montpellier, France.
INSERM U 1168, VIMA : Ageing and Chronic Diseases Epidemiological and Public Health Approaches, Villejuif, France
Université Versailles St-Quentin-en-Yvelines, UMR-S 1168, Montigny le Bretonneux, France
Euforea, Brussels, Belgium
Charité, Berlin, Germany
CHU Montpellier, 371 Avenue du Doyen Gaston Giraud, 34295 Montpellier Cedex 5, France

Josep M. Anto and Xavier Basagana
ISGlobal, Centre for Research in Environmental Epidemiology (CREAL), Barcelona, Spain

Josep M. Anto
IMIM (Hospital del Mar Research Institute), Barcelona, Spain
Universitat Pompeu Fabra (UPF), Barcelona, Spain
CIBER Epidemiología y Salud Pública (CIBERESP), Barcelona, Spain

Isabella Annesi-Maesano
Epidemiology of Allergic and Respiratory Diseases, Department Institute Pierre Louis of Epidemiology and Public Health, INSERM and UPMC Sorbonne Universités, Medical School Saint Antoine, Paris, France

Toni Dedeu
AQuAS, Barcelona, Spain

Eve Dupas
Kyomed INNOV, Montpellier, France

Jean-Louis Pépin
Université Grenoble Alpes, Laboratoire HP2, INSERM, U1042 Grenoble, France
CHU de Grenoble, Grenoble, France

Landry Stephane Zeng Eyindanga
Bull SAS, Échirolles, France

Julia Ayache and Samuel Benveniste
National Center of Expertise in Cognitive Stimulation (CEN STIMCO), Broca Hospital, Paris, France

Julia Ayache
Memory and Cognition Laboratory, Institute of Psychology, Paris Descartes University, Sorbonne Paris Cité, Boulogne Billancourt, France

Samuel Benveniste
Mines ParisTech CRI - PSL Research University, Fontainebleau, France

Nuria Calves Venturos
Direction de la Recherche, Innovation et Valorisation, Université Grenoble Alpes, Grenoble, France

Mehdi Cheraitia
Neogia, Paris, France

Yves Dauvilliers
Centre National de Référence Narcolepsie Hypersomnies, Département de Neurologie, Hôpital Gui-de-Chauliac Inserm U1061, Unité des Troubles du Sommeil, Montpellier, France

Giovanni Pau
LIP6 SU, Place Jussieu, Paris, France

Robert Picard
Conseil Général de l'Economie Ministère de l'Economie, de l'Industrie et du Numérique, Paris, France

Xavier Rodo
Climate and Health Program and ISGlobal and ICREA, Barcelona, Spain

Michael Bewick
iQ4U Consultants Ltd, London, UK

Nils E. Billo
Joensuu, Finland

Wienczyslawa Czarlewski
Medical Consulting Czarlewski, Levallois, France

Joao Fonseca
Center for Health Technology and Services Research-CINTESIS, Faculdade de Medicina, Universidade do Porto, Porto, Portugal
MEDIDA, Lda, Porto, Portugal

Ludger Klimek and Oliver Pfaar
Center for Rhinology and Allergology, Wiesbaden, Germany

Oliver Pfaar
Department of Otorhinolaryngology, Head and Neck Surgery, Universitätsmedizin Mannheim, Medical Faculty Mannheim, Heidelberg University, Mannheim, Germany

Jean-Marc Bourez
Managing Director, EIT Health France, Paris, France

Ana M. Navarro
UGC of Allergy, Hospital El Tomillar, Carretera Alcalá - Dos Hermanas km 6, 41700 Dos Hermanas, Seville, Spain

Julio Delgado
UGC of Allergy, Hospital Universitario Virgen Macarena, Seville, Spain

Rosa M. Munoz-Cano and Antonio Valero
Allergy Unit, Pneumology Department, Hospital Clinic, Institut d'Investigacions Biomèdiques August Pi Sunyer (IDIBAPS), Barcelona, Spain

M. Teresa Dordal
Allergy Service, Hospital Municipal, Badalona Serveis Assistencials, Badalona, Spain
Allergy Service, Sant Pere Claver Fundació Sanitària, Barcelona, Spain

Santiago Quirce
Department of Allergy, Hospital La Paz Institute for Health Santiago Quirce6Research (IdiPAZ), Madrid, Spain

Sangeeta Dhami
Evidence-Based Health Care Ltd, Edinburgh, UK

Ulugbek Nurmatov
Systematic Review at Decision Resources Group Abacus International, Oxford, UK

Ioana Agache
Department of Allergy and Clinical Immunology, Faculty of Medicine, Transylvania University Brasov, Brasov, Romania

Susanne Lau
Department of Pediatric Pneumology and Immunology, Charité Medical University, Berlin, Germany

Antonella Muraro
Food Allergy Referral Centre Veneto Region, University Hospital of Padua, Padua, Italy.

Marek Jutel
Wroclaw Medical University, Wrocław, Poland

Graham Roberts
The David Hide Asthma and Allergy Research Centre, St Mary's Hospital, Newport Isle of Wight, NIHR Respiratory Biomedical Research Unit, University Hospital Southampton NHS Foundation Trust, Southampton, UK
Faculty of Medicine, University of Southampton, Southampton, UK

Cezmi Akdis
Swiss Institute for Allergy and Asthma Research, Davos, Switzerland

Matteo Bonini
Sapienza University Rome, Rome, Italy

Moises Calderon
National Heart and Lung Institute, Imperial College, London, London, UK

Thomas Casale
University of South Florida, Tampa, FL, USA

Ozlem Cavkaytar
Department of Allergy and Clinical Immunology, Sami Ulus Maternity and Children Training
and Research Hospital, Ankara, Turkey

Linda Cox
Nova Southeastern University, Fort Lauderdale, FL, USA

Pascal Demoly
University and Hospital of Montpellier and Inserm Paris Sorbonnes, Montpellier, France

Breda Flood
European Federation of Allergy and Airways Diseases Patients Association, Brussels, Belgium

Eckard Hamelmann
Children's Center Bethel, EvKB, Bieledelf, Germany
Allergy Center, Ruhr-University, Bochum, Germany

Kenji Izuhara
Saga Medical School, Saga, Japan

Jörg Kleine-Tebbe
Allergy and Asthma Center Westend (AAZW), Berlin, Germany

Antonio Nieto
Children's Hospital La Fe, Valencia, Spain

Nikolaos Papadopoulos
Allergy Department, 2nd Pediatric Clinic, University of Athens, Athens, Greece

Oliver Pfaar
Department of Otorhinolaryngology, Head and Neck Surgery, University Hospital, Mannheim, Mannheim, Germany
Center for Rhinology and Allergology, Wiesbaden, Germany

Lanny Rosenwasser
Children's Mercy Hospital, Kentucky, MO, USA

Dermot Ryan
University of Edinburgh, Edinburgh, UK

Carsten Schmidt-Weber
Technische Univ and Helmholtz Center Munich, Munich, Germany

Stan Szefler
Children's Hospital Colorado, University of Colorado School of Medicine, Aurora, CO, USA

Ulrich Wahn
Department of Pediatric Pulmonology, Charite, Berlin, Germany

Roy-Gerth van Wijk
Section of Allergology, Department of Internal Medicine, Erasmus MC,
Rotterdam, The Netherlands

Jamie Wilkinson
Pharmaceutical Group of the European Union, Brussels, Belgium

Aziz Sheikh
Allergy and Respiratory Research Group, The University of Edinburgh, Edinburgh, UK

Jean Bousquet
MACVIA-France, Contre les MAladies Chroniques pour un VIeillissement Actif en France European Innovation Partnership on Active and Healthy Ageing Reference Site, Montpellier, France

INSERM U 1168, VIMA: Ageing and Chronic Diseases Epidemiological and Public Health Approaches, Villejuif, France
UMR-S 1168, Université Versailles St-Quentin-en-Yvelines, Montigny le Bretonneux, France
Euforea, Brussels, Belgium

Peter W. Hellings
UMR-S 1168, Université Versailles St-Quentin-en-Yvelines, Montigny le Bretonneux, France
Euforea, Brussels, Belgium

Clive Grattan
Dermatology Centre, Norfolk and Norwich University Hospital, Norwich, UK

Thomas Bieber
Department of Dermatology and Allergy, Rheinische Friedrich-Wilhelms-University Bonn, Bonn, Germany

Paolo Matricardi
AG Molecular Allergology and Immunomodulation, Department of Pediatric Pneumology and Immunology, Charité Medical University, Berlin, Germany

Hans Uwe Simon
Institute of Pharmacology, University of Bern, Bern, Switzerland

Ulrich Wahn
Pediatric Department, Charité, Berlin, Germany

Antonella Muraro
Food Allergy Referral Centre Veneto Region, Department of Women and Child Health, Padua General University Hospital, Padua, Italy

Peter W. Hellings
Laboratory of Clinical Immunology, Department of Microbiology and Immunology, KU Leuven, Leuven, Belgium

Ioana Agache
Faculty of Medicine, Transylvania University, Brasov, Romania

Jean Bousquet
CHU Montpellier, 371 Avenue du Doyen Gaston Giraud, 34295 Montpellier Cedex 5, France

Erik P. Rönmark, Linda Ekerljung, Roxana Mincheva, Jan Lötvall and Bo Lundbäck
Department of Internal Medicine, Krefting Research Centre, Institute of Medicine, Sahlgrenska Academy, University of Gothenburg, Box 424, 405 30 Gothenburg, Sweden

Sigrid Sjölander
ThermoFisher Scientific, Uppsala, Sweden

Göran Wennergren
Department of Paediatrics, Sahlgrenska Academy, University of Gothenburg, Gothenburg, Sweden

Eva Rönmark
Environmental and Occupational Medicine, The OLIN Unit, Department of Public Health and Clinical Medicine, University of Umeå, Umeå, Sweden

J. Bousquet
MACVIA-France, Fondation Partenariale FMC VIA-LR, CHRU Arnaud de Villeneuve, 371 Avenue du Doyen Gaston Giraud, Montpellier, France
INSERM U 1168, VIMA: Ageing and Chronic Diseases Epidemiological and Public Health Approaches, Villejuif, Université Versailles St-Quentin-en-Yvelines, UMR-S 1168, Montigny le Bretonneux, France Euforea, Brussels, Belgium

S. Arnavielhe
KYomed-INNOV, Montpellier, France

M. Bewick
iQ4U Consultants Ltd, London, UK

M. Dykewickz
Section of Allergy and Immunology, Saint Louis University School of Medicine, Saint Louis, MO, USA

R. N. Naclerio
Johns Hopkins School of Medicine, Baltimore, MD, USA

Y. Okamoto
Department of Otorhinolaryngology, Chiba University Hospital, Chiba, Japan

D. V. Wallace
Nova Southeastern University, Fort Lauderdale, Florida, USA

Suárez-Lorenzo
Postgraduate and Doctoral School, Universidad de Las Palmas de Gran Canaria, Camino Real de San Roque, 1, 35015 Las Palmas de Gran Canaria, Las Palmas, Spain

F. Rodríguez de Castro
Pneumology Unit, Hospital Universitario de Gran Canaria Doctor Negrín, Las Palmas de Gran Canaria, Spain

D. Cruz-Niesvaara
Allergy Unit, Hospital General de Fuerteventura, Puerto del Rosario, Spain

E. Herrera-Ramos and C. Rodríguez-Gallego
Immunology Unit, Hospital Universitario de Gran Canaria Doctor Negrín, Las Palmas de Gran Canaria, Spain

T. Carrillo-Diaz
Allergy Unit, Hospital Universitario de Gran Canaria Doctor Negrín, Las Palmas de Gran Canaria, Spain

Index

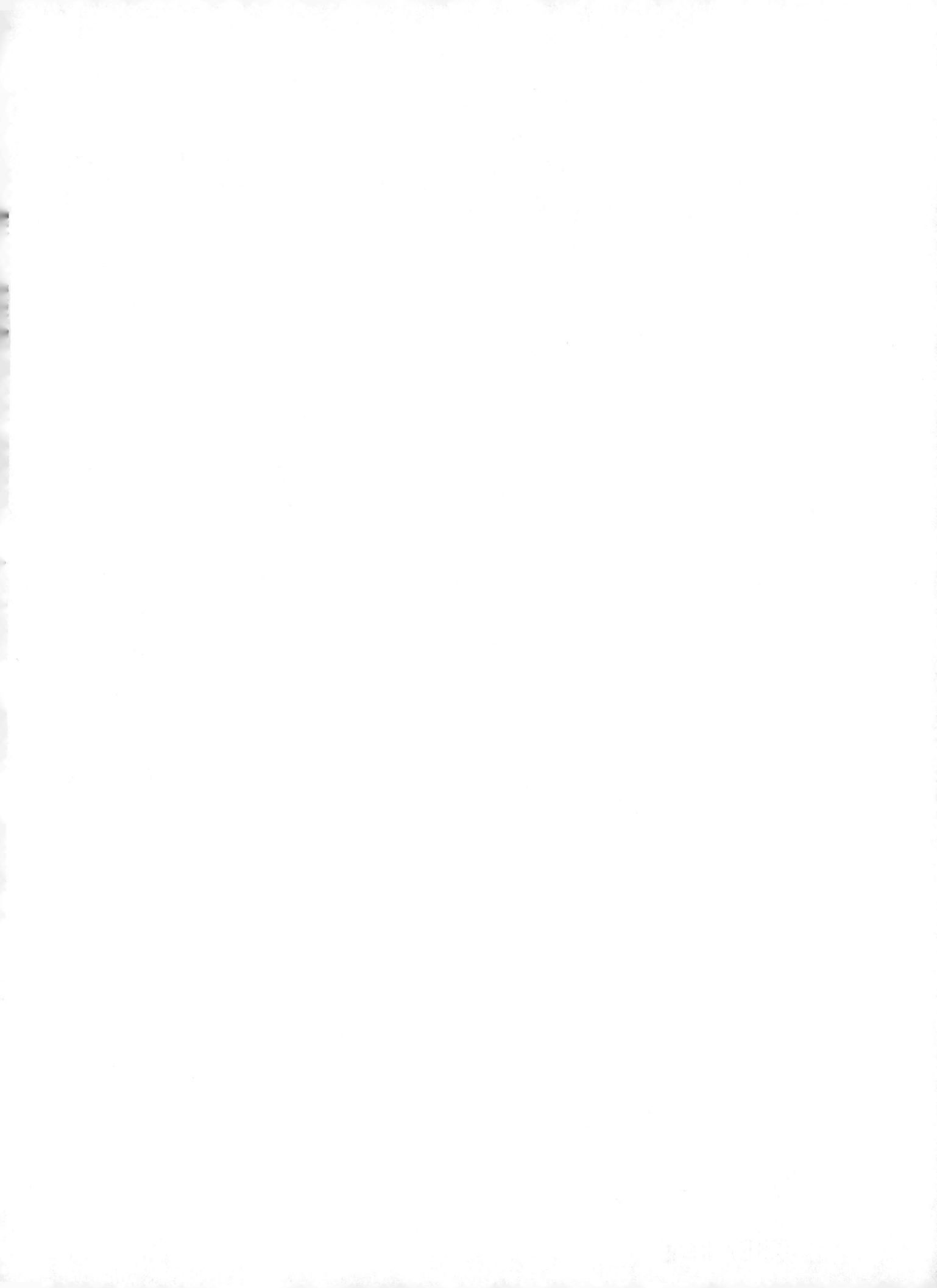

* 9 7 8 1 6 3 2 4 2 6 9 1 8 *